Fitness
After 50

It's Never Too Late to Start!

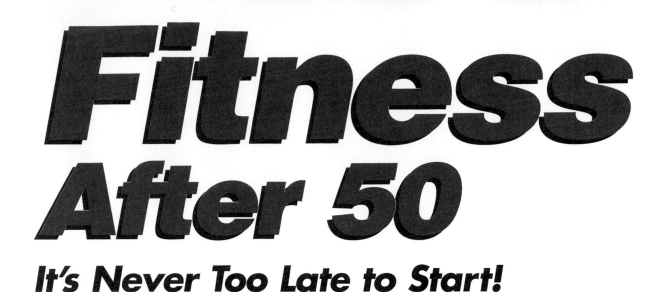

Fitness After 50

It's Never Too Late to Start!

Walter H. Ettinger, Jr., MD

Professor of Internal Medicine and Public Health Sciences
Associate Chairman, Department of Internal Medicine

Bowman Gray School of Medicine
Wake Forest University
Winston-Salem, North Carolina

Brenda S. Mitchell, PhD

Health Promotion Consultant

Fort Lauderdale, Florida

Steven N. Blair, PED

Director of Research
Director of Epidemiology and Clinical Applications

Cooper Institute of Aerobics Research
Dallas, Texas

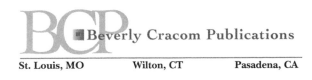

Beverly Cracom Publications

St. Louis, MO	Wilton, CT	Pasadena, CA

A joint venture between Beverly Foundation and Cracom Publishing, Inc.

BGP Beverly Cracom Publications

St. Louis, MO   **Wilton, CT**   **Pasadena, CA**

A joint venture between Beverly Foundation and Cracom Publishing, Inc.

Publisher & Editorial Director: Barbara Ellen Norwitz
Development Editor: Celia Coles
Production Editor: Colleen Clifford
Design: Mary Siener, Robert Greenhouse
Production: Robert Greenhouse

Photography: Lightworks Photography & Design, Annapolis, MD, George D. Dodson
Illustrations: Wassilchenko & Associates, Broken Arrow, OK, George Wassilchenko
Computer Illustrations: Tech-Graphics Corporation, Stoneham, MA
Cartoons: Randy Glasbergen, Sherburne, NY

Notice: The information presented in this book is intended to help you assess your current physical activity level and change your activity and nutritional habits. The life-style changes recommended in this book pre-suppose normal health and absence of heart disease or other chronic illness. If you have a chronic illness, seek medical advice before you begin to increase your physical activity. The authors and publisher of this volume disclaim any liability, loss, injury, or damage incurred as a consequence, directly or indirectly, of the use and application of any of the contents of this volume.

Library of Congress Cataloging-in-Publication Data
Ettinger, Walter H., 1951–
Fitness after 50: it's never too late to start!
Walter H. Ettinger, Jr., Brenda S. Mitchell, Steven N. Blair.
p.   cm.
Includes index
ISBN: 1-886657-05-X

1. Middle-aged persons—health and hygiene. 2. Physical fitness for the aged.
3. Exercise for the aged. I. Mitchell, Brenda S. 1946– II. Blair, Steven N. III. Title.

RA777.5.E88 1996   96-7205
613.7'044—dc20   CIP

Printed in the United States of America

10 9 8 7 6 5 4 3 2 1

Photo Credits

p. 37	Top photo courtesy of Neal Penneys, M.D.; bottom photo courtesy of the National Cancer Institute, Bethesda, MD.
p. 58	Courtesy of Peggy Woolley-Martin.
p. 64	Courtesy of Harry J. Ahearn.
p. 160	From the PhotoFile/Chris Springmann.
p. 178	Courtesy of Louisa Jacobs.
p. 188	Right photo courtesy of Nautilus Fitness System, Inc., Gaylord, MI.
p. 189	Right photo courtesy of NordicTrack, Chaska, MN.
p. 215	All courtesy of Nike, Inc., Beaverton, OR, and Reebok International, Inc., Stoughton, MA.
p. 219	All courtesy of Cannondale Corporation, Georgetown, CT.
p. 222	Courtesy of Cannondale Corporation, Georgetown, CT.
p. 232	© Winter Park Photo by Jeff Stine.
p. 234	Courtesy of Stowe Mountain Resort, Stowe, VT.
p. 235	Courtesy of Stowe Mountain Resort, Stowe, VT. © by Rick Godin.
p. 243	From Denevi & Jones Photography, San Francisco, CA.

Note From the Editor

I asked my father, aged 81, how he liked living in Florida. Answering like the traditional New Englander he is, he said, "It's okay. There are just so damn many old people here!"

I turned 50 this year—the leading edge of the baby boomer bubble. Although I've been involved with sports and fitness all my life, I've had times when, because of the demands of work and a career and a general sense that I owed myself that beer after golf or that pizza and ice cream sundae, I've varied in weight and girth.

When we were in our teens and 20s, the research in exercise was in its primitive stages. It was hard to be interested in whether rats lost weight (creepy little things), so we had little guidance regarding what we should or shouldn't do to stay fit. But now we know more, and even though there are still some contradictions, credible research indicates we should be fit and eat right.

During one of my extreme phases of physical activity, between ages 35 and 43, I was racing competitively in triathlons for my age group while running my own business. I competed in about eight events a season. I worked out 4 hours a day, 6 days a week for 8 years and burned between 2,500 and 5,000 calories a day in my workouts alone. I was the same weight I was when I was a sophomore in high school and in such excellent condition I could feel what was happening to my body during activity.

My priorities changed, as they do when we age. Between ages 43 and 49, an occasional golf game was the extent of my exercise.

I'm not sure what made me return to being more active. Maybe it was reading in my alumni newsletter that former classmates were dying from preventable problems. Or maybe it was one of my first author visits 2 years ago when we started this new publishing venture. I sat in a common area of a nursing home watching people who needed help to eat and move. I found myself thinking, "Which one is me 30 years from now?"

It took me more than a year to start exercising again. Winning races doesn't interest me anymore, and I don't want to look like a bodybuilder. But I do want to be fit and physically able to do what I want, now and when I'm 90. And I want to enjoy every day between now and then. How about you?

We write and publish books about exercise and nutrition, but we are no different from you. We've made every excuse, started to exercise and quit a dozen times in our lives, and eaten the wrong things despite knowing better. But we try to improve. We are active and exercise now because we know that it improves our chances of remaining independent and healthy. Daily exercise is like compounded interest on savings and investments. The more regularly you contribute to an active life-style, the greater the health benefits. Being physically active is a small price to pay for a healthy, productive future.

Sooner or later we approach a turning point where we realize if we don't start exercising, we never will. We hope that as you explore this book, you'll not only find your personal turning point but also have the information to help you start being physically active. That's what this publishing venture is about, and that's what this book is designed to help you do.

If it doesn't, call us at 1-800-341-0880 and let us know. We want your feedback. Tell us what you liked or didn't like, or what we could have done better. We want to continue giving you books that tell you what you *want* to know, not what we think you *should* know.

Enjoy this book. There's a lot of us, and you, and those we've known, in it.

Craig Cuddeback
Codirector, BCP

Preface

I know it's important to be fit, but I can't start exercising at my age.

I'd like to be fit, but who has time to exercise?

Do these statements sound familiar? Many Americans who are sedentary mistakenly believe that exercise requires a significant amount of time and effort to have a health benefit. They equate physical activity with high-intensity exercise that requires vigorous exertion, serious commitment of time and energy, and a disciplined, almost regimented, style. Exercise, they think, certainly can't be fun. Surely only 5 AM joggers and health club fanatics enjoy that much trouble and inconvenience. But exercise is for everyone, not just for a special breed of exercise enthusiasts. We don't have to run 3 miles or even raise a sweat to be physically active and improve our health and fitness. Ordinary, daily, routine activities, like household chores, shopping, or walking, bring lasting health benefits. This book emphasizes moderate-intensity physical activity that's easily built into everyone's life-styles. It shows you how to get started and stay with a sensible, painless, and practical exercise plan that builds physical activity into your daily life so you move more, sit less, and discover new levels of health and fitness as daily physical activity becomes natural to you.

We've been told we should exercise, but are we sure we know why? Exercise is especially important as we grow older. We have a great deal more to gain from physical activity than our younger counterparts. Research has demonstrated that, among older adults, fit individuals have lower risk than unfit individuals for many common, chronic diseases. Exercise helps us stay free from heart disease, certain cancers, stroke, and diabetes. It relieves arthritis pain and disability and helps us to recover and get back on our feet after we are sick. Physical activity is more effective than just about anything known to medical science in helping us stay healthy, live longer and better, maintain our independence, and remain in charge of our lives. If anyone should exercise, it's someone over 50.

These are strong reasons to be active. Yet the prospect of trying to change our habits makes us pause. Why? Change isn't easy. We've all tried to change our health habits in one way or another, perhaps by giving up cigarettes, eating differently, or having regular medical check-ups. We've experienced success and failure. This book builds on your experience. It begins with what you already know, asking you to understand how you made changes in other health behaviors, the obstacles you encountered, and how you overcame them. It proceeds on the premise that once you understand how you change, you can, if you want to, make changes in your physical activity patterns and stay with them.

This book acknowledges that change is difficult, that it takes energy, self-confidence, knowledge, motivation, and skill. Most of all, change takes action. For this reason, many pages in the book are designed as worksheets that invite you to complete some simple tasks designed to build on your current skills. If you'd like, take a pencil or pen and write in the book! In doing so, you'll engage actively in a process of change that positively influences how you think and encourages you to put thought into action. Often, the greatest obstacle to change is overcoming the initial inertia. We hope the simple tasks in this book will help get you up on your feet and give you momentum to stay physically active.

This book is organized so that you can either read specific chapters of particular interest or begin at the beginning and systematically read from cover to cover. The book begins by describing why fitness and exercise are important when we are older, how physical activity affects the normal aging process, and how it can protect us against disease. Next, it answers some important questions: Should you see a doctor before you start exercising? How do you measure your current activity levels? How much energy (calories) do you expend each day (and do you need to expend more)? In the core chapters (7 through 12) on the Stages of Change, you are invited to participate actively in a process whereby you change your thinking and become committed to regular exercise habits. Once you have begun to exercise, the book shows you how to tailor your exercise program to your needs and interests, whether these are walking every day at home, exercising with equipment, joining a health club, or participating in sports. Because eating right is closely allied to physical activity in maintaining your health, the last chapter provides you with nutrition information and some practical advice on eating a balanced diet and maintaining a healthy weight.

Acknowledgments

We thank our colleagues at the Bowman Gray School of Medicine and the Cooper Institute for Aerobics Research for their collaboration and stimulation over the years. The creative researchers for Project Active helped develop the life-style approach to physical activity that is featured prominently in this book. We are grateful for the leadership of a great group of interventionists involved in Project Active, especially Dr. Andrea Dunn, Dr. Bess Marcus, and Ruth Ann Carpenter.

Dr. James Prochaska, of the University of Rhode Island, originally developed the Stages of Change model, the principal theoretical model supporting the strategies for increasing physical activity presented in this book. Dr. Bess Marcus, of Brown University, applied the Stages of Change model to the field of physical activity. We acknowledge their contributions to our thinking.

Many medical, scientific, and public health organizations now recognize that the sedentary way of life most Americans follow is an important national health problem and are providing leadership in addressing this issue. We have enjoyed and continue to appreciate working with the American College of Sports Medicine; the American Heart Association; the American Alliance for Health, Physical Education, Recreation, and Dance; the National Coalition for the Promotion of Physical Activity; the Centers for Disease Control and Prevention; the National Institutes of Health; and the President's Council on Physical Fitness and Sports.

We are grateful to the National Institute on Aging and the National Heart, Lung, and Blood Institute for research support over the years. These grants have allowed us to develop our research program on the relation of physical activity and physical fitness to health and to explore new methods of helping sedentary people become more active.

For their contribution in shaping the content and thinking of this book, we thank a number of highly qualified reviewers: Dr. Patricia Dubbert; Dr. Deborah Rohm Young; Dr. Patrick Coll; Dr. Gail Dalsky; Dr. Wayne Campbell; Dr. Linda Pescatello; Dr. Roger Fielding; Dr. John Kirwan; and Dr. Bernadine Pinto. Dr. Calvin Hirsch read the entire manuscript and gave generously of his considerable experience and expertise in the combined fields of gerontology and exercise. We thank him for his valuable input.

A number of people contributed their time and expertise during the photo shoot for the book. We extend a special thanks to Mr. Joel M. Hollis, fitness instructor, of the Fitness Center, Bowman Gray School of Medicine, in Winston-Salem, North Carolina. Mr. Hollis expertly demonstrated the stretching and strength-building exercises featured in the appendices. Facilities that generously allowed us time and space to photograph organized exercise activities include the Cardiac Rehabilitation Center at the Bowman Gray School of Medicine; the Winston Lake YMCA in Winston-Salem, North Carolina; the Pinecrest Outpatient Center at Pinecrest Rehabilitation Hospital; the Delray Villas Aerobics Class in Delray Beach, Florida; and the South County Senior Center in Annapolis, Maryland.

The combined efforts of a talented team at BCP gave the book physical reality. Barbara Norwitz, publisher and editorial director, led the editorial development and extensive art program. Celia Coles, development editor, applied a strong editorial hand. Mary Siener, senior designer, was responsible for the visual design and utility of the book. Bob Greenhouse of Editorial Graphic Design & Production in Poughkeepsie, New York, implemented the design with great skill, patience, and intelligence. Photographer George Dodson of Lightworks in Annapolis, Maryland, gave the book personality by providing photographs of real people engaged in ordinary daily activities as only real people are. George Wassilchenko of Wassilchenko & Associates, Broken Arrow, Oklahoma, crafted the medical illustrations. Last, but not least, the inspired cartoons of Randy Glasbergen of Sherburne, New York, gave the book wit, humor, and grace.

Table of Contents

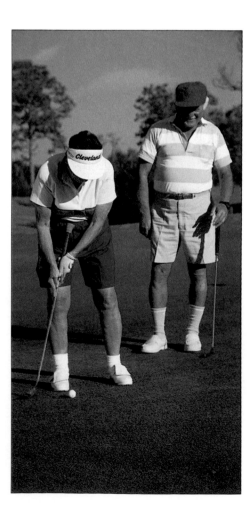

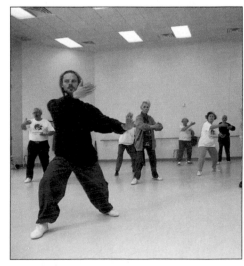

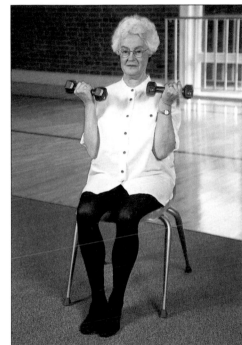

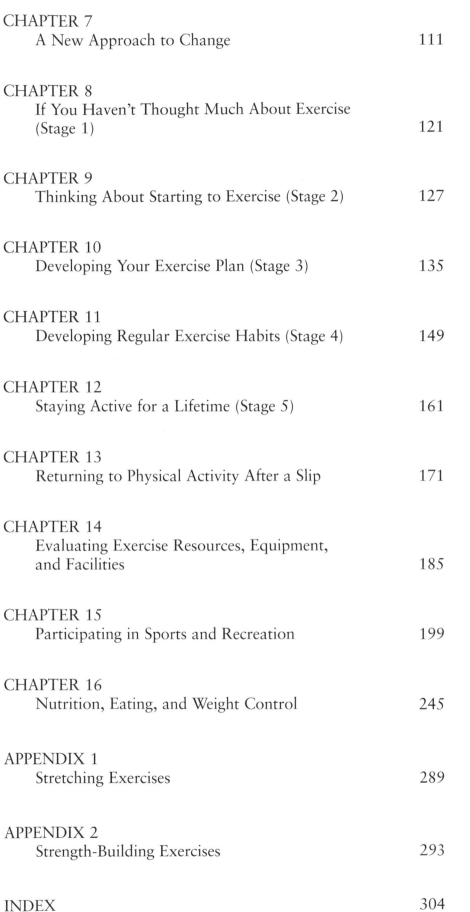

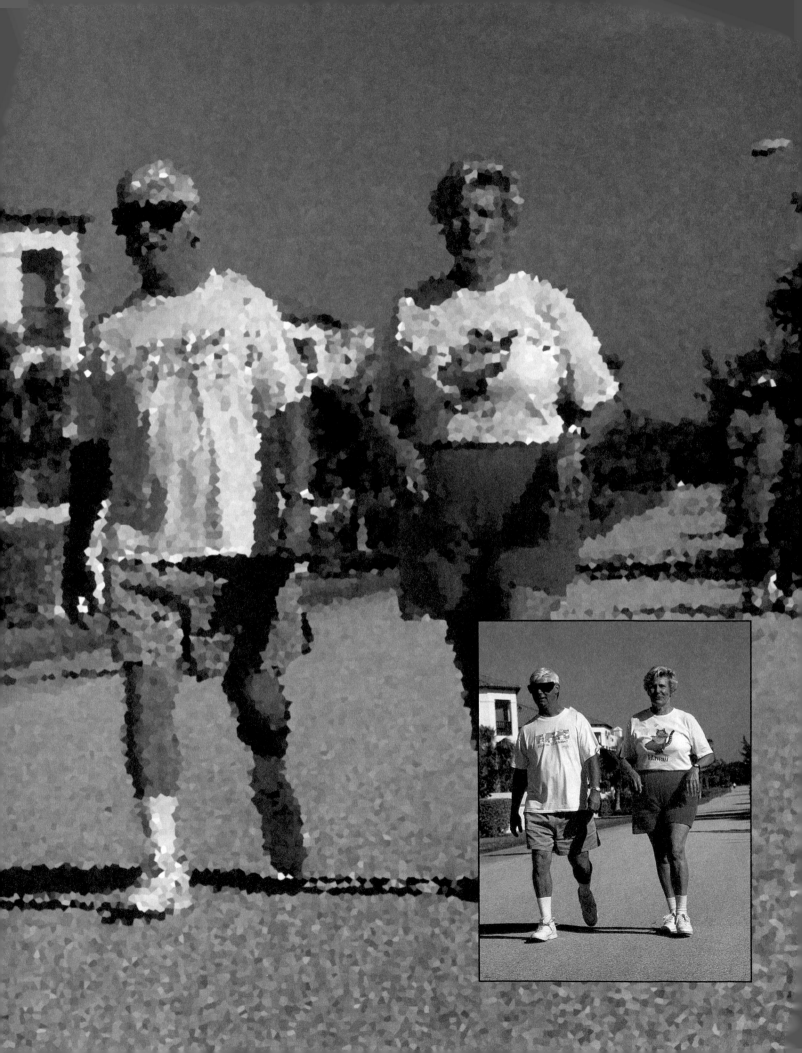

An Introduction to Fitness

*Becoming physically active means being active. We must
take charge of our daily lives and make exercise a habit.
Like money that grows when we put it with savings,
daily activity adds up to improved health and fitness
and helps secure a healthy future.*

We all wish for long life, health, and happiness, and in
some ways we're getting our wish: We're living longer
than ever before. Right now, if you're a 50-year-old
man, you have approximately 26 years of life ahead of you. If
you're a woman, you have about 31 years. That's about one third
of your life. We want to ensure that you enjoy the years after 50,
that you make the most of all you've accomplished—your job,
children, and home—and that you finally get to do the things
you've been looking forward to: traveling, playing golf and tennis,
walking, gardening, spending time with your friends and grandchildren. Quality of life in your later decades depends on keeping
your health and being able to look after yourself. We now know
that staying active greatly increases the odds of keeping our health
and independence. This book can help you stay healthy and fit by
keeping physically active. Engaging in regular physical activity is
the best protection against disease and disability and the best insurance for a healthy, independent, and productive life. These are
strong assertions, but they are true.

ACTION BOX

What Do You Want to Be Free to Do?

- Move around, look after yourself, stay healthy
- Travel
- Visit museums
- Play with your grandchildren
- Spend time with your friends
- Golf, tennis, walk, or bicycle
- Fish, dance, garden

Add your personal goals here:

_____

_____

_____

How do we know that physical activity can do all this? Research studies from major medical centers have proved it. Physical activity helps protect against the development of high blood pressure, heart disease, cancer, depression, and osteoporosis. It can help prevent disability and dependency. It reduces stress, improves sleep, and helps control your weight. Physical activity, in short, can do more than just about anything known to medical science to ensure a long, healthy, and happy life.

As this book's title suggests, it's never too late to start a physical activity program. Many people in their 50s decide that now is the time to become active. Even if you're 80, it's not too late to change your habits and enjoy a physically active life. A research study from a major university showed that men and women aged 90 and older increased their muscle strength more than 100 percent from lifting weights. Not only did they get stronger, they were able to walk better and take care of themselves better because of the exercise program. Although everyone from childhood to late adulthood can enjoy the health benefits of an active life-style, the older and more sedentary you are, the more you have to gain from becoming physically active. Now is the time to change. If not now, when? This book will help you adopt an active life-style that will enable you to enjoy the next 30 years or more. It's written with people over 50 in mind.

Why Don't We Exercise?

At this point, you're probably thinking, "I know exercise is important, but I just can't make myself do it." You're not alone. For the past 25 years, Americans have been bombarded with the message that we should exercise. Although we are told we should become more physically fit, fewer than 10 percent of Americans participate in regular exercise, and the numbers have not increased in the past 5 years. One third of Americans are very sedentary, and the most sedentary are in the over-50 age group.

So why aren't we exercising? We don't exercise partly because we think fitness is no longer a realistic goal. Moreover, we are told that the only way to be fit is to exercise vigorously. This is the "no pain, no gain" philosophy of fitness. For someone over 50, making the transition from being sedentary to exercising hard is nearly impossible. The pain and trouble of making this life-style change weighs much more heavily in the decision not to exercise than the promise of fitness down the road.

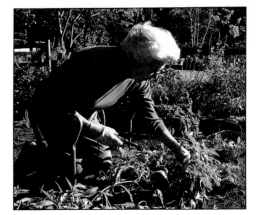

Any activity that moves the muscles and flexes the joints counts as exercise.

Fortunately, you don't need to "work out" to enjoy the health benefits of physical activity. Most health benefits of an active life-style come with moderate amounts and intensities of physical effort, so that brisk walking, gardening, housework, dancing, and bicycling can help to prolong life and prevent disability. You can spend 30 minutes each day in moderate activities and enjoy health benefits. A similar gain can be obtained from short bouts of moderately intense activities, such as using the stairs instead of the elevator, that add up to 30 minutes of exercise per day. More intense activities, such as running or playing basketball or tennis, performed for 1 hour three times a week, bring similar benefits. Activities don't have to be done all at once—they can be incorporated into your daily routine.

Indeed, physical activities should become an integral part of your daily life—true health behaviors. Health behaviors are positive actions we take to ensure health. Other examples of health behaviors include eating a nutritious diet (low in fat, high in fiber), not smoking, limiting alcohol consumption, wearing car seat belts, getting annual breast or prostate examinations, and flossing our teeth.

We know how hard it is to maintain these health habits. The difficulty in following a healthy life-style has generated a multibillion-dollar business. It is estimated, for example, that Americans spend $50 billion per year trying to lose weight, yet Americans are heavier than ever. The average weight of an American adult has risen 8 pounds in the last 10 years. Nearly everyone knows that smoking cigarettes causes cancer and heart disease, but the number of new smokers has increased over the past 5 years. Good health requires work and commitment. We are each responsible for our health and behavior. In this book, we will advise you about how to be more physically active, but ultimately the commitment to a healthy, physically active life-style comes from you. There are no quick fixes.

To change your behavior, you must know what to change and how to change it. It's easy to understand that buckling your seat belt will help prevent injury when you drive a car. But most health behaviors, especially physical activities, are complex and require knowledge, skills, adjustments to your surroundings, the support of friends and family members, and self-confidence.

The Behavioral Approach

Adopting a health behavior and incorporating it into your life isn't easy. It requires a step-by-step approach that is guided by the principles of behavioral change: analyzing your preferences and dislikes, trying a new behavior to see if you like it, formulating new plans, and trying again if you slip back into old habits. The behavioral approach to change that we advocate in this book acknowledges the struggles of a hectic life and focuses on managing time and balancing the demands of work, family, and the need for physical activity. The behavioral change theory on which we base our approach is called the Stages of Change. This theory is explained in detail in Chapter 7. The five stages of change take you through a process whereby, over about 6 months, you give up old, sedentary habits and develop new, positive health habits and behaviors. Slips and setbacks along the way will require a problem-solving approach to get you back on track. This book guides you through each stage so that you end up in Stage 5, your final destination, leading a physically active life.

Is This Book for You?

If you want to know if this book is for you, ask yourself the following questions:

- Do you want to be healthy and independent in the decades ahead?

- Are routine chores around the house harder to do than they used to be?

- Have you wanted to exercise but just couldn't get started or find the time?

- Do you have a medical condition that makes you worry about being physically active?

- Does the idea of doing moderate activities as part of your daily routine appeal to you?

If you answered "yes" to any of these questions, then this book is for you. We will help you develop a personal approach to increasing your physical activity, an approach that should help you stay active for the rest of your life.

Physical Activity and Exercise

Throughout this book, we will use the terms *physical activity* and *exercise* interchangeably. Both are behaviors—what you do. Helping you change behaviors is what this book is all about. Technically, there is a difference between physical activity and exercise. Physical activity includes all muscular activities, whereas ex-

Differentiating Physical Activity and Exercise

Physical Activity

Physical activity refers to all movement that uses energy.

Physical activities include raking leaves, vacuuming, gardening, painting the house, climbing stairs, taking the dog for a walk, even standing rather than sitting.

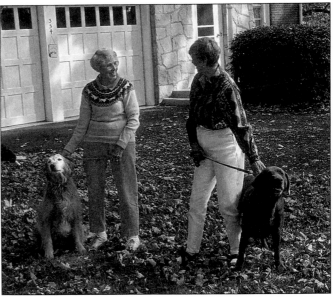

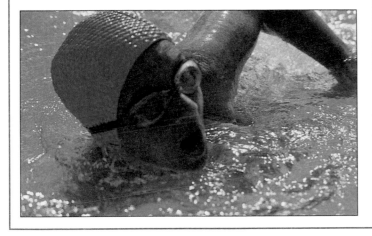

Exercise

Exercise refers to regular, repetitive, planned activity done to improve physical fitness.

Exercises include aerobic dancing classes, sports, jogging, swimming laps, bicycling, and walking.

ercise refers to traditional, repetitive activities such as swimming and running.

We believe that you can attain a more active way of life by embarking on a balanced fitness program that includes both traditional exercise and regular, daily physical activity. Balance is important to the success of any fitness program because it ensures that you spend time in activities that you enjoy.

The most common view of physical fitness is the overall ability of the body to perform physical work. Physical fitness is *what happens* in your body as a result of exercise or physical activity patterns. There are several types of physical fitness, but most important to your health and function are aerobic fitness, musculoskeletal fitness, balance, and metabolic fitness.

Aerobic Fitness

Also called *aerobic power*, *cardiovascular endurance*, *cardiovascular fitness*, or *cardiorespiratory fitness*, aerobic fitness is the maximal rate at which you can work the major muscle groups. A high level of aerobic fitness depends on the body's overall integrated ability to circulate oxygen-rich blood to the muscles. The heart, lungs, blood vessels, and muscle cells are all involved.

Although you are seldom, if ever, required to exert yourself maximally, a high level of aerobic fitness is important for several reasons. High aerobic fitness makes it easier to perform routine tasks. For example, brisk walking may require only 40 percent of maximal effort for someone who is fit, but the same walk may require nearly 100 percent of maximal effort for someone who is unfit. Every task undertaken by someone who is fit is relatively easier than the same task undertaken by someone who is unfit. That's why fit people are less likely to become fatigued from everyday activities. Moreover, people who are aerobically fit have lower rates of chronic diseases (heart disease, hypertension, stroke, diabetes, and some cancers) and are more likely to remain independent.

Musculoskeletal Fitness

Musculoskeletal fitness refers to muscle strength, muscle endurance, and joint flexibility. As you grow older, muscle strength and endurance are as important as aerobic fitness to the quality of your life and your health.

Muscle Strength

Muscle strength is required to perform the routine tasks of daily living. Every movement your body makes requires a minimum amount of strength to overcome the inertia of moving a body part (such as raising your arm) or the resistance of any load that must be lifted or moved (such as carrying a bag of groceries). Modern life does not require large amounts of muscle strength, and most people develop enough strength when they are young to perform routine tasks.

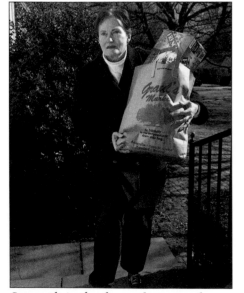

Strength is the force that muscle can exert.

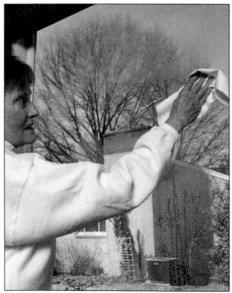

Endurance refers to the ability to perform repetitive movements without fatigue.

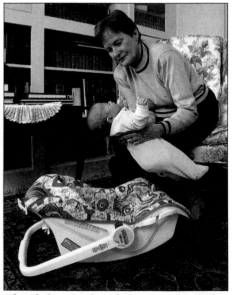

Flexibility is the ability to move the joints through the widest possible range of motion.

Muscle strength becomes problematic during the later years, however, when decades of sedentary living have caused a loss of muscle tissue. Anyone who has ever had a cast on an arm or a leg has had firsthand experience of the effect of inactivity on muscle strength. Muscles lose their size and tone. This loss, called muscle atrophy, is merely an acceleration of the same process that can result from years of little or no physical activity. If you have been inactive most of your adult life, you may have already noticed that you've lost some strength.

Sophisticated, modern screening tests such as computed assisted tomography (CAT) scanning or magnetic resonance imaging (MRI) show that many inactive older individuals have very little muscle tissue left in their arms and legs.

When older people have difficulty moving or performing simple tasks such as walking without assistance or support, their difficulty is likely caused, at least in part, by wasting of muscle tissue. Although most disability in older people is due to chronic disease, such as a stroke, arthritis, or lung disease, muscle loss due to years of sedentary habits exacerbates the disabling effects of these conditions.

Muscle Endurance

Muscle endurance, the ability to continue with a repetitive task, is related to muscle strength. You cannot sustain the effort required by a repetitive task that uses a high percentage of your muscle strength. For example, suppose that the maximal amount you can lift from your kitchen counter to a cabinet shelf above the counter is 12 pounds. Lifting a 10-pound bag of flour to the shelf would therefore require most of your strength. You could still place the flour on the shelf, but you would probably have to rest a few minutes before you could perform a similar task that required the same near-maximal exertion. If you have a maximal lifting ability of 30 pounds, placing the 10-pound bag of flour on the shelf would require only one third of your strength, and you could lift several 10-pound bags without resting. The same principle applies to climbing stairs. If you are fit enough to climb three flights of stairs without pausing, climbing one flight would be easy. If you lost most of the muscle strength in your legs, however, each step would require near-maximal exertion, and you would have to stop and rest after every step or two.

Joint Flexibility

Flexibility is a measure of the range of motion of muscles and joints. Although normally not a problem for most young people, lack of joint flexibility can become limiting after decades of inactivity and disuse. Lack of flexibility in the arms and shoulders is common. Some women are unable to fasten their bras or button their dresses in the back; others have difficulty raising their arms high enough to comb their hair. Inflexibility can become severe enough that you find it hard to turn your head and look behind

Have You Lost Muscle Strength?

- Do you find it difficult to pick up a small child?
- Is lifting a 10-pound bag of flour and placing it on a pantry shelf becoming harder?
- Do you have difficulty climbing a flight of stairs?
- Is opening a jar of pickles a challenge?
- Can you no longer move a piece of heavy furniture or turn your mattress by yourself?
- Do you have difficulty rising from a low chair or sofa without using your arms?

If you answered "yes" to any of these questions, you may have lost muscle strength. Unless you do something to reverse it, the decline in your strength will continue. You could lose more than strength; you could lose your independence!

How Flexible Are You?

- Is it difficult for you to bend over to tie your shoes or touch your toes?
- Is your range of motion limited when you try to turn your head to look behind you?
- Women—Do you avoid blouses that button in the back? Do you wear bras that hook in the front because they are easier to fasten?
- Is it difficult for you to raise your arms high enough to dry or comb your hair?

you. This problem is unimportant while you are sitting in a recliner and watching television, but it may be critical when you try to back your car out of a parking place at a crowded mall parking lot.

Low levels of musculoskeletal fitness are typically not life threatening, but they limit your ability to function. Ultimately, declines in musculoskeletal fitness result in functional limitations, which, in extreme cases, can lead to lost independence and relocation to a nursing home.

Balance

Balance is your ability to maintain your body in its upright posture, especially when abnormal stress might cause you to lose your balance—such as when you trip over an object or try to grasp at something that is just out of reach. People with poor balance tend to fall more easily during daily activities. Falling is the leading cause of accidental injury and death in people over age 65. Actor George Burns, at 100, was in good health until a fall led to his rapidly declining health and subsequent death. Even among people in their 50s, falling causes fractures. Women are especially vulnerable to fractures because their bones begin to thin after menopause.

Balance can be improved with training, and the body can adapt to the stresses of sudden movements. Although more specific research is needed to determine the best ways to improve balance, these general suggestions should help you: Develop

Test Your Balance

- Stand next to a chair and stand on your right foot. Count to 10.

  If you are able to keep your balance, try standing on the same foot with your eyes closed.

  Now change to your left foot and see if you can stand for a count of 10 with your eyes closed.

- Stand with your right shoulder to the wall. Reach forward with your right arm outstretched. Measure the number of inches that your fingertips move forward before you must take a step to prevent yourself from tumbling forward.

  People with good balance can move at least 12 to 15 inches before they must catch themselves. If you can't reach forward 12 to 15 inches, you are at an increased risk of falling.

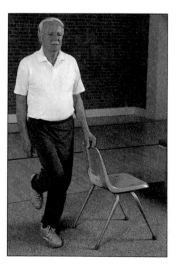
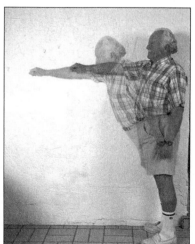

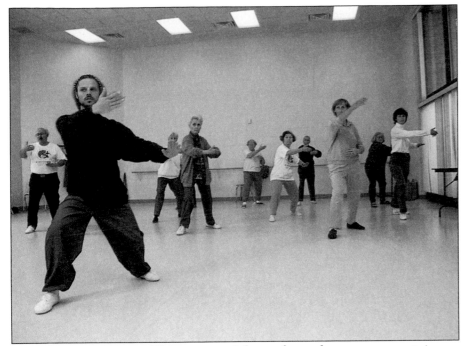

T'ai-chi is an ancient Chinese martial arts form that stresses certain repetitive, rhythmic body movements. Older adults who participated in 45-minute sessions of t'ai-chi exercises three times per week markedly improved their balance and had fewer falls. Performed vigorously, t'ai-chi is also a good aerobic exercise and leads to improved flexibility. Consider t'ai-chi as part of your overall fitness program.

strong muscles, particularly in your hips and legs and around your ankles, and perform activities that require quick movements and changes of position, such as t'ai-chi, tennis, or dancing.

Metabolic Fitness

Metabolic fitness refers to how efficiently the body burns fuel for energy. Abnormal metabolism is associated with increased risk factors such as high blood cholesterol, high blood pressure, and high or low blood sugar. Physical activity positively influences all these factors and reduces your risk of developing chronic disease.

A Balanced Fitness Program

You need a balanced fitness program to be healthy. A balanced fitness program has two components: aerobic fitness and musculoskeletal fitness. Some people focus on only one component of fitness and neglect the other. For example, it's not unusual to find avid runners who have achieved a very high level of aerobic fitness but have neglected musculoskeletal fitness. As you age, musculoskeletal fitness is as important to your health and quality of life as aerobic fitness. The type of exercise program that we advocate emphasizes both fitness components.

How to Improve Aerobic Fitness

The FIT Prescription

Since the early 1970s, scientists have prescribed an aerobics exercise program for improving aerobic fitness. You may have heard of the FIT prescription.

Frequency. *F* stands for *frequency*—how many times you exercise each week. A minimum of three exercise sessions per week is recommended.

Intensity. *I* stands for *intensity*—how hard you exercise. Aerobic exercises use the large muscles in the legs and buttocks and raise heart rate, causing a training effect as the body adapts to performing work more efficiently. Scientists have determined that to increase your aerobic fitness, you should perform aerobic exercise at an intensity that increases your heart rate into the training zone—the area where you derive the most benefit from exercise. The training zone is defined as 60 to 80 percent of your maximum heart rate. Maximum heart rate is the highest rate at which your heart safely pumps during exercise. Exercise at intensities that require your heart to beat faster than this rate are unsafe and cannot be sustained for very long.

Determine your heart rate by taking your pulse immediately after you stop exercising. You'll need a watch or a clock with a second hand or digital indicator to count accurately. Place the first two fingers (never the thumb) of your writing hand on the inside of your wrist near the thumb of your other hand. Once you locate your pulse, watch the clock. Begin counting heartbeats when the second hand or digital indicator reaches an easily distinguishable 15-second interval. Stop counting after 15 seconds. Multiply your count by 4 to calculate the heart rate you reached while exercising. You're in the training zone when your pulse count is within a 60-

---

How to Find Your Maximum and Target Heart Rates

Maximum heart rate = 220 minus your age

Example:

If you are 65 years old:

$$
\begin{array}{r}
220 \\
-\ 65 \quad \text{your age} \\
\hline
155 \quad \textbf{your maximum heart rate}
\end{array}
$$

Target heart rate = maximum heart rate x 60%

Example:

$$
\begin{array}{r}
155 \quad \text{maximum heart rate} \\
\text{x}\ 60\,\% \\
\hline
93 \quad \textbf{your target heart rate}
\end{array}
$$

Target Heart Rate by Decades

Ages	Target Heart Rate (bpm)	Maximum Heart Rate (bpm) (using the formula 220 – age)
50	102–136	170
60	96–128	160
70	90–120	150
80	84–112	140

bpm = beats per minute

to 80-percent range of your maximum heart rate. This is your target heart rate. For many people, especially those who have been inactive for most of their lives, achieving their target heart rates requires fairly vigorous exertion.

Time. *T* stands for *time*—how long each exercise session lasts. Again, scientists have been fairly specific about how much exercise you need. They recommend a minimum of 20 minutes of aerobic exercise per session.

The New FIT Prescription

Although a little complicated, the FIT prescription, if followed regularly, provides a safe and effective exercise program that can improve your aerobic fitness. Recently, however, scientists have made several discoveries and have modified the original FIT prescription.

With regard to time (*T*), studies have shown that the total cumulative time you are active is more important than doing all your exercising at one time—in one session, continuously, without stopping. A panel of experts from the Centers for Disease Control and Prevention (CDC) and the American College of Sports Medicine (ACSM) has recommended that everyone should engage in at least 30 minutes of moderately intense activity on most days of the week. Shorter bouts of activity or exercise that add up to 30 minutes of activity each day give you the same benefit as one session of the same duration.

New findings have also shown that the intensity (*I*) of the activity or exercise doesn't have to be vigorous. Moderately intense activities are beneficial. Many sedentary people who are beginning to exercise can start with less intense activities that raise their pulses to 50 percent of their maximum heart rates. Although it is wise to start at 50 percent of maximum heart rate, you should move up to 60 percent as soon as you are able in order to derive full aerobic fitness benefits. Even though you will get a greater benefit more quickly with more vigorous exercise, all activity that expends energy is beneficial. This finding is especially encouraging for those people who don't like vigorous exercise.

Borg Scale of Perceived Exertion

Level	Perceived Exertion	Physical Signs
6	Very, very light	No perceptible sign
7		
8	Very light	No perceptible sign
9		
10	Fairly light	Feeling of motion
11		
12	Somewhat hard	Warmth on cold day, slight sweat on warm days
13		
14	Hard	Sweating but can still talk without difficulty
15		
16	Very hard	Heavy sweating, difficulty talking
17		
18	Very, very hard	Feeling of near exhaustion
19		

Adapted from G.V. Borg, 1982, *Medicine and Science in Sports and Exercise, 14*, pp. 377–387.

Monitoring the intensity of your physical activity need not be complicated. We recommend using a subjective appraisal of how hard you're working. Called the Borg Scale of Perceived Exertion *(see above)*, this method of measuring exercise intensity has been used for more than 40 years and is highly reliable. To benefit from your exertions, exercise intensity should be at the "somewhat hard" to "hard" level (between 13 and 15 on the Borg Scale). At this level of intensity, on a cold day you should breathe more rapidly and your body should feel comfortably warm. On a warm day, or even at room temperature, you should breathe more rapidly and expect to sweat, at least a little. You should be able to talk without difficulty while you exercise.

The first part of the FIT prescription has been adjusted due to the modified recommendations regarding intensity and time. The frequency (*F*) of physical activity should be every day or nearly every day. If you accept that any and all activity is beneficial, regardless of intensity or duration, then being active every day seems a reasonable approach.

Which type of program is likely to work best for you? Consider the advantages of each approach. If you've tried the traditional approach and have not stayed with it, you might want to try the new FIT approach. Many people who don't like to exercise have been pleased with the results of the new FIT recommendations for increased activity through life-style pursuits. You can always use the new FIT to get started and then cross over to a

FIT Prescription for Aerobic Fitness

Choose traditional or new FIT or a combination

	Traditional FIT	New FIT
F—Frequency	Three times per week	Every day or nearly every day
I—Intensity	Within the training zone—60 to 80 percent of predicted maximum heart rate	Moderate intensity—somewhat hard or 13 to 15 on the Borg Scale of Perceived Exertion
T—Time	Minimum of 20 minutes per session	A total of 30 minutes accumulated over a day

traditional exercise program at some point. Or, you can begin with a combination of the two. Adding life-style physical activities enhances a traditional exercise program.

Advantages of the Traditional FIT Prescription

- You can complete your workout at one time.

- It may be easier for you to adhere to a single-session, scheduled exercise program.

- You are more likely to experience the euphoric feeling (sometimes called a "runner's high") that results from longer or more intense exercise bouts.

- You can achieve a fitness level that allows you to participate in competitive sports and rigorous recreational activities.

Advantages of the New FIT Prescription

- You don't have to schedule a specific time to exercise. You can be active throughout the day.

- You don't have to put on special exercise clothes or take a shower, because you aren't likely to sweat heavily.

- You don't have to learn any new exercise skills.

- You can do tasks and chores, such as gardening and housework, that you must do anyway.

- You have less chance of injury.

How to Improve Musculoskeletal Fitness

Muscle Strength and Endurance

It's not difficult to improve and maintain muscle strength and endurance. Resistance training either with calisthenics or weight training is easy to perform. Calisthenics are exercises that use the body's own weight as resistance. Push-ups and sit-ups are common calisthenic exercises. Weight training requires special equipment to pro-

How Fit Are You? Here's a Simple Walking Test

This is an easy way to monitor improvement in your aerobic fitness.

- Walk any course that takes you 4 to 6 minutes to complete. The course doesn't have to be flat, and you don't need to know the distance. You don't have to walk quickly or at any particular speed.

- Record how long it takes you to cover the course to the nearest second. Take your pulse for 15 seconds immediately after finishing the walk. Multiply by 4 to get beats per minute. Record your walking time and your heart rate. This is your baseline.

- Repeat the walking test after a few weeks of increased activity. You should see changes. Your time to walk the same course should be less or your heart rate should be lower immediately after the walk, or both responses may change.

Walk Test

Date	Time (To the Nearest Second)	Heart Rate (bpm)

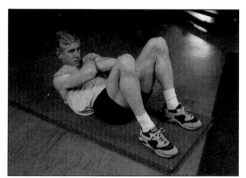

You can also do calisthenics at home on the floor.

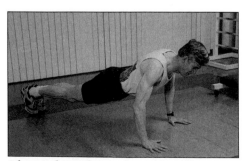

If you don't have the strength to lift your whole body, place your knees on the floor and lift only your upper body.

vide resistance. Weight-training equipment includes weight machines, handheld weights (dumbbells), or resistance rubber bands. These types of strength-building equipment are commonly found in gyms or fitness centers. (*Appendix 2 has detailed instructions for strength-building exercises.*)

Compare the advantages and disadvantages of calisthenics and weight training.

Calisthenic Exercises

Advantages

- No costs are involved because equipment is not required.

- Calisthenic exercises can be performed anywhere.

- Calisthenic exercises are easy to do.

Disadvantages

- Calisthenic exercises rarely use all the major muscle groups.

- Calisthenic exercises can be boring.

- The range of resistance is fixed by your weight. If you're heavy, exercises can be difficult.

- If you are sedentary or have physical limitations, you may not have the strength or you may be physically unable to perform this type of exercise. Also, if you have existing problems or injuries, you may cause more damage.

Handheld Weights

Advantages

- You don't have to worry about whether a weight machine fits you.

- You can easily change weights to fit your strength level.

- Weights are relatively inexpensive, and you can use them at home.

- You can use a few just to get started and add to them as you build strength.

- Weights are easy to store and transport.

Disadvantages

- If you don't use the correct technique, you may not benefit fully from the exercise or you may injure yourself.

- Some exercises require the presence of a helper or "spotter" who will assist you to safely lower a barbell or weight if your muscles are too tired to finish the exercise.

Weight Machines

Advantages

- You eliminate the need for different-sized dumbbells and weights to accommodate different abilities.

- You save time because you don't have to assemble and re-assemble equipment.

- You don't need a spotter.

- Machines are generally safer than handheld weights.

Disadvantages

- You usually need to belong to a health club to use them.

- They are expensive to buy for the home and take up a great deal of space.

If you do not want to go to a gym for a weight-training session or to use special equipment, find opportunities to exercise your muscles through daily activities. Lifting, shoving, pushing, carrying, and dragging all build muscle strength and endurance. Many people make their own weight sets. You also can perform a few calisthenic exercises at home to round out your strength-building program.

Flexibility

Flexibility is often the most neglected part of a fitness program, but it can be the easiest and most enjoyable type of exercise to perform. In time, if you exercise without stretching, certain muscles will shorten, particularly the muscles of the back, the legs, the lower back, and the hips. Muscle shortening occurs because the body favors select muscle groups. One muscle or muscle group

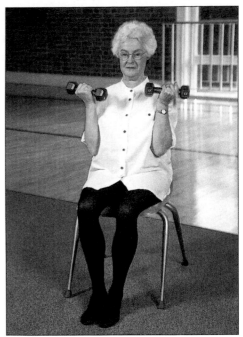

Small handheld weights are easy to use.

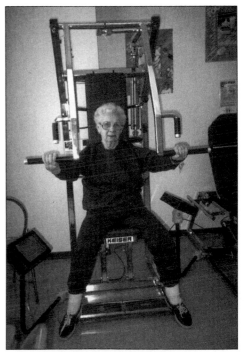

They may look a little forbidding, but when you get to know them, weight machines can be a lot of fun.

FIT Prescription for Musculoskeletal Fitness

	Muscle Strength and Endurance	Joint Flexibility (Stretching)
F—Frequency	At least 2 days per week with at least 1 day of rest between sessions.	Daily, especially as you warm up to perform other exercise activities and as you cool down after exercising.
I—Intensity	Begin at a rating of perceived exertion (RPE) of 13 on the Borg Scale. At the end of your last set of strength training exercises, you may be at an RPE of 15 or 16.	Stretch slowly and with full control—never to the point of pain—and don't bounce while the muscle is fully stretched. Inhale before the stretch and exhale during the stretch.
T—Time	Exercise should strengthen each major muscle group: chest, shoulders, arms, abdomen, thighs, calves. Do one set of 8 to 15 repetitions for each muscle group.	Gradually apply tension on the muscle, hold it for 10 to 20 seconds, and then slowly release.

Common Weight-Training Terms

Repetitions (reps). The number of times you repeat a particular exercise or lift during a set.

Set. A group of repetitions performed in sequence; a brief period of rest is allowed between sets for muscles to recover from the exertion.

Compare the Costs

Calisthenics
   Cost: $0

Dumbbells, strap-on weights, or elastic bands
   Cost: $20 to $80

Barbells
   Cost: $50 to $200

Weight machines
   Cost: $700 to $3000

Health club membership
   Cost: $150 and up per year

naturally remains stronger while another remains weaker. The rule of thumb when correcting muscle imbalance is to stretch the stronger muscles and strengthen the weaker muscles.

Stretching before an activity prepares muscles for movement and prevents tight muscles from becoming injured when they are contracted quickly. A word of caution is in order. For many years, trainers encouraged people to stretch cold muscles vigorously to "loosen up" before activity. In recent years, warm-up exercises have fallen out of favor because they have caused injuries. If you are stretching before exercise, stretch only lightly and briefly and save the heavier stretching until after you exercise. We recommend that you begin to exercise slowly at first until the muscle groups you are using have had a chance to warm up; then gradually increase your exercise intensity. Stretching after physical activity helps the muscles relax and return to their resting state. Muscles are easier to stretch after physical activity because they are looser.

You can also stretch at other times during the day—when you have been sitting for long periods or when you feel tension in your back or neck muscles. Every muscle of your body can be stretched. (*See Appendix 1 for more examples of stretching exercises.*)

Correcting Muscle Imbalance

Lack of balance between muscle groups can affect your posture and movement and even increase your chances of low back pain—one of the most widespread health problems in the United States today. Lumbar lordosis (swayback), although not the only cause of low back pain, is a frequent culprit. This condition is caused typically by strong, tight hip flexors and lower back muscles that force

Make Your Own Beginning Weight Set

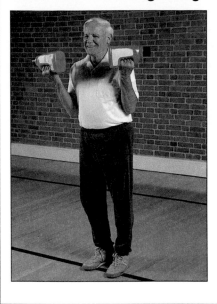

Use empty, plastic milk, juice, or laundry detergent bottles to make your own set of weights. Select containers with handles (quart, half gallon, gallon). Clean them and fill them with water or sand to the desired weight. Start lightly with two containers weighing between 2 and 3 pounds. As you grow stronger, increase the weight by adding more water or sand.

the top of the pelvis to tilt forward. Over time, this forward rotation becomes worse when weak abdominal muscles offer little resistance to the pull of the stronger muscles in the hips and back. Tight hamstrings can also contribute to swayback.

To keep your lower back healthy, your front thigh and lower abdominal muscle groups must be at least two to three times stronger than their opposing muscle group. Strengthening your abdominal muscles and improving flexibility in your lower back, hamstrings, and hip flexors will improve your posture and relieve this type of low back pain. (*See Appendix 2.*)

When you exercise similar muscle groups, try to achieve equal strength in each group. Your right front thigh and left front thigh, for example, should be equally strong. When you exercise opposing muscle groups, the goal is different. For example, when you are stretching your front thigh muscles and strengthening your back thigh muscles, the front of the thigh will probably be two to three times stronger than the back of the thigh. The same is true of your bicep and tricep muscles. Thus, if you exercise with 30 pounds of weight for your biceps, you will probably use up to 10 to 15 pounds of weight for your triceps.

A Model Fitness Program

Everyone likes to have an example to follow, so we are suggesting a model program that suits almost everyone's general activity needs. You must create an exercise and physical activity program to meet your specific needs, but this model program will get you started. The program incorporates 3 days of an aerobic activity, 2 days of resistance training activity, 1 day of a recreational activity,

Tip

If you have excessive weakness in one area or if you are recovering from surgery or illness, it's best to get help from a physical therapist—an expert in muscle function—who will prescribe appropriate exercises.

Times to Stretch

- **Before activity—but BE CAREFUL!** Stretch lightly and briefly to prevent injury.
- **After activity—to relax the muscles and return to the resting state.**
- **Anytime—to relieve tension and relax.**

Did You Know?

There are more than 430 skeletal muscles that appear in pairs on opposite sides of your joints. Fewer than 80 pairs are responsible for the common movements you make during exercise.

Exercises for Muscle Strength and Balance

Stretch the Stronger Muscles	Strengthen the Weaker Muscles

Calf or back of lower leg (gastrocnemius)

Stretch the calf: In a standing lunge with both feet pointed forward, straighten your rear leg to cause a stretch.

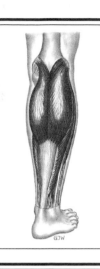

Shin or front of lower leg (tibialis anterior)

Strengthen the shin: Lift the toe toward the shin. Add resistance to gain more strength—use weights or rubber bands.

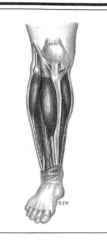

Front of thigh (quadriceps)

Stretch the front of thigh: Lie face down on the floor and lift the heel of one leg toward the buttocks. Grasp the ankle with either hand. Gently pull the heel out and back until you feel the stretch.

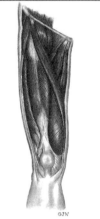

Back of thigh (hamstrings)

Strengthen the hamstring: Lie face down on the floor and lift the heel of one leg toward the buttocks against resistance—use weights, rubber bands, one leg against the other (cross at ankles), or furniture.

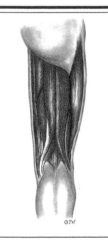

Inner thigh (adductors)

Stretch the inside thigh: In a straddle sitting position, lean forward into the stretch from the hips.

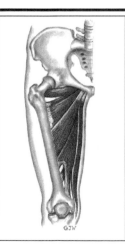

Outer thigh (abductors)

Strengthen the outside thigh: Lie on one side with your head resting on your hand. Lift the top leg to work the outer thigh. Repeat with the other leg. As strength increases, add resistance—use weights or rubber bands.

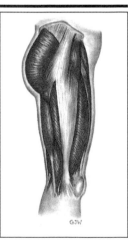

Exercises for Balance and Flexibility

| Stretch the Stronger Muscles | Strengthen the Weaker Muscles |

Lower back (erector spinae)

Stretch the low back: In a sitting position with the legs extended, slowly flex the trunk forward from the hips.

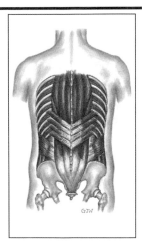

Lower stomach (abdominals)

Strengthen the abdominals: Lie face up on the floor with your knees bent and your arms across your chest. Slowly curl the head and shoulders off the floor approximately 6 to 8 inches. Keep the knees bent while lifting.

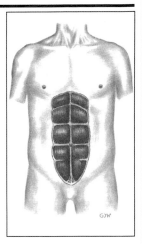

Chest (pectorals)

Stretch the chest: Face into a corner and stand about 2 feet away. Place one hand on each wall and slowly press into the corner until you feel the stretch.

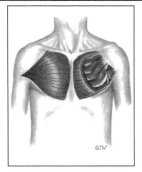

Upper back (rhomboids)

Strengthen the upper back: Raise the arms to shoulder level and bend the elbows. Press the arms backward to stress the upper back muscles. Use weights if possible.

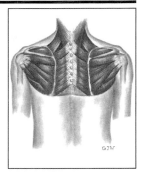

Front of arm (bicep)

Stretch the biceps: Generally, lack of bicep flexibility is not a problem.

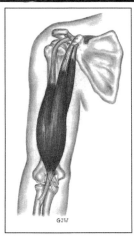

Back of arm (tricep)

Strengthen the triceps: After the elbow has been flexed, extend the arm back to stress the tricep. Add resistance—use body weight (push-ups or chair dips) or hand weights.

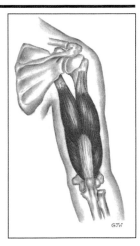

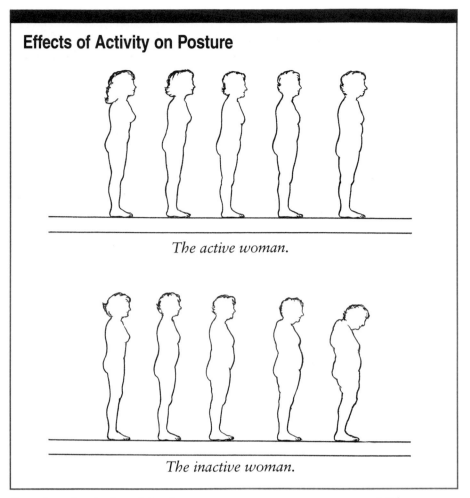

Effects of Activity on Posture

The active woman.

The inactive woman.

Regular physical activity improves posture at every age and life stage.

and flexibility exercises on each of these 6 days. This balanced fitness program can help you achieve and maintain all aspects of physical fitness.

If you are applying the "new" FIT program, you may want to take a morning walk every day, beginning slowly and gradually increasing speed as your body warms up.

A Model Walking Program

We thought it would be helpful to provide a model walking program for the person who has not exercised regularly and must ease into an active life-style. You can apply the following model to other activities, such as bicycling, that do not require a high level of fitness. Activities such as jogging, cross-country skiing, and skating that require a higher level of fitness and skill are less appropriate if you're just starting to exercise.

- *Equipment and clothing.* No special equipment or clothing is required to start a walking program. To start, you should wear comfortable shoes. Athletic or walking shoes provide excellent support for the bones and tendons in your feet. Once you start walking longer distances, you may want to invest in a pair of walking shoes.

- *Time of day.* It doesn't matter what time of day you walk. Set aside time when it's most convenient. Vary the time of day if necessary. Also, remember you can break up the designated walking time into two or three sessions per day.

- *Location.* You can walk almost anywhere. Initially, you may want to choose a location where you can do laps, such as a high school track, a park, or a circuit around a city block, so that if you tire you are not too far from your starting point. When you're ready, vary the setting in which you walk. Walk in a hilly area to increase the work done during your walk. If the weather is unpleasant, walk indoors at a gymnasium or a mall. Many malls open their doors early to allow people to walk in safe, pleasant environments.

- *Technique—warm up (Phase 1).* Your walk should have three phases: warm up, fitness, and cool down. For the first 5 minutes of your walk, warm up by walking at your usual speed and emphasize arm movements. Your posture will change according to the pace of your walk.

- *Fitness (Phase 2).* After you warm up, begin the fitness portion of your walk. Increase your walking pace until you can feel yourself breathing rapidly but not so hard that you can't talk. You should be working "somewhat hard" on the Borg Scale of

There's No Rush

Remember, you're making a commitment to be more physically active for a lifetime and, although you may feel refreshed, more energetic, and less stressed within a week or two of starting your walking program, the major health benefits of physical activity accrue over many months to years. Therefore, you don't need to rush. Set realistic goals, and gradually increase your walking time as you become more fit. It may take you 3 to 6 months or more to reach your goal. That's perfectly okay. The important thing is to start slowly, warm up and cool down, be flexible, and keep at it.

Reasons to Walk

- It's easy to do. No special skills are required to get started.
- No special equipment is needed, except for a comfortable pair of shoes.
- You can do it most anytime and anywhere—outdoors or indoors at a mall, a gymnasium, or an airport.
- It's a safe, low-impact activity. You're not likely to get injured.
- You can increase your intensity as you improve your fitness level.
- It's a weight-bearing activity that can help build strong leg muscles and bones.
- You can burn additional calories by increasing the intensity (walk faster) or the duration (time) of your walk.
- You can do it alone or with a partner or group.
- You can participate in special walking events and competitions.
- It can help reduce stress.
- Walking offers important health benefits.

Walking Posture and Pace

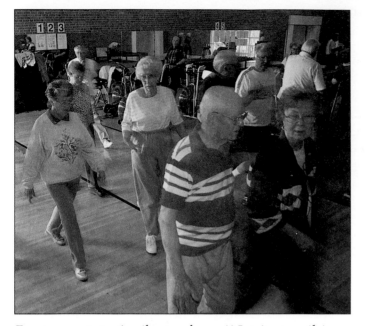

For paces up to 4 miles per hour (15-minute mile), walk with your body erect and arms fully extended, alternating with each stride. Your feet should roll forward from heel to toe.

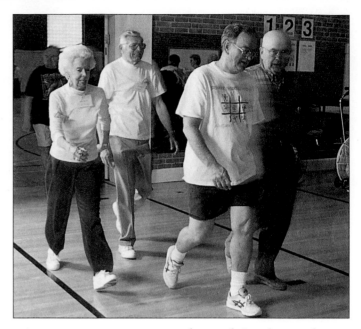

As you increase your pace beyond 4 miles per hour, convert to a bent-arm swing with your arms at a 90-degree angle, forming loose fists with your hands.

Perceived Exertion (*see p. 14*). On a cold day, your body should feel comfortably warm while you walk. On a warm day, you should expect to sweat at least a little while walking. Sweating is one of the body's mechanisms for getting rid of the heat your muscles generate while they are working and indicates that your body is adapting to the exercise. Continue walking at this pace for up to 15 minutes. If you can't walk continuously for 15 to 20 minutes at a "somewhat hard" level of work without tiring, start at a level at which you are comfortable and slowly work up to the goal of 30 or more minutes a day. Begin by walking for 10 minutes in Phase 2 and increase your time by 5 minutes every 2 weeks.

- *Cool down (Phase 3)*. After 15 minutes in Phase 2, slow down and walk at your warm-up pace for 5 more minutes.

- *Stretch*. Finish by doing the stretching exercises listed on pp. 20–21 and in Appendix 1. If it's inconvenient to stretch immediately, wait until you return home. Your leg muscles may feel stiff and sore for a week or so after you begin. Starting your program slowly and doing the stretching exercises will help to minimize the soreness. Remember that this type of muscle soreness is normal and will resolve on its own.

- *Schedule*. Repeat your routine 3 or 4 days a week either on consecutive days or with rest days in between. Increase Phase 2 of your walking by 5 minutes every 2 weeks. At this rate, you'll be walking 30 minutes per day in 6 weeks.

A Balanced Fitness Program

Day of the Week	Activity	Length of Times (Minutes)
Monday	Flexibility exercises	5 minutes
	Aerobic exercises	20 minutes
	Flexibility exercises	10 minutes
Tuesday	Flexibility exercises	5 minutes
	Resistance training	30 minutes
	Flexibility exercises	10 minutes
Wednesday	Flexibility exercises	5 minutes
	Aerobic exercises	20 minutes
	Flexibility exercises	10 minutes
Thursday	Flexibility exercises	5 minutes
	Resistance training	30 minutes
	Flexibility exercises	10 minutes
Friday	Flexibility exercises	5 minutes
	Aerobic exercises	20 minutes
	Flexibility exercises	10 minutes
Saturday or Sunday (or both)	Dancing, yard work, tennis, canoeing, or other recreational activities of your choice	60 minutes

Incorporating Exercise Into Your Daily Routine

Look for ways to incorporate exercise into your daily routine. Walking can be done while you shop. Stretching can be done while you clean the house. For example, if you are cleaning windows, use slow motions and extend your arms in a circular pattern so that you feel the stretch in your arm, shoulder, and side and back muscles. Resistance exercises can include digging in the garden or lifting boxes (use your legs, not your back) as you clean the attic. Every activity that moves or stretches the muscles and burns calories counts as exercise, even the most mundane.

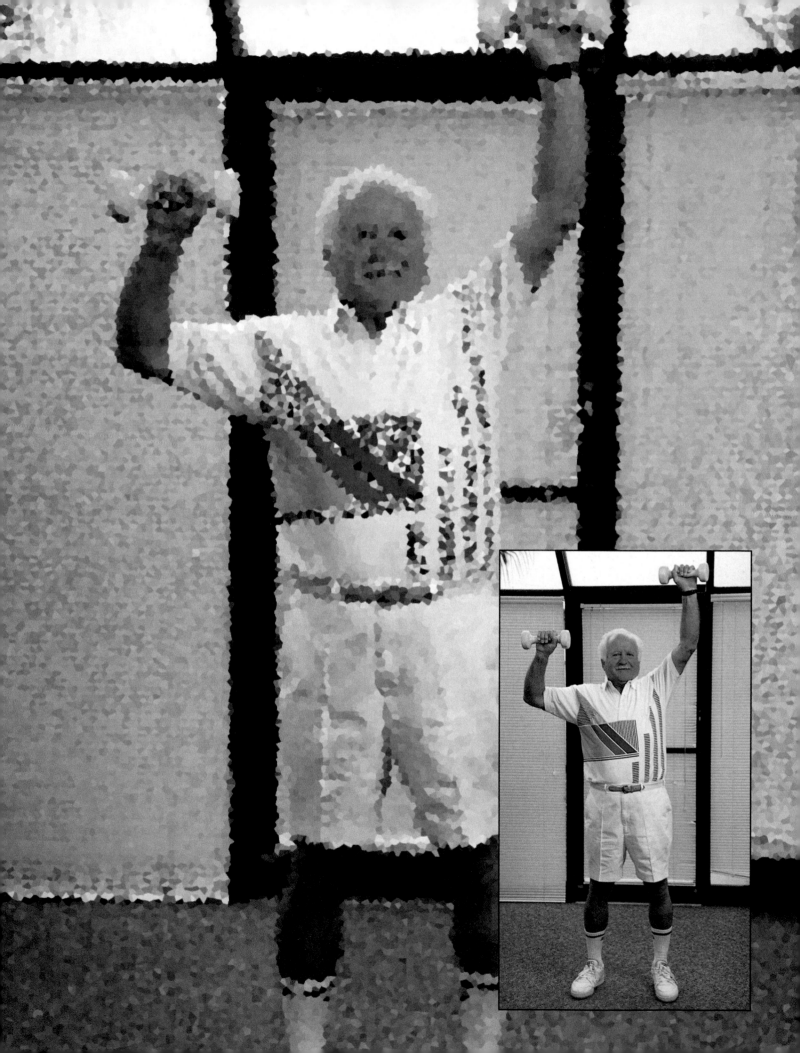

CHAPTER 2

The Aging Process

In response to a birthday greeting, a 65-year-old man said, "It's great to be 65, considering the alternative!" Aging is a natural process that begins at birth and continues throughout life. If you think about it, all the alternatives to aging are bad!

Signs of Aging

The earliest signs of aging are easy to recognize:

- Our hair may begin to thin in our 20s. Gray hair appears in our 30s or 40s. By our 70s, our hair is usually completely gray.

- Weight appears in all the wrong places. How often have we heard the lament, "I used to be able to eat whatever I wanted, but now I put on 15 pounds at the drop of a hat!" Women usually gain weight in the hips or thighs (especially after child-birth); men develop "beer bellies" or "love handles."

- In our 40s, our skin begins to sag and lose its elasticity. Wrinkles become more prominent.

- Flexibility begins to decline in our mid-20s, and muscle strength declines after our late 30s or early 40s. We notice we're sore and stiff from gardening or a weekend game of soft-ball. As muscle mass and strength decline, we burn calories less efficiently and store food as fat more easily. Mobility may become a problem.

Selecting Your Doctor As You Age

As you grow older you may want to consult a geriatrician—a physician who is an expert in the care of older people. Choose a doctor who possesses these characteristics:

- Interest and expertise in caring for people over 50

- Emphasis on prevention, wellness, and quality of life

- Good communication skills, explains, answers questions, and listens

- The eye lens changes shape, becoming thicker and less pliable, making it more difficult to see close objects. By age 50, nearly everyone requires glasses to read the newspaper or use a telephone book.

- Our sense of taste diminishes as we age.

- Our mouths and eyes may become dryer.

- Our bones lose calcium and become more brittle. Women, more than men, lose bone density, especially after menopause.

- In our 70s, we lose height when thinning vertebrae shrink.

Although we cannot prevent aging, we can control the pace of these changes with exercise and nutrition. Research in aging has made great strides in these areas, so we can take advantage of what we now know to ensure both a longer and better quality of life.

Two Types of Aging

Although the visible signs of aging are easily recognized, the biological processes that cause aging are largely unknown and are a topic of hot debate among gerontologists (scientists who study the aging process). The experts agree on two things, however:

- Biological aging is the result of predictable changes that occur in our cells, organs, and body systems over time. These changes are normal and happen to everyone.

- Pathological aging is caused by abnormal processes that increase our susceptibility to fatal and disabling diseases, such as heart disease, stroke, cancer, arthritis, and diabetes. These abnormal processes are less predictable than normal aging and affect only certain individuals. Fortunately, pathological changes can be prevented.

In this chapter, we will discuss only the normal changes of biological aging.

Biological versus Pathological Aging

Biological Aging

- Normal

- Predictable changes that occur in the cells, organs, and body systems

- Affects everyone

- Probably can't be controlled

Pathological Aging

- Abnormal

- Leads to heart disease, cancer, diabetes, and arthritis

- Affects only certain individuals

- Many diseases can be controlled or prevented

Can the Aging Process Be Altered?

Does aging lead inevitably to physical frailty, disability, and dependence? Is the normal aging process programmed and predictable—locked by a master biological clock in our genes? Or is aging the result of wear and tear from exposure to the physical environment? Aging is an outcome both of genetic and environmental factors.

Genetic Factors

There is strong evidence that many aging processes are genetically controlled. Gerontologists are finding that at the cellular level, our genes program certain biochemical processes that turn on or turn off at various stages of cell life, and these chemical changes control how well the cells work and how long they survive.

The Hayflick Phenomenon

Normal cells taken from skin and grown in a test tube divide (reproduce) a fixed number of times and then stop. The genes control this process of cell division. The number of cell divisions depends on cell age. Cells from younger animals divide more often than cells from older animals. There is almost a one-to-one correlation between an animal's age and the number of times its cells divide. This relationship, called the Hayflick phenomenon, is one of the strongest arguments for the genetic control of aging.

Because cells make up every part of the body, biochemical changes in the cells occur in the organs as well. The eye, for example, is affected by cell changes that occur with aging. The lens of the eye is composed of flexible and clear materials which allow you to focus on objects both near and far. As we age, the lens becomes thick and less flexible, resulting in a need for reading glasses. The proteins in the lens may also darken and eventually impair your vision—a process that may result in cataracts.

Environmental Factors

Not only genetic changes, but also the environment—the sun's ultraviolet light and cigarette smoke—can influence the development of cataracts. Thus, although many genetically determined cellular changes that contribute to aging are beyond our control, we can control environmental and life-style factors—the air we breathe; the water we drink; what we eat; our physical activity level; our use of drugs, alcohol, and tobacco; and our exposure to sunlight— and thus we can control the aging process.

Life Span versus Life Expectancy: What's the Difference?

Life span potential refers to how long the longest-lived member of an optimally protected population of a specific species survives.

Scientists know that the rate of aging varies markedly across animal species. In mammals, for example, life span varies from 2 or 3 years in rats to more than 101 years in humans. Life span is the same for all members of a species, is fixed, and, as far as we can tell, has not changed in humans since the beginning of time.

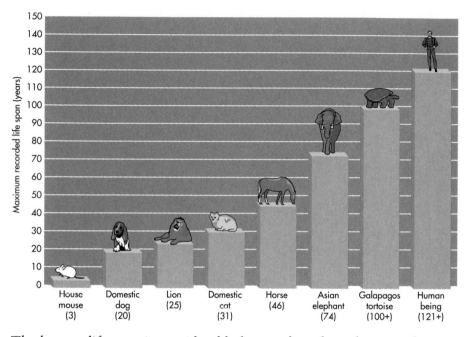

The human life span is considerably longer than that of many other species.

Life expectancy is the average length of time one expects to live and is always less than the life span potential. In the United States, the life expectancy is currently 74 years for men and 80 years for women. Over the past two centuries, life expectancy in the United States has increased substantially. In the 18th century, for example, the life expectancy for U.S. citizens was approximately 25 years. Life expectancy increased to 50 years at the beginning of the 20th century and will approach 85 years in the early part of the 21st century. Life expectancy of persons living in underdeveloped countries today is much the same as it was in the United States in the early part of the 20th century. As living standards in these countries improve, citizens of these countries will live longer.

Life expectancy is an outcome of several factors including environmental conditions, sanitation, medications, exercise, nutrition, and industrial safety. As our environment improves, as new drugs are discovered and we learn more about curing and preventing disease, and as our nutritional and exercise habits improve, the longer we will live and the closer we will come to the maximal life span potential of more than 121 years. The fastest growing segment of our population is the over-80 group, and among these individuals, many will live to be 100.

The increased life expectancy in the United States over the first 150 years after 1800 was largely due to improvements in the environment and standard of living:

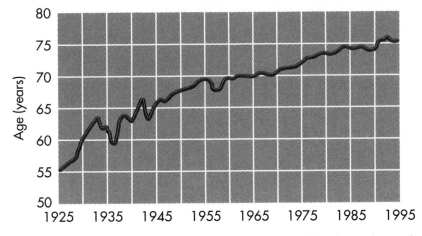

Life expectancy in the United States has risen steadily throughout the 20th century, reaching a high of more than 75 years in 1995.

- Improved sanitation and advances in medical care lead to reduced death rates, especially among children, from infectious diseases such as diphtheria, measles, and pneumonia.

- A more abundant and safer food supply improved the population's general health.

Increased life expectancy in the second half of the 20th century is due to fewer deaths from chronic diseases, such as heart disease, stroke, and cancer. These diseases mostly affect middle-aged and older people. The reduced death rate from these diseases comes from improvements in life-style:

- Reduced cigarette smoking

- Reduced consumption of fatty foods

- Improved control of high blood pressure, high blood cholesterol, and diabetes

- Increased participation in exercise and physical activity

The environment in which you live and the way you live—both modifiable factors—affect how quickly or slowly you age.

Theories of Aging

There are dozens of theories of aging, none of which adequately explains the aging process. Although each theory has some scientific evidence to support it, none can explain all the age-related changes observed in humans. Proponents of these different theories have used them to support the use of one antiaging nostrum or another.

Even though some antiaging measures may be part of a healthy approach, none is a panacea. Supporters of the free radical theory, for example, advocate using vitamin E and other antioxidants to prevent aging. Although antioxidant vitamins may help reduce the risk of certain diseases such as heart attack, there

Popular Theories of Aging

- *Free Radical Theory.* Highly reactive by-products of metabolism called free radicals react with key parts of the genetic structure of the cell (DNA, the building blocks of genes) to cause damage and interfere with cellular function. The proponents of this theory suggest that if you maintain high levels of antioxidants such as vitamins C, E, and beta carotene, these antioxidants will combine with free radicals before they have a chance to damage DNA.

- *Glycosylation Theory.* Sugar attaches to protein and other molecules to form advanced glycosylation end products (AGE), which cause dysfunction in aging cells.

- *DNA Repair Theory.* The rate and ability of DNA repair varies among species (and perhaps among people). Animals that live longer have better and more rapid repair of DNA than shorter-lived animals.

- *Antitoxin Theory.* The body's ability to eliminate toxins such as carcinogens (chemicals that cause cancer) decreases with longevity.

is no scientific evidence that they are a "fountain of youth" or can slow the normal aging process. The evidence that suggests that such antiaging nostrums can slow or prevent aging is called "anecdotal," because it comes from anecdotes or reports of a number of people whose collective accounts appear to confirm that something occurs. Although anecdotal evidence is not scientific, it may later be proved accurate in scientific studies.

The Only "Fountain of Youth"

Among the hundreds of purported "fountains of youth," only one intervention has been proven to slow the aging process—caloric restriction. Maximal life span potential has been extended as much as 30 to 40 percent in mice and rats that were fed one third to one half fewer calories than rats that were allowed to eat at will. Restricting calories appears to slow the normal biological processes of aging and reduces susceptibility to disease. The greatest improvement in longevity is seen in animals whose caloric intake has been restricted from birth. Substantial effects both on longevity and on physiological measures of aging can also be seen in rodents placed on low-calorie diets in mid-life.

It is not yet known whether similar levels of caloric restriction will delay age-related changes in higher mammals such as primates. Experiments are being carried out in monkeys—a species genetically very similar to humans—to determine the effects of caloric restriction on the aging process.

The benefits of caloric restriction may be offset by some unwanted side effects. In rodents, caloric restriction also led to

---

How Do You Know What's True?

"Consumer beware" is good advice when evaluating health resources and products, especially those that claim to halt the aging process. You should be able to answer "yes" to these questions:

- Has the theory been tested in humans?

- Were experiments done at a major university?

- Has the theory been verified by more than one study? And have the results been duplicated by others who have performed the same study?

- Is the evidence published in a respected scientific journal?

If you answered "yes" to these questions, you should still be cautious and ask:

- Was the research paid for by an organization that stands to gain financially from the results?

- Does it sound too good to be true?

If you answered "yes" to these questions, you have reason to be skeptical of the claims being made.

---

stunted growth and decreased sexual function. Nonetheless, understanding the biochemical and physiological basis of caloric restriction will have profound implications for gerontology and might well have implications for public health.

Aging, Function, and Capacity

Aging is characterized by a slow loss of capacity in all body systems beginning in early adulthood and progressing throughout adult life. Many age-related changes that occur in the major organ systems have important implications for physical health and independence. These changes, by themselves, do not result in debilitating decline or lost independence, but age-related changes do cause concern when they accelerate because of a sedentary life-style or when they interact with disease to cause loss of function. How does aging interact with disease?

Decrease in Maximal Capacity

With time, an organ system loses its capacity to perform its work. This reduced functional capacity reduces our ability to handle the stress of illness, accident, or surgery. For example, we lose maximal muscle strength (capacity) with age. After age 50, healthy, sedentary people experience a steady decline in muscle strength. This slow loss of strength usually does not prevent us from performing daily activities, but recreational activities become more and more difficult (loss of function). Eventually, we reach a threshold where essential activities such as standing up from a low chair

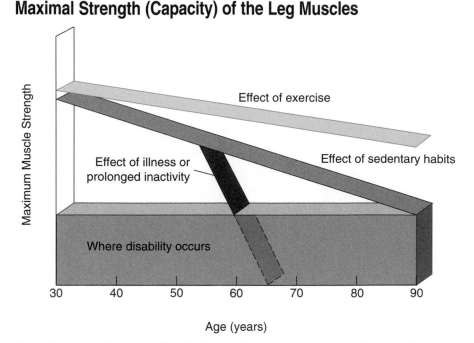

Maximal Strength (Capacity) of the Leg Muscles

Maximum Muscle Strength

Effect of exercise

Effect of illness or
prolonged inactivity

Effect of sedentary habits

Where disability occurs

30   40   50   60   70   80   90

Age (years)

Muscle strength gradually declines after age 30 and accelerates if we are sedentary. With less muscle mass, we are less able to withstand the stresses of illness and immobility. Our muscles can become so weak we may lose our ability to move, shop, eat, clean, or look after ourselves.

or climbing stairs require almost 100 percent of our strength reserves. If we then became ill with pneumonia, or if we broke a hip or a leg, which resulted in prolonged bedrest, we would lose muscle strength at an accelerated rate. We might become so weak that we couldn't get out of a chair or walk without assistance (loss of function and decreased capacity).

Can we prevent the loss of muscle strength that occurs with age? Through regular exercise and physical activity we can slow, but not stop, the age-related loss in maximal muscle strength and therefore prevent potential disability. The longer we stay stronger, the greater the odds of keeping our independence and freedom to move, get about, shop, cook, eat, clean, and manage our lives.

Change in Maximal Capacity

The maximal capacity and rate of change in any organ system varies from person to person. An 80-year-old person can have an organ system with a greater capacity than the same organ system of a 30-year-old. Consider cardiovascular power—the ability of the heart and lungs to supply the cells with oxygen. A measure of cardiovascular power is maximal heart rate (the highest rate your heart can beat). This value declines with age. A simple formula to predict maximal heart rate is 220 minus your age. Thus, the predicted maximal heart rate of a 60-year-old is 160 (220 minus 60), and the predicted maximal heart rate of a 30-year-old is 190 (220 minus 30). Studies have shown, however, that the actual maximal

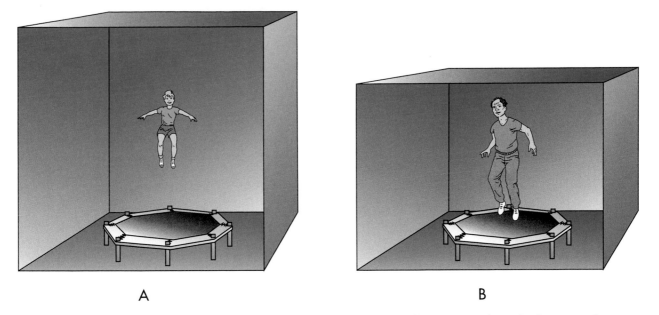

A   B

Reserve capacity (sometimes called functional reserve) is a term researchers use to describe how much capacity a system has to handle extra workload. A room with a movable ceiling and floor provides an analogy for reserve capacity. The space within the room represents the area within which the body can function well. In the first room (A), this space is large; the young adult in this room has a high reserve capacity and is able to function well across a wide range of activities. In the second room (B), the ceiling and floor have compressed. The older adult in this room, while still able to function well within a narrower area, now has a lower reserve capacity for extra activities.

heart rate for 60-year-olds is 145 to 185 and for 30-year-olds is 175 to 215. In other words, some 60-year-olds who have heart rates of 185 actually have more capacity than some 30-year-olds whose heart rates are 175!

Changes in Body Composition

Our body composition changes with aging. When scientists refer to changes in body composition, they are referring to changes in both total and relative amounts of fat, muscle, vital organs, and bone.

Even if our body weight stays the same over time (a rare event indeed!), between the ages of 30 and 70 the amount of muscle decreases and the amount of fat increases. The accelerated loss of muscle that occurs with aging affects the efficiency of our metabolism and prevents the body from burning fuel efficiently. Muscle is the most metabolically active tissue in the body and uses most of the energy (calories) we get from food. The more muscle mass we have, the more calories we burn. As we age, we have less muscle to burn energy, and thus we store more fat. The decreased muscle and increased fat account for much of the weight gain that occurs with aging.

Although these changes are a normal part of aging, much age-related change in body composition is due less to normal aging than to an inactive life-style. As we age, we eat the same amount

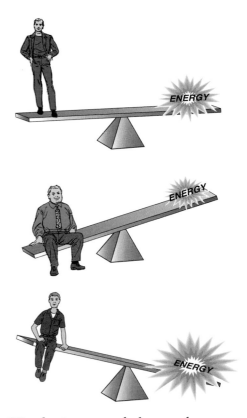

We obtain energy balance when we burn the same number of calories as we take in. Imbalance occurs when we burn fewer or greater calories than we take in every day.

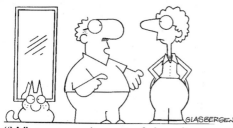

"Who says we're out of shape? We've got lots of shape!"

of food but exercise less and burn fewer calories. Excess calories are stored as fat.

The increased fat and lower amount of lean body mass (muscle) have another consequence—they reduce the body's energy needs. Fat is not metabolically active like muscle and doesn't require energy to work. Fat cells are passive receptacles for storing extra energy. Because the relative amount of fat increases, and the amount of muscle decreases with age, we need fewer calories to maintain body weight.

The excess weight that is acquired with aging has adverse health consequences. Being overweight can cause or worsen high cholesterol, diabetes, and high blood pressure. Excess weight results in greater wear and tear on the weight-bearing joints, particularly the knees and lower back. Obesity is a contributing factor in osteoarthritis, the most common cause of painful knees. When an overweight person puts stress on the knee joints, the pain precipitates a downward spiral. Pain deters the person from physical activity. With increased immobility, the person burns fewer calories and stores more fat. Larger stores of fat put more stress on the joints, which exacerbates the pain of arthritis and leads to further immobility.

People who acquire fat as they age store it in different places. People who have "pear-shaped" bodies (usually women) store fat around the hips and thighs. People who have "apple-shaped" bodies store fat around the midsection or abdomen. People who are "apple shaped" are at greater risk of serious health problems such as diabetes, high cholesterol levels, and heart disease than those who are "pear shaped."

Aging of Body Systems

It is important to understand how each body system ages and how physical activity and exercise affect the aging process. Although we don't understand what causes the changes that occur with aging, we know what is likely to occur.

Skin

As we age, the skin becomes discolored, thinner, and less elastic. Most changes in the skin's appearance are due to chronic exposure to ultraviolet radiation from sunlight. This process, known as photoaging, differs from intrinsic or normal aging. The most common effect of photoaging is both fine and coarse wrinkling on exposed areas such as the face, arms, hands, and neck. People who have spent a lot of time in the sun—farmers, avid golfers, or sailing buffs—have deeply wrinkled skin. Sun-induced wrinkling is made worse by cigarette smoking. Smokers often have deep furrows in their foreheads and around their eyes.

Sunlight also causes mottling or uneven coloring of the skin and the development of brown age spots (maculas). Thinning of

Slip, Slap, Slop

To protect your skin at the beach or pool:

- **Slip on a shirt**
- **Slap on a hat**
- **Slop on some sunscreen**

Recommendation from the American Cancer Society.

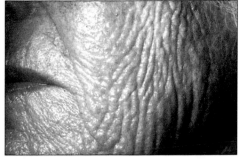

Skin damaged by sun.

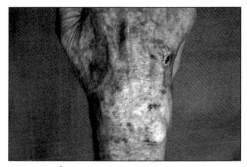

Actinic keratoses.

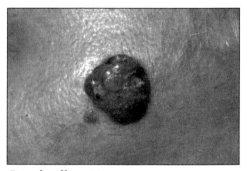

Basal cell carcinoma.

Cosmetic Surgery

Many people choose to have their wrinkles removed by surgery, which can cost $2,500 or more depending on what they have done. Some people have wrinkles removed by laser surgery; others have their entire faces "lifted" to tighten the skin. We don't take a position for or against cosmetic surgery. Just remember that whatever you have done will be temporary, and whether you have surgery or not, exercise will tone your body and make you look and feel better.

the skin's subcutaneous layers combined with sun damage can lead to bleeding into the skin, or purpura. Serious, long-term sun exposure can lead to rough, red, precancerous lesions called actinic keratoses or to skin cancer itself.

Americans spend millions of dollars each year on skin care products. Is it worth it? Do these products keep old age at bay? We cannot say, but here are some facts for you to consider. As we age, our skin will wrinkle, lose its tone and sag, and become thinner and more translucent. You can take the following steps to keep your skin looking and feeling as good as possible:

- Stay out of the sun, especially between 10 AM and 2 PM.

- Protect your skin from the sun.

- Use a sunscreen with an SPF of 15 or more.

- Wear a brimmed hat and a long-sleeved shirt and pants.

- Use inexpensive creams to keep your skin moist.

- Exercise and eat a healthy diet.

- Don't smoke cigarettes!

Although there is no evidence that exercise has any effect on the aging of skin, by improving circulation and toning the muscles, exercise will make you feel and look better.

Sweat Glands

Sweat gland activity declines as we grow older. Sweat glands are the body's cooling system. Secreted sweat evaporating on the skin's surface carries off excess heat, cooling the body. Because sweat glands cool the body less effectively as we age, we may not be able to tolerate high heat and humidity as well as when we were young. Use caution, therefore, if you are exercising in very hot or humid conditions, especially if you have not adjusted to the climate.

Hair

Hair is an appendage of the skin. The most familiar sign of aging is graying hair. Hair loses its color and begins to turn gray in about

50 percent of persons by age 40. Also, progressive hair loss begins in the second or third decade in men. By age 80, some 80 percent of men are substantially bald. As far as we know, none of these events can be prevented. Exercise, although it improves circulation, will not affect your baldness. However, the overuse of chemicals can dry and damage the hair, aggravating hair loss.

Hearing

Hearing may decline with age. Hearing loss of some sort affects about one third of all adults between 65 and 74 years of age and about half of those between 75 and 79 years. Poor hearing can adversely affect quality of life and the ability to live independently.

The most common type of hearing loss in older people is called presbycusis ("hearing loss due to aging") and is due to dysfunction of both the sensory elements in the inner ear and the nerve fibers that carry signals from the ear to the brain.

The exact cause of age-related hearing loss is unknown, but exposure to loud noise appears at least in part responsible. Usually, men are more severely affected than women, probably due to more noise exposure over their lifetimes. Initially, presbycusis affects only very high sound frequencies and does not interfere with understanding speech. Progressive hearing loss, however, affects your ability to hear and understand conversation, especially if you are talking to someone in a room with a lot of background noise.

Many different kinds of hearing aids are available to fit individual needs. If you experience hearing loss, request a complete evaluation by a licensed audiologist or physician who specializes in ear problems to rule out any disease process or drug reaction. Only then should you be fitted for a hearing aid by a professional who will ensure that you get the best possible fit for your life-style and needs.

There is no evidence that exercise has a positive or negative effect on hearing.

Eyes

Sight may diminish with age because of changes in the eyes. The most common change in the aging eye is presbyopia, or the need for reading glasses. To bring into focus an object that is closer than 1 to 2 feet, the lens must increase its thickness. With presbyopia, the lens becomes less flexible and can't make this adjustment. Near objects appear blurred, and we need reading glasses to read or decipher small objects.

Tear production also declines, affecting the surface moisture of the eye. The iris, or colored part of the eye, regulates pupil size and reaction to light. With age, the pupil becomes smaller, which allows less light to reach the lens so that objects do not seem as bright. The iris also reacts more sluggishly to changes in light, so that we might have difficulty adjusting to bright light and shadow.

We may be dazzled when we go outdoors into bright sunlight or blinded a little when we come back into a dimly lit room. We may also have difficulty seeing at night. Poor night vision is very common in people from age 50 on.

To our knowledge, none of these aging changes can be prevented. If you have difficulty seeing in the dark or in dim light, you should take this into account if you exercise at dusk. We do not recommend that anyone, whether he or she has impaired or perfect night vision, run or walk on the open road at night. This practice is dangerous and puts both pedestrians and drivers at risk.

A common condition in the aging eye is cataracts. The lens becomes less clear with age. After age 40, pigments may appear that impair vision and that may develop into cataracts. Because age is the major risk factor for developing a cataract, almost anyone who lives

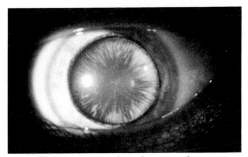

When cataracts develop in the eye, a gray-white film can be seen in the lens behind the pupil.

How to Select Sunglasses

If you wear prescription glasses

- Have sunglasses made according to your prescription. Clip-on shades are generally not as effective as custom-made sunglasses.

If you wear contact lenses or have normal vision

- Select a quality pair of nonprescription sunglasses. Expensive designer sunglasses are no guarantee of quality.

If you've had cataract surgery

- Your eye-care professional will recommend special-purpose lenses. Cataract surgery removes the eye's ultraviolet light-absorbent lens.

If your occupation or recreational activities keep you in very bright sunlight (reflected off water, sand, or snow)

- See an eye-care professional to prepare special-purpose lenses that provide maximal protection.

Selecting Sunglasses for Maximal Protection

- Do they conform to American National Standard Institute (ANSI) standards for ultraviolet light absorption? Glasses that comply with this standard have Z-80.3 printed on their frames.
- Do they have a "transmission factor" of less than 25 percent? This means that they block at least 75 percent of the visible light.
- If no "transmission factor" is stated, can you see your eyes when you look in the mirror while wearing the glasses? If the glasses are dark enough, you won't be able to see your eyes.
- Do they block most blue light? Blue light may be damaging to the macula, an area of the retina. Lenses that absorb instead of block blue light are tinted yellow, brown, or amber. Avoid sunglasses with brown lenses.
- Are the lenses large enough to protect against light coming in from the sides? Consider wraparound sunglasses.
- Do they fit snugly to your nose? Sunglasses that slip can let in ultraviolet rays.
- Do the lenses distort color? Gray and green lenses are better because they distort color the least. Check color accuracy outdoors.
- Do the lenses distort the image? Hold the glasses at arm's length and look at a straight line in the distance. Slowly move the lenses across the line. If the line bends, the lenses are imperfect.

Glass versus Plastic Lenses

Glass Lenses	Plastic Lenses
Heavier	Lightweight
Resist scratching	Scratch easily
Break easily	Resist fogging
	May be impact resistant

long enough will develop one. Fortunately, cataract surgery is common and very safe. If your vision becomes impaired, check with your eye doctor to determine whether surgery is indicated. The risk of developing cataracts increases from exposure to ultraviolet rays of the sun and from smoking. Of the million cataracts removed each year in the United States, as many as 100,000 may be related to sun damage and could be prevented. While exercise does not directly impact the development of cataracts, exercising in bright sunlight will. To protect your eyes, use sunglasses that filter ultraviolet light. To further reduce your risk of cataracts, don't smoke.

Taste

The ability to taste and differentiate foods declines somewhat with age. So does saliva production. However, these changes rarely interfere with the enjoyment of food or eating. A more pronounced inability to taste, a persistent bad taste in the mouth, and dry mouth can interfere with eating, but these changes are more likely to be due to diseases and medication effects rather than aging. Some antidepressant, antihypertensive, and antihistamine medications cause dry mouth and interfere with taste and saliva production. If you experience problems with taste, discuss them with your physician because they may be due to medications.

Cardiovascular and Respiratory Systems

The cardiovascular and respiratory systems include the heart, blood vessels, blood, and lungs. These systems provide oxygen and nutrients to body tissues and remove the major by-products of metabolism.

Oxygen is taken into the blood by the lungs and is pumped by the heart to the vital organs and muscles where it is used for normal metabolism. Waste products (in particular carbon dioxide) are filtered by the blood through the lungs, where they are excreted when we exhale.

How efficiently our bodies deliver and use oxygen and get rid of carbon dioxide determines how much work we can do. The rate and efficiency with which the body takes up and uses oxygen determines how quickly we become breathless when we walk briskly, climb stairs, or play sports. This type of fitness is referred to as cardiovascular endurance. The better our cardiovascular endurance, the more work our bodies can do.

For reasons that are not completely understood, the ability to use oxygen efficiently (cardiovascular endurance) declines with age. It is well documented that lung capacity declines modestly with age and that the heart's pumping function also declines somewhat. The work of the heart is a product of heart rate and the amount of blood pumped by each heartbeat. One of the most noticeable changes that occurs with age is a decline in the maximum heart rate, the highest rate at which the heart will beat. These

Primary Risk Factors for Cardiovascular Disease

- Smoking cigarettes
- Physical inactivity
- High blood pressure
- High blood cholesterol
- Overweight
- Diabetes
- Family history of cardiovascular disease
- Stress
- Gender—Men over age 45 and women over age 55 (after menopause)

Changes to the Cardiovascular System with Aging

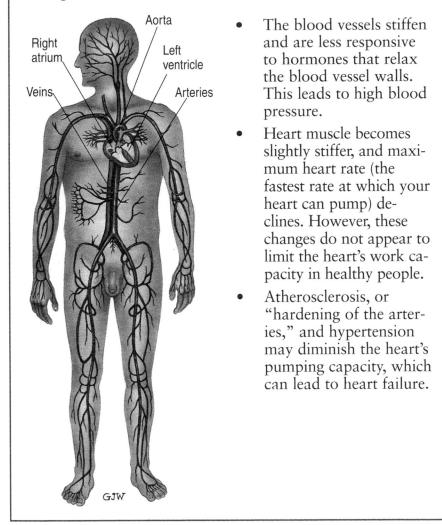

- The blood vessels stiffen and are less responsive to hormones that relax the blood vessel walls. This leads to high blood pressure.

- Heart muscle becomes slightly stiffer, and maximum heart rate (the fastest rate at which your heart can pump) declines. However, these changes do not appear to limit the heart's work capacity in healthy people.

- Atherosclerosis, or "hardening of the arteries," and hypertension may diminish the heart's pumping capacity, which can lead to heart failure.

changes in heart and lung function, however, are limiting only at very high levels of work and rarely impact our ability to perform normal activities. A more important cause of the decline in work efficiency is the loss of muscle mass that occurs with aging. The efficiency with which the body uses oxygen depends not only on how well the lungs extract oxygen and how well the heart pumps blood, but also on the efficiency with which the muscles extract oxygen during physical exertion. Loss of muscle mass seems to be as important as any change in heart function in lowering the efficiency with which we use oxygen. Not only is there less oxygen-rich blood being pumped from the heart, there is also less muscle for extracting and burning oxygen efficiently.

Fortunately, cardiovascular endurance can be maintained at very high levels well into later life with regular physical activity. And it's never too late to improve fitness and work capacity. People who have low endurance because of inactivity can regain much of their work capacity by becoming physically active. Those who have the lowest endurance have the most to be gained from increasing their activity. A very modest program of walking, bicy-

Work Capacity Depends On:

- The lungs' capacity for taking in oxygen (respiratory function)

- The heart's capacity for pumping blood (cardiac output)

- The muscles' capacity for removing oxygen (metabolism)

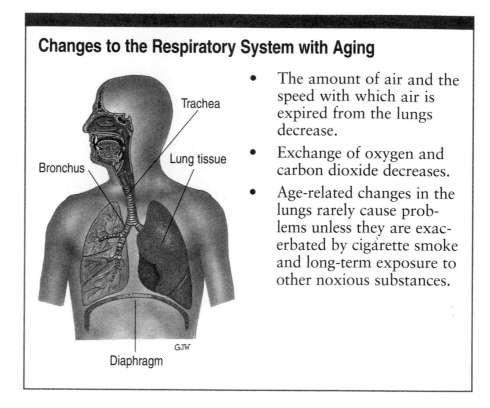

Changes to the Respiratory System with Aging

Trachea

Bronchus

Lung tissue

Diaphragm

GJW

- The amount of air and the speed with which air is expired from the lungs decrease.

- Exchange of oxygen and carbon dioxide decreases.

- Age-related changes in the lungs rarely cause problems unless they are exacerbated by cigarette smoke and long-term exposure to other noxious substances.

cling, or other activities that raise the heart rate will quickly improve physical endurance by increasing both the heart's capacity for pumping blood and circulating oxygen and the muscles' capacity for extracting it.

Blood Pressure

Blood pressure depends on the heart's capacity for pumping blood and the blood vessels' capacity for moving blood throughout the body. Blood vessels have a natural elasticity that enables them to dilate (open and close) to provide resistance or pressure and thus control the flow of blood through the vascular bed. Blood flow is also regulated by hormones that relax the muscles in the blood vessel walls.

These important properties change with aging. Blood vessels become stiffer due to the loss of normal elastic tissue in the blood vessel walls. Moreover, the vessels lose their sensitivity to hormonal changes that regulate blood flow. Deposits of fat and cholesterol in the artery walls further impede the flow of blood through the blood vessels. This is due to the disease process of atherosclerosis, called "hardening of the arteries." All these age-related changes in the blood vessels increase the resistance of the blood moving against the artery walls so that blood pressure rises.

High Blood Pressure. Why is high blood pressure important? The higher our blood pressure, the greater our risk of stroke, heart attack, and kidney failure. Even within the so-called normal range of blood pressure (less than 140/90 mm Hg), a higher blood pressure is associated with a greater risk of these events. This relationship is what scientists call "continuous risk." For example, a person

What Do the Numbers Mean?

- *Systolic blood pressure* (**the top or high number**) Gives the pressure of the blood against the artery walls when the heart muscle contracts to pump blood into the arteries.

- *Diastolic blood pressure* (**the bottom or low number**) Gives the pressure of the blood against the artery walls when the heart is at rest (between beats).

Both numbers are important. A normal resting blood pressure indicates that the heart is generating the proper amount of force to push the blood into the arteries and also that the artery walls are not excessively stiff.

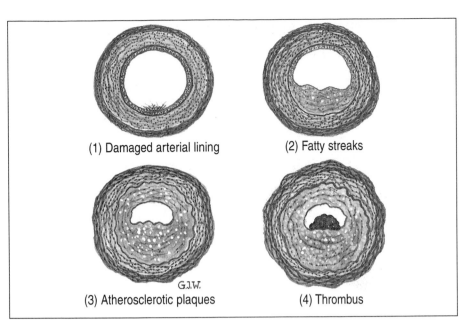

(1) Damaged arterial lining   (2) Fatty streaks

G.J.W.

(3) Atherosclerotic plaques   (4) Thrombus

The progression of atherosclerosis in an artery. In the initial stage, fatty streaks develop within the arterial lining (2). Over time, fats and calcium are deposited in the arterial wall, causing atherosclerotic plaques to develop within the artery (3). The channel through which blood flows eventually becomes so narrowed that obstruction by a blood clot (thrombus) may occur (4).

with a blood pressure reading of 120/80 mm Hg (which is within the normal range) has a greater risk for a heart attack than a person with a blood pressure reading of 110/70 mm Hg.

Like many other age-related changes, high blood pressure is not inevitable and appears to be largely related to life-style, particularly physical activity. Persons who are physically active have lower blood pressure levels and are less likely, over time, to have their blood pressure reach the levels that require drug treatment. Furthermore, physical activity seems to be effective in lowering high blood pressure. Along with a low-sodium diet and weight loss, exercise is one of the first therapies that doctors recommend for people with high blood pressure.

Low Blood Pressure. Low blood pressure, or hypotension, is not a problem for most people. A condition known as postural hypotension troubles some people. They may experience a short period of dizziness when they quickly change from a reclining to a standing position. This condition is usually transient and causes most concern in the frail elderly.

Taking Your Blood Pressure

Avoid caffeine, nicotine, over-the-counter drugs, and vigorous activity on the day your blood pressure is measured. If possible, have it measured twice, because blood pressure fluctuates from day to day.

Tips About Blood Pressure

- There are no symptoms for high blood pressure. That's why it's called the "silent killer." You could have high blood pressure and not know it. If left untreated, it could lead to stroke, heart attack, or kidney failure.

- Know your numbers. Get your blood pressure checked by a health care professional at least once every year, even if all previous readings were normal. Make a note of your blood pressure and keep track of any changes.

- Be active, avoid cigarettes, maintain an appropriate body weight, and limit your intake of sodium and alcohol to help keep your blood pressure within a normal range.

- If you take blood pressure medication, take it as prescribed by your doctor. Don't change your medication dose or schedule without talking with your doctor first.

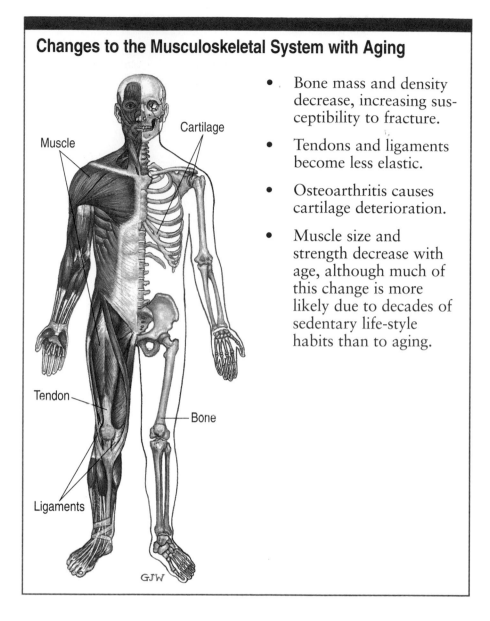

Changes to the Musculoskeletal System with Aging

- Bone mass and density decrease, increasing susceptibility to fracture.

- Tendons and ligaments become less elastic.

- Osteoarthritis causes cartilage deterioration.

- Muscle size and strength decrease with age, although much of this change is more likely due to decades of sedentary life-style habits than to aging.

Musculoskeletal System

The musculoskeletal system comprises the skeletal muscles, bones, tendons, ligaments, and joints.

Muscle

Some degree of muscle atrophy (muscle shrinkage) is a normal part of aging, but loss of muscle mass accelerates with inactivity. Muscle loss begins in the mid-40s and, unchecked by exercise, proceeds at a rate of approximately 1.5 percent per year. Over a 20-year period, about 30 percent of your original muscle mass may be lost through loss of muscle tissue.

Muscles work by contracting (shortening). The force of the contraction across the joints sets us in motion. To demonstrate the role of muscle in moving the joints, sit in a chair and extend your leg, raising your foot off the ground. Feel your thigh muscle as it contracts or shortens to pull your leg straight at the knee. Both the strength and the speed with which the muscle shortens decline with age.

The loss of muscle that occurs with aging rarely affects our ability to accomplish daily tasks. When we enjoy good health, we rarely need our maximal muscle strength to accomplish routine daily activities such as housecleaning, shopping, and cooking. We also enjoy leisure activities—gardening, golf, or swimming—without maximal exertion. If, however, we develop a medical problem such as heart disease, pneumonia, or arthritis, the immobilizing effects of these conditions accelerate muscle loss. If we have good reserves of maximal muscle strength before illness, the muscle losses due to enforced immobility are not enough to prevent us from resuming normal activities when illness resolves. We continue to shop, cook, clean, and play golf, even if more slowly. But if we have allowed our muscles to waste from years of sedentary life-style habits, the enforced immobility that accompanies illness will have a much greater impact on muscle strength and fitness, and we will be less able to cope with the stresses of illness or make timely recoveries. The inability to resume normal daily activities may result in lost independence and diminished quality of life.

Physical activity can protect against the loss of muscle mass that accompanies aging. Several research studies have shown that older people, even those in their 90s, can increase muscle mass and strength through weight training. Physical activity can slow the physiological changes of aging and preserve our ability to stay healthy, live independently, recover from illness, and manage our lives.

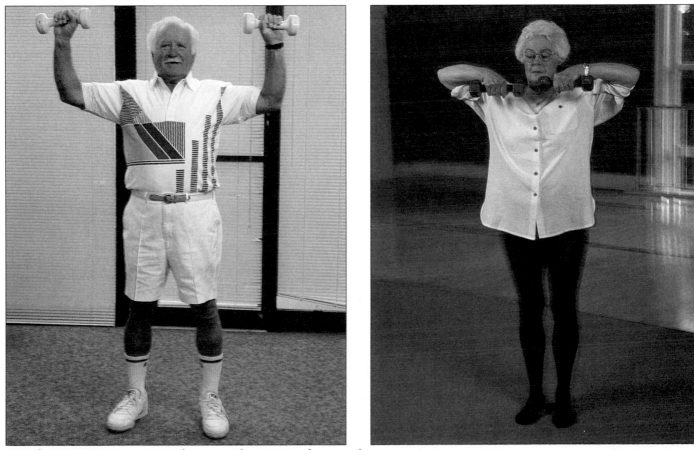

Weight training can restore lost muscle mass and strength.

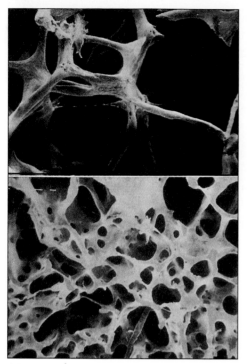

Tissue of osteoporotic (top) and normal bone (bottom).

Bones

Bone is made of collagen and calcium. Under normal circumstances, bone is constantly being remodeled. The body uses the bones as a reservoir for calcium to assist in many vital body functions. In proportion to how much calcium the bones give up, new bone is formed. Both diet and aging affect bone remodeling. When calcium stores are low, the body breaks down more bone than it can remake. For this reason, maintaining a high-calcium diet is important to keep the bones strong and supple. Also, with age, the bones lose their capacity for remodeling. Over time, bone tissue loses density, becomes thin, brittle, and susceptible to fracture. This process is caused both by natural aging and by osteoporosis, a disease that accelerates loss of bone tissue.

The degree and prevalence of bone loss differs according to race and sex. African-Americans have more bone mass than whites, who have more bone mass than Asians. Women have less bone mass to start with than men. During menopause, the ovaries stop producing estrogen, which protects against bone loss. After menopause, at around age 50, bone loss in women accelerates. Men don't usually experience significant bone loss until their 80s.

Untreated, bone loss progresses to a "fracture threshold," the point at which the bones break when they are subject to even mild stress or trauma. Osteoporosis is the leading cause of bone fractures in the older population, causing an estimated 1.5 million fractures a year in the United States. The most common sites for fractures are the spine, hips, lower legs, wrists, and vertebrae. Approximately one third of women and one sixth of men who live to be 90 will experience a hip fracture. Vertebral fractures,

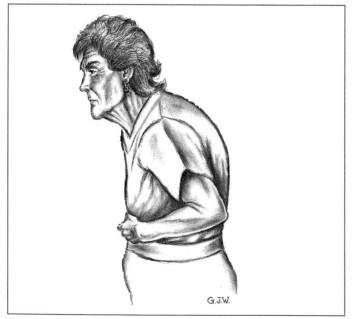

Dowager's hump is caused by multiple fractures of the vertebrae and occurs in 40 percent of women who have osteoporosis.

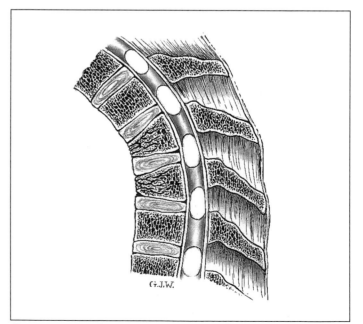

Compression fractures occur in soft, weakened bone when stress is placed on the spine. Fractures can occur from mundane activities such as opening a window or lifting a heavy bag of groceries.

tiny hairline breaks in the spine, are associated with severe, debilitating pain. Sometimes, more than one vertebrae are affected. Multiple fractures commonly lead to shortening of the spine, which can reduce height by as much as 15 to 20 percent. A hump develops in the upper portion of the spinal column, bringing the head and shoulders forward. This condition, called kyphosis or dowager's hump, affects 40 percent of women who have osteoporosis.

The rate of bone loss can be slowed by regular physical activity, adequate intake of calcium, and, in women, the use of estrogen replacement therapy after menopause. Numerous studies have shown that walking, strength training, and participating in sports slow the rate of bone loss and help prevent fractures and changes in stature.

Joints

There are two types of joints in the body. Diarthrodial joints are the joints between two long bones, such as those in the legs, feet, arms, and hands. These joints allow almost all free movement through a wide range of motions. Amphithrodial joints connect the bones by fibrous tissue and are mostly found between the vertebrae in our spines. These joints allow flexibility and stability through a more limited range of motions.

Important parts of the joints are:

- *Ligaments.* Fibrous bands that hold the joints together.

- *Bursae.* Sacs of fluid that allow the skin and muscles to slide over joints and bones.

- *Tendons.* Attach muscles to bone.

- *Cartilage.* Smooth tissue on the ends of the bones that allow the joints to move easily.

Little is known about the normal aging of joints, but it appears that most joints maintain full function well into later life. A decrease in joint range of motion, however, occurs with age due to decreased elasticity of ligaments and tendons. We can maintain range of motion of the joints (flexibility) with regular physical activity, especially stretching. Flexibility is an important and often neglected component of physical fitness.

Unfortunately, joint inflammation and cartilage degeneration due to arthritis occur frequently as we age. In fact, problems with muscles and bones are the leading causes of disability in people over 60. Although people with rheumatoid arthritis and other musculoskeletal problems often think that physical activity and exercise are harmful, nothing could be further from the truth. Modest physical activity lessens joint pain and improves flexibility and function. Stretching, walking, swimming, and water aerobics are all excellent ways to exercise without causing further joint damage or injury. During arthritis flare-ups, you may want to lessen activity until stiffness subsides.

Who Is Susceptible to Osteoporosis?

Are you:

- Female?
- Postmenopausal?
- Fair skinned?
- Of Asian or Scandinavian origin?
- Of small body frame?
- Of low body weight or underweight?
- Inactive?
- A smoker?

The more "yes" responses you make, the greater your risk of developing osteoporosis.

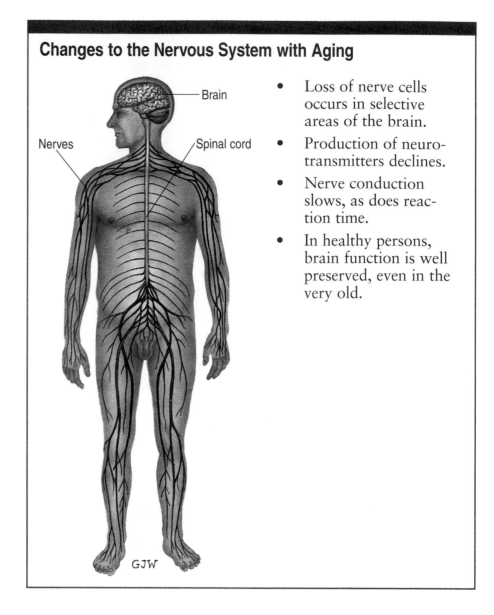

Changes to the Nervous System with Aging

Brain

Nerves

Spinal cord

- Loss of nerve cells occurs in selective areas of the brain.
- Production of neurotransmitters declines.
- Nerve conduction slows, as does reaction time.
- In healthy persons, brain function is well preserved, even in the very old.

GJW

Nervous System

The nervous system comprises the brain, spinal cord and nerve branches, and neurotransmitters, chemicals that send nerve signals across the spaces separating nerve fibers. Studies of the aging brain show that the brain shrinks slightly with age. Apart from slowed reaction times, temporary forgetfulness, and altered sleep-wake patterns, normal changes do not significantly affect our thinking or behavior, and brain function is preserved well into old age. Reaction time slows, probably due to delayed conduction of impulses along nerve fibers or delayed transmission of messages across the spaces (synapses) between nerve fibers. Slowed reaction times are exacerbated by stress.

Memory, Sleep, and Mood

Memory. Many people find that they have trouble remembering little things as they get older, such as the names of friends or where they left their car keys. The speed of recall may slow with age, but this benign memory loss rarely causes problems. And, fortunately, we can usually remember what we forgot! Difficulty remembering things is probably related less to aging than to fatigue, stress, too much caffeine, and the demands of a busy life. More serious and permanent memory loss is generally associated with age-related diseases, such as Alzheimer's disease or small strokes. Some medications may cause a loss of memory. If you experience memory problems, consult your physician.

Sleep. Curiously, we need less sleep as we get older. Many older people sleep only 5 to 6 hours per night, whereas they needed 8 to 9 hours of sleep per night 20 years ago. We also experience lighter sleep and awaken more frequently during the night, but these patterns are more likely due to age-related health conditions and medications rather than to changes in neurological function. Both men and women find that they must get up during the night to urinate as they grow older. Pain from arthritis or shortness of breath from lung disease may also disrupt normal sleep patterns.

Mood. There seems to be little change in mood with age. Clinical depression, a common and disabling condition throughout life, occurs no more often in people over 50 than it does in the general population. However, as we age, we often have to deal with many serious life events and crises, such as the death of a parent or spouse or the loss of financial security. Many people in their 40s and 50s belong to the "sandwich generation"—they find themselves raising their children (probably teenagers!) while also caring for their elderly parents. The stress from looking after both children and parents can lead to depression, anxiety, and loss of well-being.

Does physical activity affect these changes in mental well-being? The answer is "yes." Studies have shown that:

- People who are more physically active can recall facts more quickly than those who aren't active.

- People who incorporate regular physical activity into their daily routines report that they fall asleep more easily at night and that their quality of sleep is better.

- Exercise reduces stress, probably by reducing the hormones released by the autonomic nervous system. The body is better able to cope with stress, so the response to stress is less marked.

Digestive System

The digestive system consists of the esophagus, the stomach, the small intestine, the large intestine or colon, the liver and gallbladder, and the pancreas. The digestive system absorbs nutrients and works efficiently into advanced age, but several important changes may occur.

Changes to the Digestive System with Aging

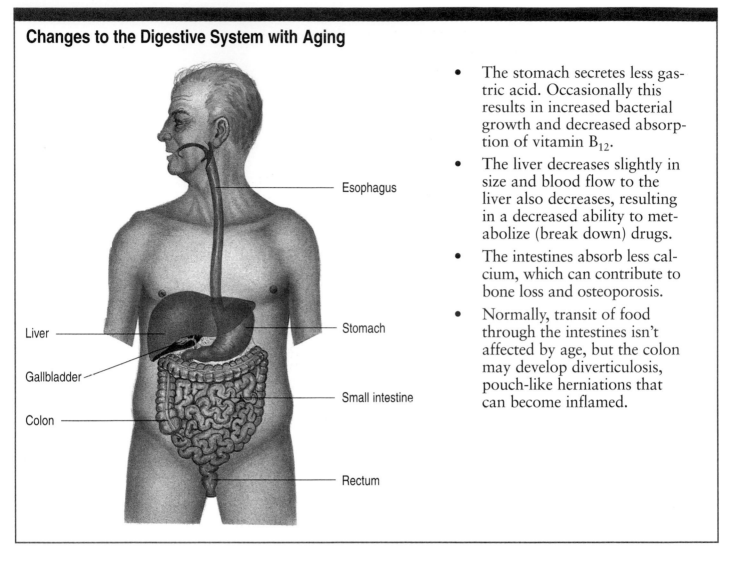

- The stomach secretes less gastric acid. Occasionally this results in increased bacterial growth and decreased absorption of vitamin B_{12}.

- The liver decreases slightly in size and blood flow to the liver also decreases, resulting in a decreased ability to metabolize (break down) drugs.

- The intestines absorb less calcium, which can contribute to bone loss and osteoporosis.

- Normally, transit of food through the intestines isn't affected by age, but the colon may develop diverticulosis, pouch-like herniations that can become inflamed.

Stomach

Decreased secretion of stomach acid can occasionally result in increased bacteria growth in the intestine and decreased absorption of vitamin B_{12}. Vitamin B_{12} is necessary for the production of red blood cells and for maintaining neurological function. Deficiency of vitamin B_{12}, called pernicious anemia, can cause confusion and difficulty walking.

Liver

The liver controls energy expenditure and cholesterol metabolism and breaks down many of the body's wastes. The liver has an important function in metabolizing medications. Blood flow to the liver and the ability to oxidize or metabolize drugs decline with age. Thus, older people may require lower doses of certain medications.

Intestines

In general, the movement of food through the intestines is not dramatically affected by age. The small intestines absorb less calcium, which can result in the loss of bone density and osteoporosis. Although constipation is a common complaint, reduced intestinal motility (the inability to move food through the intestines) is likely due to lack of dietary fiber, inactivity, medication use, and over-reliance on laxatives. Research has shown that regular physical activity and a diet high in fiber prevent constipation and help to maintain intestinal function and normal bowel movements.

Urinary System

As we age, the kidneys shrink by as much as one quarter to one third. Blood flow through the kidneys decreases by as much as 10 percent per decade beginning in our mid-40s. This decrease is accompanied by a progressive decline in the rate at which the kidneys filter substances in the blood.

Age-related changes affect the urinary system in several ways. Bladder capacity, the ability to postpone urination, and urinary flow seem to decrease in both men and women, and urinary patterns also change. As we grow older, we get up in the night, more frequently to urinate. Nocturia, excessive urination at night, is a normal part of aging and only occasionally indicates kidney disease or other conditions such as congestive heart failure.

It is not known whether physical activity has any effect on the urinary system. Physical activity, by strengthening the pelvic muscles, may help bladder control.

Changes to the Urinary System with Aging

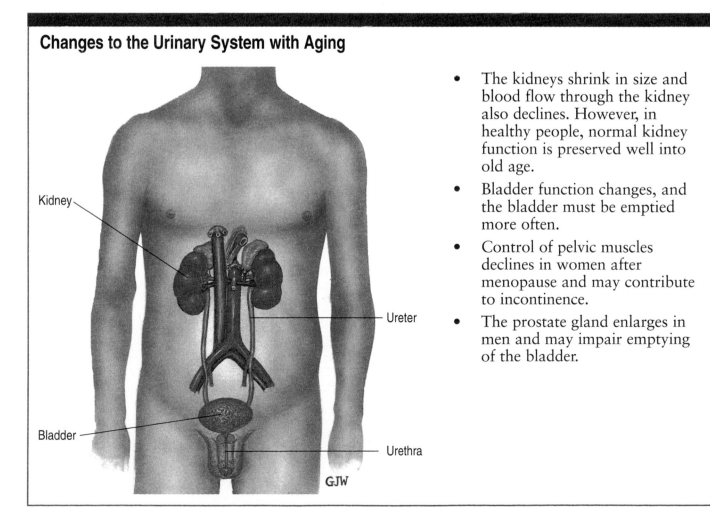

Kidney
Ureter
Bladder
Urethra
GJW

- The kidneys shrink in size and blood flow through the kidney also declines. However, in healthy people, normal kidney function is preserved well into old age.

- Bladder function changes, and the bladder must be emptied more often.

- Control of pelvic muscles declines in women after menopause and may contribute to incontinence.

- The prostate gland enlarges in men and may impair emptying of the bladder.

Endocrine System

The endocrine system comprises a complex network of glands and structures that secrete hormones directly into the blood to regulate a number of important functions, among them fat and sugar metabolism and reproduction.

Pancreas

The pancreas regulates metabolism. *Metabolism* is a broad term encompassing all the mechanisms the body uses for burning fuel (sugar and fat) for energy. After we eat, the pancreas secretes insulin (a hormone) that allows the cells in muscle tissue to take up glucose (sugar) from the bloodstream and use it as fuel for their work. If we don't take in enough food, the body runs out of glucose and uses reserves of energy stored in fat. Glucose can be converted to energy more quickly than fat.

The efficiency of these processes declines with age. The aging body's cells are less sensitive to the effects of insulin and need more of it to convert glucose to energy. This abnormal requirement for more insulin is called "insulin resistance." Insulin resistance becomes more pronounced as the amount of muscle decreases and the amount of fat increases.

What Causes Diabetes?

Diabetes can be classified as Type I or Type II.

Type I (Insulin-Dependent Diabetes Mellitus)

In Type I diabetes, the pancreas stops producing insulin. The Type I diabetic thus needs to take insulin, which is available commercially for administration via injection or insulin pump.

Only 10 percent of diabetics have Type I, which is also known as juvenile or juvenile-onset diabetes because it is most common in children and young adults.

Type II (Non-Insulin-Dependent Diabetes Mellitus)

In Type II diabetes, the body has developed a resistance to insulin. Unlike Type I diabetics, those with Type II can produce insulin, but more insulin is needed to maintain normal glucose levels. Type II diabetes is usually managed through a combination of diet, exercise, and hypoglycemic drugs, such as the sulfonylureas and metformin. Sometimes, people who have Type II diabetes stop producing insulin and then require insulin injections.

Type II diabetes is also know as adult-onset or stable diabetes, because most people who develop it are over 40. Numerous research studies suggest that Type II diabetes in older adults is related to a lifetime of overeating and physical inactivity.

Who is susceptible to Type II diabetes?

Are you:

- Over 50?
- Overweight?
- Inactive?
- "Apple shaped?"

The more "yes" responses you make, the greater your risk of developing diabetes.

Signs of Diabetes

- Fatigue
- Increased thirst
- Increased urination
- Blurred vision
- Rapid weight loss
- Recurrent infections

Changes to the Endocrine System with Aging

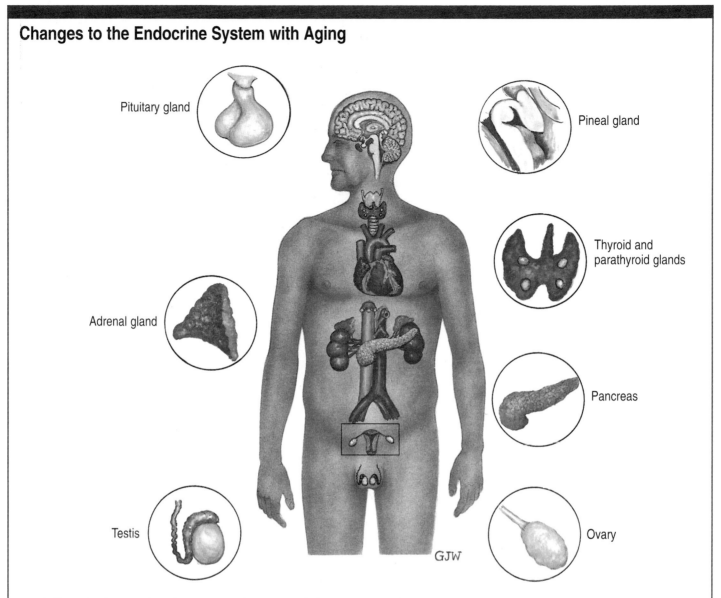

Pituitary gland

Pineal gland

Thyroid and parathyroid glands

Adrenal gland

Pancreas

Testis

Ovary

GJW

- **The pituitary gland** secretes the growth hormone. Decreased levels of growth hormone may contribute to age-related declines in muscle and bone strength, thinning skin, and increased fat.

- **The pineal gland** secretes melatonin. Decreased levels of this hormone may be responsible for changes in the sleep-wake cycle.

- Secretion of the thyroid hormone by the **thyroid gland** does not change with age.

- The **pancreas** secretes insulin. With age, muscle cells become "resistant" to insulin and are unable to use it efficiently to pick up glucose in the blood stream and use it for energy. The pancreas responds by secreting more insulin. Initially, we may have too much insulin in the blood—a condition known as hyperinsulinemia, but eventually the pancreas may wear out. Then we need insulin injections.

- **The adrenal glands** secrete cortisol and DHEA. Levels of cortisol remain constant with aging, but DHEA secretion declines significantly and may affect immune and cardiovascular function.

- **The ovaries** secrete estrogen. Estrogen production declines significantly in women after age 50, leading to bone loss and increased risk of heart attack.

- **The testes** secrete testosterone and dyhydrotestosterone. Modest declines in these hormones may in part be responsible for decline in muscle strength. They are not associated with changes in sexual activity.

Hormones and Aging

- *Estrogen*—Female hormone that helps maintain healthy bone and prevents heart disease. Levels decrease markedly after menopause.

- *Testosterone/dyhydrotestosterone*—Male hormone necessary for normal sexual functioning that helps maintain healthy muscle and bone. Levels of the hormone decrease slightly with age.

- *Insulin*—Hormone necessary for metabolizing sugar. Older, overweight adults become resistant to insulin and can develop diabetes.

If left unchecked, insulin resistance develops into diabetes. Diabetes is common in people over age 50, affecting between 15 and 20 percent of people in this age group. In its early stages, this type of diabetes, called Type II or adult-onset diabetes, is associated with too much rather than too little insulin in the blood. However, people with adult-onset diabetes may eventually require insulin therapy. Over time, the pancreas cannot produce enough of the hormone to compensate for the cells' inability to use insulin for converting glucose. Eventually, the pancreas simply wears out. The insulin resistance syndrome can lead to the development of serious problems including high blood pressure, atherosclerosis, heart disease, and stroke. Diabetes is a major risk factor for cardiovascular disease. We can protect against insulin resistance and these serious problems that follow in its wake by controlling our weight and staying physically active.

Ovaries

The ovaries regulate female reproductive processes by secreting the female sex hormones estrogen and progesterone. Secretion of hormones begins to decline in the mid-30s and 40s and stops at menopause. The average age of onset of menopause has remained at around 50 years for several centuries. Loss of estrogen is associated with several physiological and clinical changes, including accelerated bone loss, increased risk of heart disease, and changes in the reproductive organs, particularly thinning of the vaginal walls. Hot flashes occur in about half of postmenopausal women.

While exercise has no effect on the onset of menopause, it has a positive effect in avoiding some of the symptoms of menopause. Exercise increases muscle and bone mass and, when combined with a daily calcium intake of 1,000–1,500 mg per day (equivalent to 4 cups of milk per day), protects against calcium loss and osteoporosis. Exercise also improves balance and coordination, reduces the risk of falling and injury, and helps to ensure continued mobility and independence.

Testes

The testes secrete the male sex hormones testosterone and dyhydrotestosterone. Although studies show a modest age-related decline in the level of these hormones, there is not an abrupt change as there is in women. Many elderly men, even in their 90s, have testosterone levels that are not significantly different from those of middle-aged men.

Most men and women maintain sexual function well into late life. Over 75 percent of healthy men over age 70 have sexual intercourse at least once a month, and 25 percent of men over age 78 engage in regular sexual activity. The numbers are lower in women, in large part due to the absence of suitable partners. Sexual activity in later life correlates with the degree of sexual activity in earlier life, as well as with general good health.

Schedule of Preventive Exams for Healthy People After Age 50

Disease/Condition	Test	Frequency of Test
Hypertension	Blood pressure	Yearly
High cholesterol	Blood cholesterol level	At least every 5 years
Coronary heart disease	Stress electrocardiogram Electrocardiogram (ECG)	Recommended before starting a vigorous exercise program
Obesity	Weight and height measurement	Yearly
Breast cancer	Breast exam Mammogram	Yearly Every 1 to 2 years
Cervical cancer	Pap smears	Yearly; may discontinue at 65 if adequate screening has occurred at younger ages
Vision	Eye exam including test for glaucoma	Routinely by eye specialist every 2 years
Hearing	Hearing exam (audiometry)	Only if evidence of impariment
Colorectal cancer	Test stool for blood Sigmoidoscopy Colonoscopy	Yearly Every 5 to 10 years For high-risk individuals only
Skin cancer	Observation during physical exam	Yearly
Prostate cancer	PSA test Digital rectal exam	Yearly, but this is controversial
Thyroid disease	Thyroid-stimulating hormone	Once
Osteoporosis	Dual absorptiometry to measure bone mineral content	May be clinically useful in high-risk women after menopause

With aging, sexual response becomes delayed, and greater stimulation is required to produce the male erection. Furthermore, there is a longer refractory period after ejaculation and before another erection. No correlation has been documented between levels of male sex hormones and sexual activity. Although there is no research to support the claim, many people who exercise report that they feel better about themselves and are more sexually active.

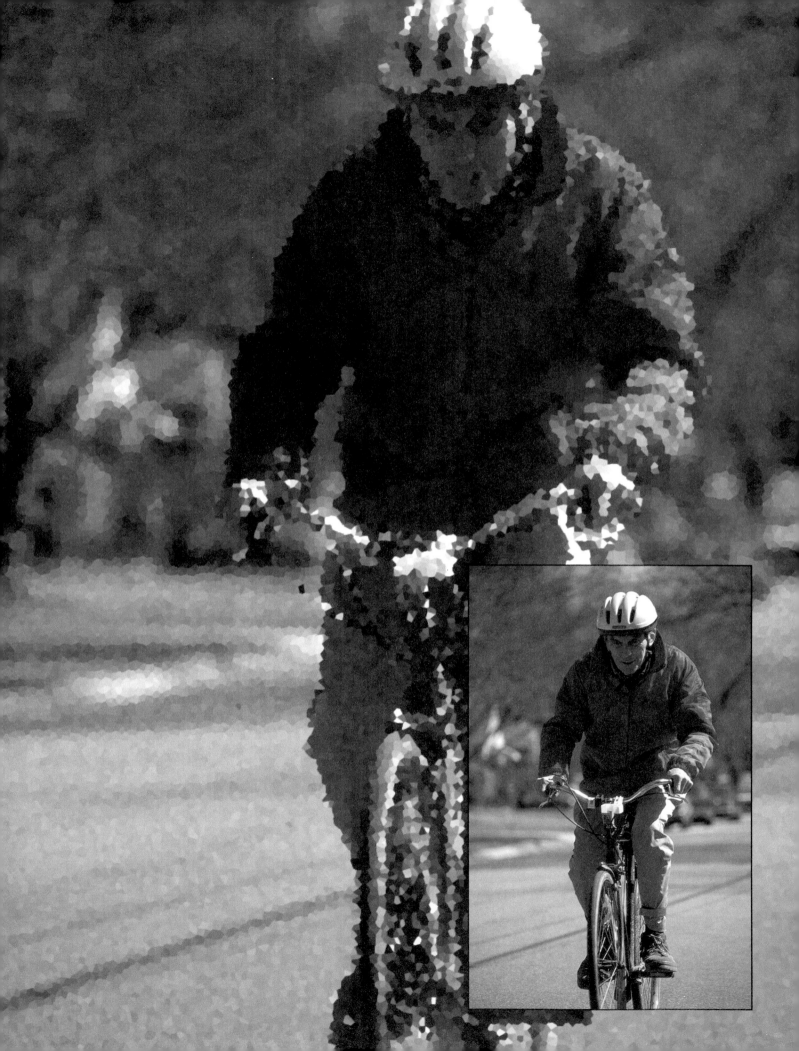

CHAPTER 3

The Many Benefits of Physical Activity

Physicians and philosophers of ancient Greece wrote about the health benefits of physical exercise, but until recently we really didn't know just how good activity is for us. Scientific study of how regular physical activity affects health did not begin in earnest until the mid-1950s. Over the past 40 years, thousands of research studies published in the world's scientific literature have documented the numerous benefits of being active.

This chapter briefly reviews what is known about the connection between physical activity and health and describes the health benefits we can expect from leading fit and active lives, especially as we grow older. And, if the scientific evidence is not persuasive enough, you'll meet several men and women who enjoy the benefits of active life-styles.

Health Benefits of Regular Physical Activity

Human beings are not well adapted to life in highly developed societies. We evolved as hunter-gatherers on the grassy plains of the temperate zones of our planet. For more than 99 percent of human history our ancestors lived in small nomadic bands, ate diets low in fat and calories, were very active, and were not exposed to many environmental pollutants. We do not advocate a return to a Stone-Age way of life, but understanding the way our ancestors lived throughout most of human existence helps us appreciate the rationale for emulating their healthful life-styles.

Fitness Profile

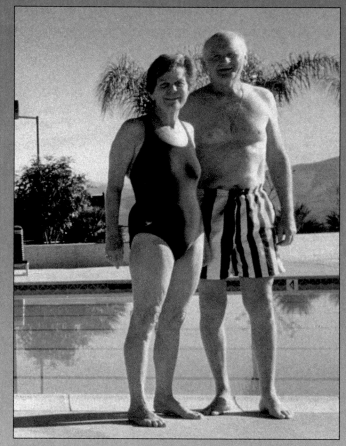

Peggy Woolley-Martin, aged 79, and James Martin, aged 74, enjoy a physically active life that Peggy says helps her "do everything my kids do." Activities they enjoy include walking, bicycling, hiking, swimming, and cross-country skiing. They start each morning with an exercise program that includes a workout on a Health Rider or a Nordic Track, jumping rope, and calisthenics.

Peggy and Jim travel extensively and currently participate in the Friendship Force, an international organization that grew from a program called People to People, which Miz Lillian Carter developed after her son Jimmy left the Presidency. Participants in the program live with families in the foreign countries they visit. Peggy describes these experiences as a great way to meet people and learn about different cultures. She and Jim continue their exercise program while they are abroad, and Peggy, who has traveled widely throughout her life, notes, "I've jogged in almost every country of the world."

Exercise and fitness are so well integrated into their lives that she and Jim never think twice about whether they want to exercise when they get up in the morning. They feel good when they wake up, ready for the physical rigors and intellectual challenges of another day. "It's a habit for us," says Peggy, who exercises every morning as many of us might eat breakfast or watch morning news programs.

"It's good for the mind, too," explains Peggy, who teaches music at a local nursery school. "It keeps me thinking young as well as feeling young." The only change she has made in her fitness regimen over the years has been to switch from jogging to walking, "because the running can be hard on the knees!"

Physical Fitness and Cardiovascular Disease

The importance of physical activity in preventing death from cardiovascular disease is seen in data from the Aerobics Center Longitudinal Study, which was conducted at the Cooper Clinic in Dallas, Texas. The study followed 10,224 men and 3,120 women for 8 years after a clinical examination that included a maximal exercise test on a treadmill. Treadmill test performance is determined primarily by a person's physical activity habits and is taken as the best measure of overall physical fitness. Study participants were assigned to physical fitness categories by their treadmill test results. The least fit 20 percent of men and women were classified as low fit, the next 40 percent of the fitness distribution were called moderately fit, and the most fit 40 percent were assigned to the high fitness category.

During the 8-year follow-up, 240 men and 43 women died. Individuals with low levels of physical fitness at the initial examination were much more likely to die during the follow-up than were men and women who were moderately or highly fit. Cardiovascular disease death rates also were much higher in the low fitness group. As the top figure shows, fewer men and women in the moderate fitness category died than did those in the low fitness category. There was a further decline in risk for men and women in the high fitness category, but the greatest difference was between the low and moderate fitness groups. *This study shows the great benefit of being even moderately active. The study suggests that you do not have to train as if for the Olympics to improve your longevity and health substantially.*

What would have happened to the low fitness group had its members improved their fitness? Would their risk have been reduced? A follow-up study answered this important question. There were 9,777 men who were assessed by the treadmill test twice over a 5-year period. The men were then followed for 5 more years, during which time 223 men died. Of the 994 men who were unfit at the first examination, 638 became fit by the second examination. As

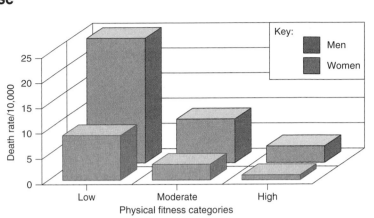

Effect of fitness on risk of death from cardiovascular disease.

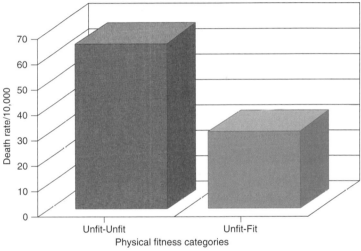

Effect of fitness—unimproved and improved—on risk of death from cardiovascular disease.

the bottom figure shows, the cardiovascular disease death rate was much lower in the men who improved their fitness than it was for those who remained unfit.

Men who were physically fit at both examinations had the lowest death rate (14/10,000), suggesting that it is better to be fit and stay fit. Nonetheless, men who improved their fitness from one examination to the next benefited substantially. Furthermore, the pattern was present in all age groups. Men who were 60 or older cut their death rate in half if they improved from unfit to fit. *This study shows that it is never too late to increase your physical activity, improve your fitness, and reap the health benefits. The reduction in risk associated with improving fitness compares with the reduction in risk observed for smokers who stopped smoking.*

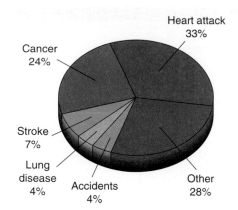

Causes of death in the United States, 1992.

How Important Are These Health Benefits to You?

- Increased longevity
- Reduced risk of heart attack
- Reduced risk of stroke
- Reduced risk of high blood pressure
- Reduced risk of kidney failure
- Lower blood pressure
- Lower blood cholesterol
- Reduced risk of adult-onset diabetes
- Reduced risk of some cancers
- Improved joint function
- Stronger bones
- Improved muscle strength and flexibility
- Improved function
- Less depression
- Improved sense of well-being
- Better weight control

In modern industrialized countries, the major causes of disability, illness, and death are lifestyle-related diseases and conditions such as heart attack, stroke, hypertension, cancer, diabetes, obesity, lung disease, accidents, and osteoporosis. Physical inactivity is an important contributor to many of these health problems. In the United States, diseases of the heart and vascular system are the leading cause of death. In addition, these health problems account for much disability, time away from work or usual activities, and health care expenditures.

A physically active life-style reduces your risk of developing several types of cardiovascular disease, including heart attack, stroke, and hypertension.

Controls High Blood Pressure

The most common cardiovascular disease in the United States is high blood pressure. The American Heart Association (AHA) estimates that more than 60 million people in the United States have high blood pressure.

High blood pressure, or hypertension, has serious consequences, including an increased risk of heart attack, stroke, and kidney failure. High blood pressure is a chronic disease, and once the condition develops, treatment can last for the rest of one's life. There are effective drug treatments, but all have side effects. Often, exercise and a low-sodium diet can control mild hypertension or reduce the number of medications required to effectively treat high blood pressure. But the best defense against high blood pressure is to avoid developing the condition.

The major risk factors for developing high blood pressure are obesity, physical inactivity, and a diet high in fat and salt. Sedentary, unfit individuals are about 50 percent more likely to develop high blood pressure than their more active and fit counterparts. So staying active is a good way to avoid developing this chronic disease.

Reduces Adult-Onset Diabetes

For most people, the term *diabetes* conjures up images of insulin injections. Juvenile-onset diabetes commonly develops early in life and always requires insulin therapy because the pancreas cannot produce the insulin needed to metabolize blood sugar. Contrary to common understanding, this form of diabetes accounts for only about 10 percent of cases.

Most diabetes develops in the middle or later years and is called "adult-onset diabetes." It is characterized by high rather than low levels of insulin in the blood. Adult-onset diabetes is the leading cause of blindness in adults, is an important risk factor for heart attack, and leads to a number of other serious health problems, including kidney failure. Adult-onset diabetes typically develops in sedentary, overweight individuals. Few cases are seen in

Physical Fitness and Cancer

Data from the Aerobics Center Longitudinal Study show lower rates of cancer with higher levels of physical fitness. More than 25,000 men and more than 7,000 women were followed for an average of 8 years after a preventive medical examination that included a treadmill exercise test to measure physical fitness. Study participants were assigned to five physical fitness categories, with *1* being the lowest fitness level and *5* the highest.

During follow-up, 179 men and 44 women died of cancer. Analysis of cancer death rates across fitness categories revealed a downward trend, as the figure to the right shows. *This study shows that maintaining a program of regular physical activity improves your odds against getting cancer.*

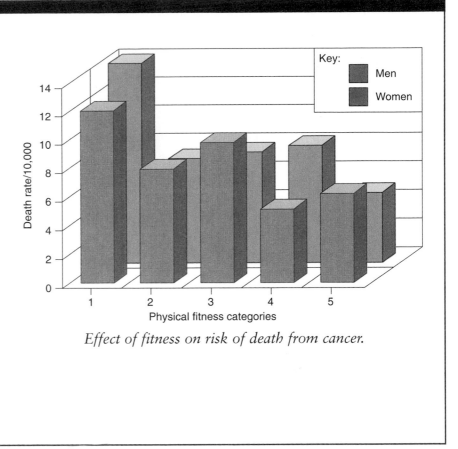

Effect of fitness on risk of death from cancer.

middle-aged and older men and women who maintain normal weight and regular physical activity programs.

Reduces Risk of Some Cancers

Cancer is the second leading cause of death in the United States. It is perhaps the most feared disease because of the high death rate after diagnosis, the unpleasant treatment options, and the wasting nature of the disease. Cancer is a broad category of diseases that differ according to their causes. Smoking causes more cancers than any other single factor, including other poor health habits and pollution.

Lack of exercise is emerging as an important risk factor for cancer. There is now considerable evidence that inactivity is associated with increased risk for colon cancer and lung cancer in both men and women, breast cancer in women, and prostate cancer in men. These are the most common and most feared cancers, and they account for a sizable proportion of cancer deaths each year.

Prevents Osteoporosis

Osteoporosis, a condition that weakens the bones, is common in older people, especially women. Elderly men are susceptible to osteoporosis, but the condition tends to occur later in men than in women. Osteoporosis may affect the spine, leading to "crush fractures" of the vertebrae, which cause the characteristic "dowager's

Fitness Profile

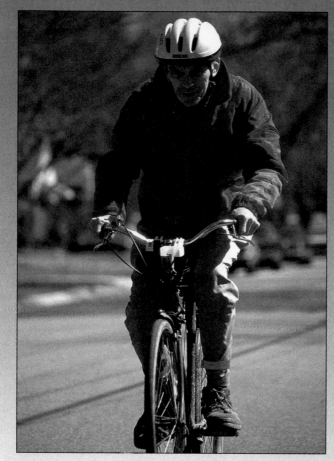

Dr. Michael Potter, aged 72, remembers an experience from medical school that has influenced his activity habits for his entire life. When Dr. Potter was a student, a distinguished professor of cardiology and author of a cardiology textbook was featured in a newspaper photograph riding his bike to work. Impressed by the photograph, Dr. Potter, now a respected physician and researcher in his own right, adopted the same habit and has ridden his bike to and from work at the National Cancer Institute every day for the past 25 years.

Recalling the words of the cardiology professor, Dr. Potter says, "It's important to do a little bit of something every day that takes you outside and keeps the body active." The 1-mile ride from his home to the Institute takes him through a park and makes the journey a little easier. "I ride most of the way through Rock Creek Park," he says, "but there's a long downhill ride just before the Institute, and I have the uphill portion on the way home."

Dr. Potter doesn't rely on an 18-speed bike to help him up the hill, preferring an old 3-speed model he purchased about 23 years ago after its predecessor—an "old, beat-up model that no one would ever think of stealing"—was stolen from his front porch. He rides to work in all kinds of weather, driving only when the snow is too deep.

hump" sometimes seen in older women. Osteoporosis is responsible for almost all hip fractures in older men and women. The outcome may be disastrous, with extensive disability and high death rates in the first few weeks or months after the fracture.

The best protection against osteoporosis is to develop a high bone mass early in life. Some bone loss is inevitable with aging, but if we start with higher masses, bone loss takes longer to reach a critically low threshold. A diet high in calcium and plenty of exercise while we are young is the best way to ensure a high peak bone mass. If we have been habitually sedentary, however, there are still things we can do to maintain our bone health.

Estrogen is the most critical factor for preserving bone in women. After menopause, estrogen levels decline precipitously, and bone loss is very rapid in the first few years after menopause. Estrogen replacement therapy is increasingly prescribed, and it clearly benefits bone health. Like any medication, it has side effects, and each woman must make this important medical decision in consultation with her physician.

Both men and women can preserve bone as they age by following diets with plenty of calcium and vitamin D and by being physically active. Physical activity, in fact, is essential to protect against bone loss. Weight-bearing exercise places stress on the bones, which respond by laying down more bone cells and thereby become stronger. Any weight-bearing activity such as walking is beneficial. Activities in which you change direction seem to be more beneficial than straight-ahead walking. Folk and square dancing and racket sports are highly recommended activities. Even greater benefits come from strength-building exercises (*see Appendix 2*). These can include calisthenics, weight lifting, or doing heavy labor such as digging and working in the garden.

Improves Joint Function and Arthritis

Arthritis is a common disease among older adults and is the leading cause of disability in the United States. Arthritis of the hip and knee is especially debilitating. The pain and stiffness associated with these conditions can have far-reaching effects on mobility and function. Individuals who have these conditions may become more and more sedentary, rarely leaving their homes. Progressively sedentary habits lead to weight gain, which increases the stress on the hips and knees, further damages the joints, and further limits the ability to move and get about. Weight gain and inactivity then combine to worsen existing clinical conditions, such as high blood pressure, high cholesterol, and diabetes. Eventually, the spiraling effects of inactivity due to arthritis can lead to lost personal independence and reliance on others to meet basic needs.

Many people who have arthritis believe that exercising arthritic joints increases damage to cartilage and bone. But rest and inactivity are the worst things you can do for arthritis. Exercise, in fact, is the mainstay of care, improving joint function, strengthening the joints' supportive structures, relieving stiffness, and improving mobility. At the same time, increased physical activity improves overall health.

We are not suggesting that men and women who have arthritis of the hip or knee take up running or strenuous sports. We are recommending regular moderate intensity exercise, such as walking or swimming, for the important health benefits such exercise confers on arthritis patients. If you have arthritis, consult your physician about increasing your activity.

Improves General Well-Being

Physical activity—even very short periods of activity—make us feel good. Inactivity is so unnatural to us that being forced to sit for prolonged periods, perhaps on airplanes or during long car rides, can be almost painful. Getting up, moving about, stretching, bending, or taking short walks always refreshes us.

Exercise and Arthritis

A research study at the Bowman Gray School of Medicine of Wake Forest University documented the benefits of exercise for people with arthritis. More than 400 people over age 60 who had arthritis of the knees were divided into three groups. One group participated in a walking program 3 days per week, a second group lifted weights 3 days a week, and the third group did not exercise. After 18 months, the adults who walked and those who lifted weights had improved their fitness. More important, they had less pain and were better able to carry out daily activities than the adults who didn't exercise. *This study shows that regular, moderate exercise improves symptoms and fitness in people with arthritis.*

Fitness Profile

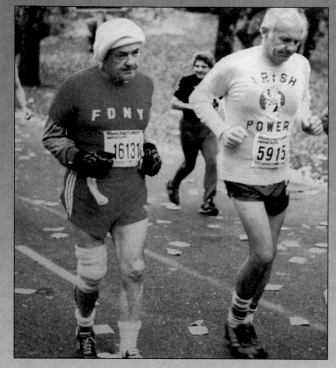

Harry Ahearn, aged 83, shown at far left, is a retired New York City firefighter and novelist who ran his first marathon at age 60. By age 80, he had added 17 more marathons to his resume, finishing the race each time.

"I began running after watching one of my sons in the New York City marathon, held each fall," Harry explains. *"I started running in nearby Marine Park, in Brooklyn. First I ran from one lamppost to another and added a lamppost each day until I was able to run the entire 1-mile track."* He trained for the marathon the same way, adding an extra mile to his course each month of the year before the race. He would rest for 1 month after every marathon, not running at all until beginning his training in December for the next year's race.*

He remembers his first marathon well, due in part to his son's companionship. "He [Harry's son] would start cramping up because of my slow pace, so he would run ahead of me, then double back to check on my progress. The crowd of spectators were all yelling to my son, 'You're going the wrong way!'" Harry recalls with a chuckle.

A competitive athlete in his youth and early adult years, Harry has discovered a different attitude among those who run. "Runners are friendlier," he notes. "I've made a lot of friends among the people who run and walk in the park. We look out for each other and check on people if we don't see them for a while." Harry was recently one of the "missing" when he underwent surgery to replace a faulty heart valve. But, he says, his doctors attribute the ease of the operation and the speed of recovery to the extra efforts he has made to stay fit.

There appear to be long-term psychological benefits from regular physical activity. Several controlled studies show improvements in overall feelings of general well-being in individuals who change from sedentary to active ways of life, largely because activity reduces feelings of tension and anxiety. Activity may also help reduce depression. Many psychologists and psychiatrists use exercise to treat individuals with clinical anxiety and depression. If we want to feel better, a little physical activity may be just what the doctor ordered.

Physical Activity and Weight Gain

In the Aerobics Center Longitudinal Study, men and women who decreased their physical activity were 40 to 80 percent more likely to gain 10 pounds over 5 years than individuals who maintained constant levels of physical activity. Persons who increased their activity were considerably less likely to gain this amount of weight than those who maintained or decreased their activity patterns. *This study shows that if you're active, you'll be less likely to gain weight as you age.*

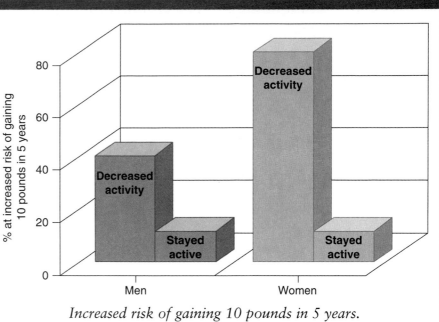

Increased risk of gaining 10 pounds in 5 years.

Helps Control Body Weight

C. Everett Koop, former U.S. Surgeon General, in announcing the Shape Up America! campaign, said, "Too many Americans are too big." The percentage of adult Americans classified as overweight by the National Center for Health Statistics increased over the past decade from about 25 percent to about 33 percent. This enormous increase in the overweight population is unprecedented and indicates a growing public health problem.

Being overweight is common in all age groups but is more common in those over 50. Approximately 40 to 50 percent of men and women aged 50 and older are considered overweight. Excess weight in older people is mostly due not to age but to a lower level of physical activity. Active men and women seem less likely to gain weight as they age.

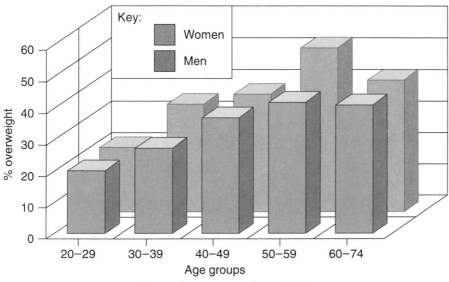

Percent of people overweight at different ages.

Physical Fitness and Obesity

Data from the Aerobics Center Longitudinal Study indicate that being overweight is not particularly harmful if you are physically fit. Researchers followed 25,389 men for approximately 8 years after an examination at the Cooper Clinic. Body weight and physical fitness were measured at the initial examination. Men who were obese but who also were physically fit had no higher death rates than fit men of normal weight. The physically fit obese men had lower death rates than unfit normal-weight men. *This study shows that you can be fat **and** fit. If you are, your mortality risk is comparable to fit, normal-weight people. Your blood pressure, cholesterol, and glucose levels can also be normal if you are physically active.*

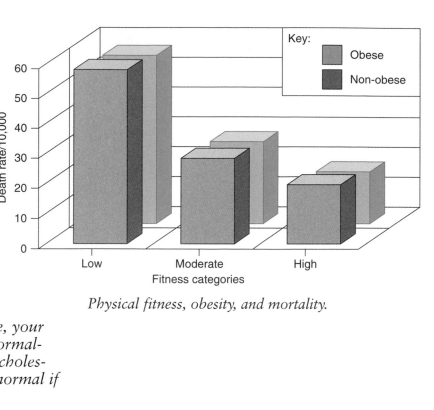

Physical fitness, obesity, and mortality.

Being overweight is more serious in people over 50 because they are more likely to have other health problems, such as high blood pressure or arthritis, that are exacerbated by excess weight. Thus, if you are over 50 it is important to maintain a desirable body weight.

Physical activity contributes to weight loss. Several controlled experiments show that if we are active and watch our diets, we'll lose more weight than if we rely on dieting alone. On average, people who exercise as well as diet lose about 4 or 5 pounds more than people who diet without exercising. Another benefit of adding exercise to dieting is that a greater percentage of the weight lost is from fat. With dieting alone, a high proportion—about 25 to 30 percent—of the weight lost comes from lean muscle or other active tissue. This loss of tissue from the muscles and vital organs may be harmful, especially in older individuals. Weight lost through physical activity is almost entirely from fat stores. Combining exercise with diet also prevents loss of lean tissue.

Perhaps the greatest value of incorporating regular physical activity into a weight loss program comes after the weight is lost. Whereas we rapidly regain weight lost by dieting, we are more apt to keep off weight lost from exercising. Increased activity therefore should be integrated into any dietary weight loss plan.

Maintains Muscle Strength and Function

The problem of low levels of muscle strength is more acute in the later years. Decades of sedentary living can cause a loss of muscle tissue. Lost muscle strength can impinge on functional capabilities required for daily living. Ultimately, declines in function may lead to loss of independence and relocation to a nursing facility.

Activities of Daily Living

Which of the following activities will you want to do when you are 90?

- *Moderate recreational activities.* Leisure bicycling, fishing, ballroom dancing

- *Strenuous recreational activities.* Jogging, cross-country skiing, tennis, team sports

- *Light household activities.* Cooking, ironing, painting inside

- *Moderate household activities.* General carpentry, cleaning, raking

- *Strenuous household activities.* Digging in garden, mowing, shoveling snow

- *Moderate personal care activities.* Bathing, going to the toilet, dressing, getting in/out of bed/chair/bathtub

- *Activities requiring dexterity.* Writing, turning key, buttoning

Risks of Physical Activity

For most people, the risks of most kinds of physical activity are quite low, and the benefits of being physically active outweigh the

Physical Fitness and Function

In a study of men and women between 40 and 90 years of age, approximately 19 percent of the men and 33 percent of the women reported at least one limitation on the "Activities of Daily Living" assessment. Men and women who were in the moderate and high categories of physical fitness were much less likely to report limitations than those in the lowest fitness categories. Highly fit men and women in their 60s were no more likely to have functional limitations than unfit men and women 20 to 25 years younger. *This study shows that physical activity and fitness can help you maintain function and live independently for as long as possible.*

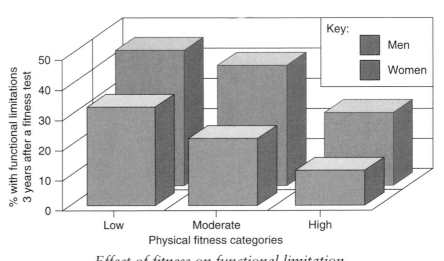

Effect of fitness on functional limitation.

risks. Risk is based on probability—the chance, on average, that an adverse event will occur as a result of being physically active. Three categories of risks are associated with physical activity:

- The risk of heart attack or sudden death during exercise

- The risk of injury to bones, joints, ligaments, and muscles

- The risk of injuries specific to certain types of physical activities

Risk of Sudden Cardiac Death During Exercise

Death that results from physical activity is rare. However, when someone dies of a heart attack during a recreational or sporting activity, this event receives much more attention than if someone dies sitting at a desk or watching television. In one large study conducted over a 5-year period, only 38 deaths occurred in over 33 million hours of exercise. This means that a person who exercises 3 hours per week over a period of 1 year has less than a 1 in 10,000 chance of dying while he or she is exercising.

Although it is true that a person who participates in regular activities has a greater risk of dying while exercising than while not exercising, the regularly active person has a much lower overall risk of heart attack or sudden death than a person who is inactive. A physically active person doubles his or her risk of a heart attack during heavy physical exertion, while a physically inactive person increases his or her risk up to 50 times. Your risk of a heart attack while moving furniture, changing a tire, or shoveling snow is much greater if you are inactive.

The risk of heart attack is also directly related to the level of physical exertion. High levels of physical exertion—when the heart is working at its maximal capacity, such as when shoveling snow—increase the risk of heart attack. Moderate intensity activities, such as walking or bicycling, are associated with a very small risk of heart damage, even among sedentary people and among those with heart disease.

A study documents the low risk of cardiac death during exercise in 51,303 cardiac patients in 167 rehabilitation programs over a 5-year period. During this time, the patients participated in more than 2.3 million hours of exercise, with only three sudden cardiac deaths reported. At this rate, a person would have to go to the rehabilitation program three times a week for more than 5,000 years before experiencing sudden death.

You can feel confident that the moderate level of physical activity this book recommends is safe for almost everyone.

Musculoskeletal and Other Risks Associated with Exercise

Muscle soreness and stiffness are common when you start a physical activity program or resume exercising after a long layoff. These are not permanent injuries, but rather natural reactions to overusing muscles you don't use regularly. Expect to feel some soreness when you start an exercise program or when you change or increase your activity routine. This soreness is temporary and will pass as you exercise more regularly.

You can also strain muscles, tendons, or ligaments while exercising. These types of overuse injuries come from long sessions of physical activity or from sudden overstretching of muscles or joints. The risk of these injuries increases with the intensity of the activity.

The most serious musculoskeletal injuries are sprains, fractures or broken bones, torn ligaments, and torn muscles. Broken bones generally occur from falling and usually are associated with activities, such as skating or skiing, that result in high-impact falls. On rare occasions, physical activity can cause a stress fracture—a minute crack in a bone. These fractures occur from repetitive pounding on a weak area of the bone, usually in the foot, lower leg, or hip. The major symptom of a stress fracture is persistent pain. A stress fracture is difficult to diagnose because a standard X-ray does not show any abnormality, and diagnosis requires a special X-ray or a bone scan. Sprains commonly occur in the ankle, knee, and shoulder. Severe sprains or tears of the ligament result from injuries where excessive force or torque is applied at the joint.

Severe joint injuries (tears to ligaments or cartilage) tend to increase the risk for arthritis or arthritis pain as you grow older or when you engage in certain activities and movements. The previous injury causes the arthritis, however, not the current activity.

Although musculoskeletal injuries appear to increase with age, you can protect against them by achieving the appropriate level of fitness for an intended activity and by using proper technique and equipment.

Other risks associated with specific physical activities are discussed in Chapter 15. Good judgment and caution are the keys to low-risk physical activity.

Regular participation in physical activity is one of the best things you can do for yourself and your health. Human beings were meant to lead active lives. If you aren't active, you may be at increased risk for numerous health problems. Sedentary habits increase your risk for several types of cardiovascular disease, including heart attack, stroke, and high blood pressure. Inactivity also puts you at greater risk for adult-onset diabetes, certain cancers (colon, prostate, breast, and lung), osteoporosis, arthritis, and obesity.

Staying active and fit protects against the development of these diseases, improves the quality of life, preserves function, and extends the period of independent living as we age. For most people, this last benefit is the greatest of all.

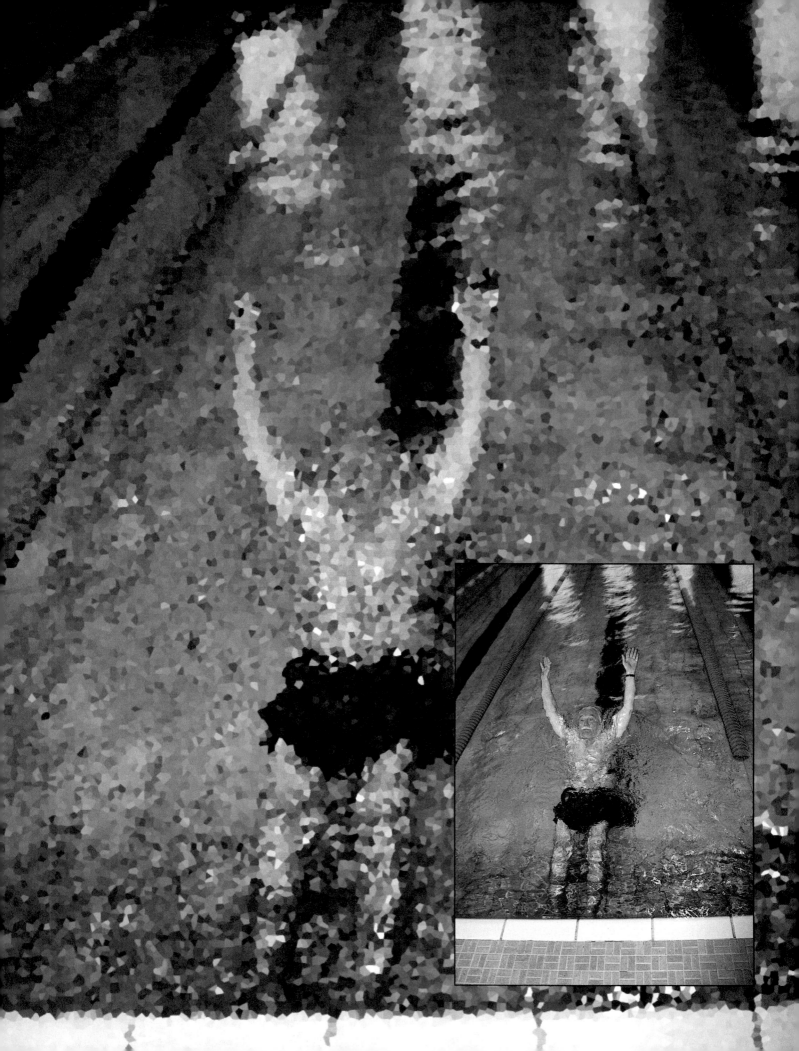

Should You See a Doctor Before You Start Exercising?

any people over age 50 ask if they should see their doctors before starting exercise programs. There is no clear-cut answer. It depends on several factors:

- Your health

- Your environment

- The type and intensity of your activity

- Your personal view of the risk/benefit ratio of becoming more active

Some people want a risk-free existence; others are ready to sue for any bad thing that happens. Their attitude seems to be that someone (but not them) must be at fault for all misfortunes. With this in mind, it is easy to understand why advice about exercise is often prefaced with, "Check with your doctor before starting an exercise program." This cautionary statement is frequently made on the advice of an attorney, and although it may be sound advice from a legal perspective, we think it is bad public health policy.

Is a Medical Evaluation Necessary?

There are several reasons we believe it is not necessary, or even desirable, to recommend a thorough medical evaluation for all individuals who plan to increase their physical activity levels.

- *Low risk of physical activity.* Physical activity will not cause any serious medical problem in the vast majority of healthy individuals, especially the moderate amount and intensity of physical activity we recommend for sedentary people starting activity programs. In fact, sudden cardiac death is rare even in cardiac patients participating in exercise rehabilitation programs.

- *High risk of sedentary living.* It is well established that sedentary habits, not physical exercise, cause health problems, from loss of function to increased risk of heart disease, stroke, diabetes, obesity, and certain cancers. (*See Chapter 3.*)

- *Medical examinations as barriers to activity.* Many adults have difficulty becoming and staying physically active. The cost in time and money of obtaining a medical examination may further deter people from changing their activity patterns. If we calculate the cost/benefit ratio of requiring every sedentary person to obtain a medical evaluation before starting an activity program, we must weigh the number of deaths that might have been prevented by a medical examination against the number of deaths occurring in people who never exercise.

- *Cost of a medical examination.* An estimated 40 to 50 million adult Americans have a twofold to threefold increased risk of death because of their sedentary life-styles. The cost of providing all these individuals with even minimal medical examinations is very high and would be much higher if exercise tests were part of the evaluation. Each examination and exercise test would cost $250 to $500, for a total outlay of $10 to $25 billion. This is clearly impractical. In addition, perhaps another 60 to 70 million individuals are somewhat active but could lower their risk of dying by 20 to 30 percent if they increased their activity to optimal levels. Thus, the burden on the medical care system, in terms of time and costs, would be prohibitive if everyone received medical examinations before starting activity programs. Furthermore, there is little evidence that such screening would reduce the number of deaths and injuries that occur during exercise.

- *Too much emphasis on scientific and medical approaches to a normal and routine behavior.* Exercise scientists and physiologists frequently talk about physical activity as if it were complicated, dangerous, and unusual. The opposite is true. Being active is natural to human beings. For thousands of years our ancestors led physically active lives. Indeed, they needed high levels of activity to survive. We recommend that you try to recapture some of the basic activity habits and functions for which your body was designed. Becoming active does not have to be complicated. You do not need to know your target heart rate or a lot of other exercise physiology. You only need to go for a walk, and most of you do not need to have your cardiologist go with you.

In summary, we believe that the benefits of physical activity far outweigh the risks and that widespread medical screening is not needed to clear men and women for exercise programs. This advice is consistent with positions taken by health and medical groups such as the American College of Sports Medicine (ACSM), the American Heart Association (AHA), and the Centers for Disease Control and Prevention (CDC).

Screening Before Starting an Exercise Program

Although very few sedentary adults need extensive medical evaluations before starting physical activity programs, you should review your health status before increasing your physical activity to determine if you should seek medical advice. Consider the type of physical activity you plan to do. If you plan gradual increases in moderate-intensity activities such as walking, you are less likely to need a medical evaluation than individuals who plan to take up vigorous sports or jogging.

Individuals with known serious diseases, major physical limitations, or symptoms of cardiovascular problems may need medically supervised exercise programs. A few simple screening questions can effectively sort individuals into these two categories.

The principal purpose of screening is to identify those few people with known diseases that might make physical activity unwise or unsafe. The primary concern is for people who have risk factors for coronary heart disease.

Most sudden deaths occurring during exercise are in people who have advanced heart disease. In other words, their disease killed them, not their exercise. When sudden cardiac death occurs in persons under 35, this event is most often an outcome of a condition called cardiomyopathy, in which the heart's walls have thickened and the heart has enlarged. In persons over 35, cardiac death is usually due to atherosclerotic disease of the coronary arteries and, rarely, heart valve abnormalities, especially aortic stenosis.

Screening Recommendations

There are no hard-and-fast answers regarding how much and what type of screening you need before starting a physical activity program. The ACSM has considered this issue for 20 years. Its current recommendations regarding pre-exercise medical evaluations provide reasonable advice, and we support them.

The first step in the ACSM recommendations is to identify your current health status. In which of the following groups do you belong?

- *Apparently healthy individuals* have no known chronic disease and have no more than one of the risk factors for coronary heart disease.

Risk Factors for Coronary Heart Disease

- High blood cholesterol levels
- High blood pressure
- Diabetes
- Cigarette smoking
- Obesity
- Sedentary life-style

Common Chronic Diseases in People Over 50

- Hypertension (high blood pressure)
- Coronary heart disease
- Peripheral vascular disease
- Valvular heart disease (aortic stenosis)
- Congestive heart failure
- Stroke
- Diabetes
- Chronic obstructive pulmonary disease (emphysema, chronic bronchitis)
- Asthma
- Arthritis
- Chronic low back pain
- Osteoporosis
- Cancer

Symptoms Related to Exercise

- Chest pain or discomfort
- Shortness of breath with mild exertion
- Dizziness or fainting
- Swelling of the ankles
- Skipped heartbeats
- Leg pain with walking

- *Higher-risk individuals* have two or more of the risk factors for coronary heart disease. This category is further subdivided into those with symptoms and those without symptoms of major chronic diseases.

- *Individuals with disease* have diagnosed cardiovascular, lung, or metabolic disease.

Canadian public health and exercise science authorities have developed an excellent screening questionnaire—"**The Physical Activity Readiness Questionnaire (PAR-Q)**"—to identify persons who may benefit from medical evaluations before starting exercise programs (*see following page*). Read it carefully and complete it as the first step in preparing to become more physically active. Although the PAR-Q is designed for people up to age 69, we believe it is an effective screening tool also for people 70 and over.

Do You Need an Exercise Stress Test?

Research shows that persons who have electrocardiographic abnormalities during exercise are more likely to have heart disease or

Physical Activity Readiness Questionnaire—PAR-Q
Revised 1994

PAR-Q & YOU
(A Questionnaire for People Aged 15 to 69)

Regular physical activity is fun and healthy, and increasingly more people are starting to become active every day. Being more active is very safe for most people. However, some people should check with their doctors before they start becoming much more physically active.

If you are planning to become much more physically active than you are now, start by answering the seven questions in the box below. If you are between the ages of 15 and 69, the PAR-Q will tell you if you should check with your doctor before you start. If you are over 69 years of age, and you are not used to being very active, check with your doctor.

Common sense is your best guide when you answer these questions. Please read the questions carefully and answer each one honestly: Check "Yes" or "No."

		Yes	No
1.	Has your doctor ever said that you have a heart condition and that you should only do physical activity recommended by a doctor?		
2.	Do you feel pain in your chest when you do physical activity?		
3.	In the past month, have you had chest pain when you were not doing physical activity?		
4.	Do you lose your balance because of dizziness or do you ever lose consciousness?		
5.	Do you have a bone or joint problem that could be made worse by a change in your physical activity?		
6.	Is your doctor currently prescribing drugs (for example, water pills) for your blood pressure or heart condition?		
7.	Do you know of *any other reason* why you should not do physical activity?		

If You Answered "YES" to One or More Questions

Talk with your doctor by phone or in person BEFORE you start becoming much more physically active or BEFORE you have a fitness appraisal. Tell your doctor about the PAR-Q and to which questions you answered "Yes."

- You may be able to do any activity you want—as long as you start slowly and build up gradually. Or, you may need to restrict your activities to those that are safe for you. Talk with your doctor about the kinds of activities you wish to participate in and follow his/her advice.

If You Answered "NO" to All Questions

If you answered NO honestly to all PAR-Q questions, you can be reasonably sure that you can:

- Start becoming much more physically active—begin slowly and build up gradually. This is the safest and easiest way to go.
- Take part in a fitness appraisal—this is an excellent way to determine your basic fitness so that you can plan the best way for you to live actively.

DELAY BECOMING MUCH MORE ACTIVE

- If you are not feeling well because of a temporary illness such as a cold or a fever—wait until you feel better; or
- If you are or may be pregnant—talk to your doctor before you start becoming more active.

Please note: If your health changes so that you then answer "YES" to any of the above questions, tell your fitness or health professional. Ask whether you should change your physical activity plan.

Informed Use of the PAR-Q: The Canadian Society for Exercise Physiology, Health Canada, and their agents assume no liability for persons who undertake physical activity, and if in doubt after completing this questionnaire, consult your doctor prior to physical activity.

You are encouraged to copy the PAR-Q, but only if you use the entire form.

NOTE: If the PAR-Q is being given to a person before he or she participates in a physical activity program or a fitness appraisal, this section may be used for legal or administrative purposes.

I have read, understood, and completed this questionnaire. Any questions I had were answered to my full satisfaction.

Name _____ Date _____

Signature _____ Signature of Parent or Guardian _____

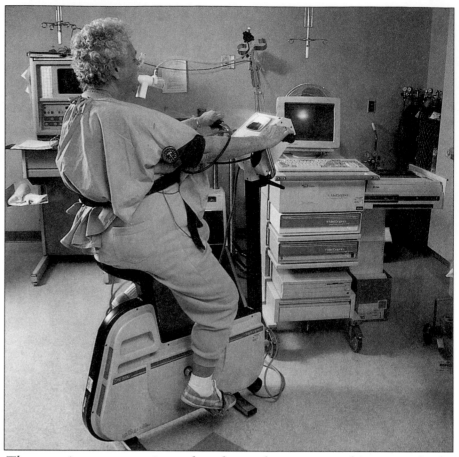

The exercise stress test is used to detect the presence of coronary heart disease. Testing equipment usually consists of a treadmill or stationary bike. During testing, the patient's heart rate, blood pressure, and electrocardiac activity are closely monitored to determine the level of stress that produces symptoms of heart disease. The speed of the treadmill or bike is increased so that the workout becomes progressively more demanding.

heart attacks over the next few years than patients who have normal exercise electrocardiograms. The exercise stress test is a more sensitive indicator of unknown heart disease than the standard electrocardiogram taken with the patient resting.

In addition to helping diagnose heart disease, the exercise test provides a good measure of a person's endurance level. Low endurance itself is an important risk factor for cardiovascular disease, some cancers, obesity, and diabetes. The exercise test thus provides important health information beyond diagnosing heart disease.

Exercise testing has some limitations. First, as with other medical tests, it is not perfectly accurate. Tests may misclassify patients. For example, the test may incorrectly indicate that an individual has a disease. In this case, the test is said to be false positive. A test may show that a person does not have a disease when in fact he or she does. This test is said to be false negative. False-positive tests cause unnecessary concern and often lead to additional and perhaps expensive testing or therapy. False-negative tests give inaccu-

Recommendations for a Medical Examination and Exercise Stress Test for People Over Age 50

Type of Activity	Current Health Status			
	Apparently Healthy	Higher Risk, No Symptoms	High Risk, Symptoms	With Chronic Disease
Moderate exercise	No	No	Yes	Yes
Vigorous exercise	Yes	Yes	Yes	Yes

Reproduced from *ACSM's Guidelines for Exercise Testing and Prescription*, 5th ed., by the American College of Sports Medicine, 1995, Baltimore: Williams & Wilkins.

rate assurance that an individual is healthy and thus may delay possibly helpful treatment.

In low-risk groups such as individuals with no symptoms or known disease, the number of false-positive exercise stress tests often exceeds the number of true-positive tests. This is the primary reason groups like the American College of Cardiology, the AHA, and the ACSM recommend against mass exercise stress test screening in apparently healthy individuals. In addition, there is the time and expense involved with the procedure, with the subsequent burden on the medical care system.

We are not opposed to all exercise stress testing. There are many situations when it is appropriate or even desirable *(see table above)*. However, we do not believe that all sedentary persons need exercise stress tests before they begin to increase their physical activity. In other words, they do not have to get tests before they decide to go for walks after dinner.

Should You Exercise If You're Sick?

It is generally not advisable to exercise or engage in other strenuous physical activities during an acute illness. An acute illness is one that comes on suddenly and usually ends in a few days to a few weeks. It is cured when the illness is over.

As we grow older, we become more susceptible to both acute (short-term) and chronic (continuing) illness. The unexpected onset of illness or injury may interfere with regular physical activity. Chronic illnesses that affect the heart, lungs, joints, bones, or neurological system may make certain activities more difficult. The most common types of acute illness are infections. These can range from simple illnesses such as a cold to more serious infections, such as a kidney infection or pneumonia, that require antibiotic treatment and even hospitalization.

Avoid strenuous physical activity during an acute illness so that your body can direct its energy to fighting the illness and to repairing itself. Rest is an essential part of the healing process.

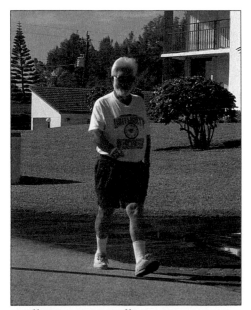

Walking is an excellent way to regain stamina and strength after an illness.

If You Have a Fever

Don't exercise. Wait until you have been free of fever for at least 24 hours before resuming exercise.

Common Acute Illnesses in People Over 50

- Infections caused by a virus (cold, flu, and upper respiratory infections) usually go away with time; no medication indicated

- Infections caused by bacteria (sinusitis, pneumonia, bladder infection) are more serious and require antibiotics

- Acute heart problems (heart attack, congestive heart failure, arrhythmia)

- Lung problems (acute asthma attack, worsening of emphysema, acute bronchitis)

Once the illness is over, you may resume your regular activity program at a level that is compatible with your strength and stamina.

In general, the more serious and long lasting an acute illness, the less you will tolerate physical exertion and the more you will need to reduce the intensity and amount of physical activity. For example, let's assume you take a 45-minute walk every day or nearly every day. If you developed pneumonia and were hospitalized for 5 days, your strength and stamina probably would not return to normal for 4 to 6 weeks.

How would you adapt your exercise program? Two weeks after you returned home, you could begin walking again for 10 to 15 minutes per day at a slower pace. You would gradually increase the length of your walks over the next 4 to 6 weeks until you could resume your usual 45-minute walk at your previous pace.

Always talk with your doctor about what types and levels of physical activity are possible after an acute illness or after surgery. Certain types of physical activity may interfere with the healing of an incision. Physicians used to recommend long periods of bedrest and inactivity after acute illness. That approach has been proved wrong. In many cases, bedrest can delay recovery of your previous level of physical activity. Resuming light activities, such as getting out of bed and walking to the bathroom as soon as possible, is an important part of the healing process. The objective is to get back to a normal level of activity as quickly and safely as possible.

What Should You Do If You're Injured?

Although exercise and physical activity are quite safe and the benefits far outweigh the risks, you could experience a minor injury, such as a strained muscle or sprained ankle. Follow a commonsense approach using the PRICE method to treat minor injuries:

P—Protection: You may need to apply a protective device to prevent further injury and provide support. Examples include slings, splints, and braces. Elastic bandages provide too little support for a joint and, if applied too tightly, may impede circulation.

R—Rest: Rest the injured area. The amount of rest varies from complete rest to reduced participation depending on the severity of the injury. With most minor injuries, it's safe and actually hastens healing to continue physical activity at a lower intensity level.

I—Ice: Apply ice to the injured area. Cold reduces tissue swelling and bleeding, reduces inflammation, and decreases firing of the pain-nerve receptors. Don't apply ice directly to your skin. Wrap the ice or ice pack with a cloth or apply with a bandage. A general rule is to apply ice for 20 minutes (maximum of 30 minutes) followed by at least 30 minutes without cold packs. You can repeat this process three times a day.

C—Compression: Gentle pressure used with ice helps to limit swelling. Apply compression with an elastic bandage wrapped with consistent, even pressure. Do not wrap the bandage so tightly that it constricts and reduces the blood flow. During the early stages when swelling is severe, loosen the wrap every half hour, then reapply it.

E—Elevation: At first, elevate the injured part above the level of your heart, even while sleeping, until the swelling subsides. Gravity prevents the pooling of blood and other fluids, enhances blood flow, and reduces swelling.

In addition to following these guidelines, you can use acetaminophen, ibuprofen, aspirin, or other mild pain medication to provide comfort. Resume physical activity gradually as the injury or pain improves.

What Should You Do If You Have Symptoms During Exercise?

Be aware of normal and abnormal responses to exercise. Listen to your body. Pay attention to what's going on inside your body while you are exercising. Probably, your heart beats faster, you breathe more deeply and more often, and you may perspire heavily. These responses are normal and to be expected. Remember what is normal and establish norms for yourself. When something is different, or if things aren't normal, stop. If you perceive a problem, seek help and get medical advice.

Although nobody enjoys pain, it is our bodies' way of telling us something is wrong. If you experience pain during exercise, or

**Important—
See a Physician
Immediately If:**

- **The pain is severe**
- **You can't move the injured part**
- **The injury does not seem to heal after reasonable home treatment**

Symptoms During Exercise

What's Normal	*What's Not Normal*
• Faster pulse	• Chest pain, pain down your arm, heaviness in chest (angina)
• A few skipped heartbeats	• Persistent palpitation or uneven heartbeat
• Breathing deeply	• Extreme breathlessness with light to moderate activity (not necessarily exercise)
	• Wheezing, inability to catch breath
• Breathing faster	• Lightheadedness
• Sweating	• Nausea
	• Extreme fatigue
	• Numbness
	• Pain of any kind

Early Warning Signs for Heart Attack

- *Angina or chest pain.* Pain or pressure in the chest radiating up the neck or jaw or down the arm. Pain develops during exercise and is relieved when you stop and rest. If you experience this kind of pain, call your physician. If the pain continues or worsens even when you are resting, call for emergency medical service or have someone take you to the emergency room.

- *Skipped heartbeats.* You may notice "skipped heartbeats" during or after exercise. We all experience some skipped beats, and most are not of concern. However, if you have many and frequent skipped beats, call your physician.

- *Shortness of breath.* Increased rate and depth of breathing is a normal response to exercise. However, if you notice extreme breathlessness, especially with mild exercise, check with your physician.

- *Other warning signs.* Other signs that may warrant further review by your physician are extreme fatigue that persists after exercise, lightheadedness, or nausea, especially if these conditions occur after mild or moderate physical activity.

if pain continues after exercise, evaluate it and determine if you need to seek medical attention. For example, if you begin to experience joint pain, you probably need only to reduce the intensity of exercise and rest the joint. If you still have pain the next time you exercise, you may want to take acetaminophen or ibuprofin and rest for a few days by doing exercises that don't involve that joint. However, if you experience chest pain or pain radiating down your arm, or numbness, or dizziness, immediately stop exercising and seek medical attention.

Although the risk of heart attack during exercise is quite low, heart attack is possible. The odds of such an event are greater for older individuals, men, and people with major risk factors such as high cholesterol, high blood pressure, cigarette smoking, and diabetes. However, a heart attack could happen to anyone, so everyone should be aware of what the AHA calls "Early Warning Signs."

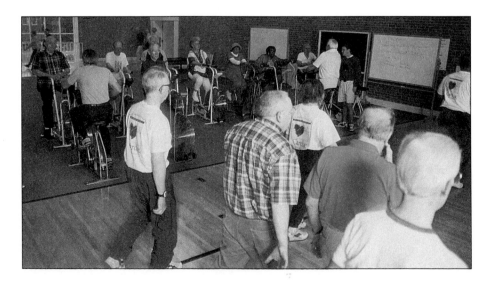

Cardiac rehabilitation programs often include walking and riding exercise bicycles.

What Should You Do If You Have a Chronic Illness or Condition?

Chronic illnesses or conditions are those that are long standing or continue for months or years *(see following page)*. Chronic illnesses are more common in people over age 50. It is estimated that two thirds of people 65 and older have at least one chronic condition. Fortunately, most common chronic conditions that occur with age don't necessarily prevent participation in physical activity. In fact, an active life-style may reduce symptoms of chronic conditions and prevent complications.

People with chronic conditions stand to gain more from being physically active than people without chronic conditions. A person with a chronic illness is at greater risk for complications and is more likely to be helped by preventive measures. Scientists call this "secondary prevention."

For example, if you've had a heart attack, you are three to five times more likely to have another than someone who has never had one. A regular walking program reduces the risk of a second heart attack more than it reduces the risk of a first heart attack. This principle applies to preventing complications from all chronic conditions. Having a chronic condition gives you more, not less, reason to exercise.

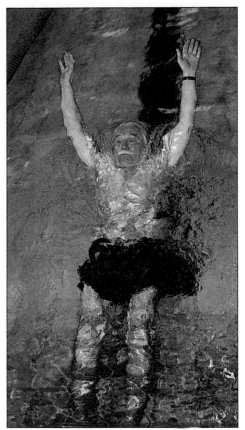

The aerobic benefits of swimming can be especially useful if you have high blood pressure or coronary heart disease.

If You Have Hypertension

- Aerobic exercises, such as walking, cycling, and swimming, not only prevent high blood pressure but help lower blood pressure when it becomes elevated.

- People with severe high blood pressure (greater than 180/110 mm Hg) should be treated with medication and have their blood pressure under control before starting exercise programs. Blood pressure medication will not interfere with physical activity. Occasionally, patients taking beta-blockers (a class of drugs that slow the heart) complain of tiring easily during exercise. If excessive fatigue interferes with exercise, discuss the problem with your doctor to determine if you can modify the dose or take an alternative medication.

- Avoid weight lifting with very heavy weights if you have high blood pressure. The extra strain on the muscles may raise blood pressure to very high levels during the activity itself. Choose a strength-building program with the guidance and supervision of an exercise therapist or certified trainer who can design a safe program for you and monitor your blood pressure during the weight-training sessions. *(See Appendix 2 for examples of strength-building exercises.)*

Common Chronic Diseases in People Over 50—Causes and Symptoms

- *Hypertension.* Blood pressure over 140 (systolic—top number) and/or 90 (diastolic—bottom number) millimeters of mercury. Hypertension is caused by atherosclerosis (hardening of the arteries) and by the blood vessels' diminished elasticity and inability to dilate (open and close). It usually does not cause symptoms, but if left untreated it can lead to stroke, heart attack, and kidney failure.

- *Coronary heart disease.* Inadequate blood supply to the heart muscle. The most common cause is atherosclerosis, or blockage of the blood vessels by fat and cholesterol. The symptoms are angina (heart pain with exercise) or heart attack. People who have had coronary artery bypass surgery (surgery to bypass blockages) or angioplasty (a catheterization procedure that opens blocked blood vessels) also are considered to have coronary heart disease.

- *Peripheral vascular disease.* Caused by blockage of the arteries that carry blood to the legs. The most common symptom is pain in the calves, thighs, or buttocks occurring with exercise. A person with peripheral vascular disease frequently has coronary heart disease.

- *Valvular heart disease.* Conditions in which the heart valves are either blocked or leak. Aortic stenosis, a thickening of the valve separating the heart from the aorta and other blood vessels, is the most common valve problem in people over 50. It limits the amount of blood the heart pumps out and prevents an adequate blood supply from reaching the rest of the body.

- *Congestive heart failure.* Inadequate or abnormal pumping of the heart. Congestive heart failure causes fluid to back up into the lungs. The major symptom of congestive heart failure is shortness of breath.

- *Asthma.* An allergic condition in which the bronchial tubes become inflamed and constricted, causing wheezing and shortness of breath. Asthma affects people of all ages.

- *Chronic obstructive pulmonary disease (COPD).* Usually caused by smoking cigarettes for more than 25 years. The smoke from cigarettes inflames the lungs and eventually destroys normal lung tissue. The symptoms are shortness of breath, especially during activity, and chronic coughing. People with COPD get frequent respiratory infections, especially during the winter. In severe cases, the lungs' performance is so compromised that the level of oxygen in the blood drops to critical levels, a condition called hypoxemia. This extremely dangerous situation can lead to organ damage and even death. Some people with this disease must use supplemental oxygen to maintain adequate blood levels of oxygen.

- *Osteoarthritis.* Affects the spine, hips, knees, feet, and small joints of the hands. Osteoarthritis occurs when cartilage in the joints degenerates. Symptoms include pain and stiffness, especially when you use the joint. Osteoarthritis is the most common form of arthritis in people over age 50.

- *Low back pain.* Most often caused by strain to the back muscles and ligaments. Occasionally, more serious problems such as spinal compression, fractures, spinal stenosis, or tumors may cause persistent low back pain.

- *Osteoporosis.* Thinning of the bones, which occurs with aging. There are no symptoms unless the bones become so thin that they break. Most commonly, fractures from osteoporosis occur in the spine, hip, lower leg, and wrist. Women have more severe osteoporosis than men because their bones are thinner and lose density after menopause.

- *Type II diabetes.* Occurs when the body's cells become resistant to insulin's effects and levels of blood sugar and insulin go up. Symptoms include fatigue, excessive thirst and urination, blurred vision, rapid weight loss, and recurrent infections.

If You Have Coronary Heart Disease

- Request a complete evaluation by a physician. An exercise stress test will help your doctor determine at what intensity it is safe for you to exercise.

- If you have had a heart attack or a surgical procedure for the heart, you should participate in a supervised cardiac rehabilitation program for the first 12 weeks after the event. Most cardiac rehabilitation programs include aerobic exercise, resistive training with low weights, and education programs to help manage and cope with heart disease.

- People with coronary heart disease should avoid activity in hazardous environmental conditions such as high temperatures, high humidity, and high altitudes.

If You Have Peripheral Vascular Disease

- Request a thorough medical evaluation to confirm the diagnosis. The symptoms of peripheral vascular disease can be confused with arthritis or nerve damage to the legs. People with peripheral vascular disease often also have coronary heart disease.

- Aerobic exercises such as walking and cycling have been shown to lessen the pain and lengthen the distance you can walk without pain.

If You Have Other Heart Problems

- Exercise can be dangerous for people who have aortic stenosis (thickened aortic valves) and can cause fainting or even death. If you have aortic stenosis or other valvular heart disease, consult your doctor or a heart specialist before engaging in any physical activity program.

- For persons with congestive heart failure, physical activity and, in particular, exercise may produce abnormal stress on the heart and worsen symptoms. All physical activity programs should be undertaken only with careful supervision in a cardiac rehabilitation program after a thorough medical evaluation.

If You Have Asthma

- Nearly all people with asthma can exercise safely. Exercise may trigger asthma attacks even in nonasthmatic individuals who have allergies. This condition is called "exercise-induced asthma."

- Exercise in warm and more humid conditions, use a face mask or scarf in cold weather, and breathe slowly through your nose.

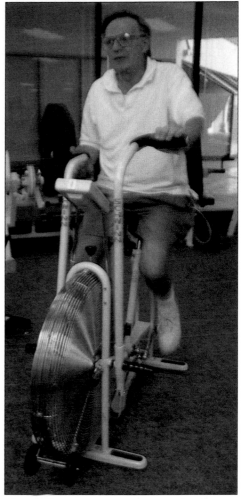

Your physician may recommend aerobic exercise as a means of restoring cardiovascular fitness after a heart attack.

Even Competitive Athletes Have Asthma

Eight percent of the 1988 American Olympic team had asthma, including gold-medalist Jackie Joyner-Kersey.

Symptoms and Factors in Exercise-Induced Asthma

Symptoms

- Excessive breathlessness
- Coughing, wheezing, and mild chest discomfort during or immediately after a bout of physical activity

Factors

- High level of exertion
- Cool air
- Low humidity
- High degree of air pollution

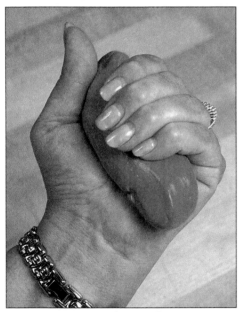

Exercising your fingers by squeezing putty is often recommended if you have arthritis.

- Use caution if you exercise during times of increased air pollution or high pollen counts.

- Take medications if necessary. Several types of safe, inhaled medications are useful to prevent asthma attacks. These medications are inhaled 15 to 30 minutes before exercise or physical activity.

If You Have Chronic Obstructive Pulmonary Disease

- Request a medical evaluation before beginning an exercise program.

- Enroll in a supervised pulmonary rehabilitation program. Some of the symptoms of chronic obstructive pulmonary disease (COPD) can be improved through a regular aerobic exercise program.

- Strengthening exercises for the arm, chest, and back muscles may help you breathe more easily.

If You Have Arthritis

- Regular exercise reduces the pain and disability from osteoarthritis without further damaging the affected joint.

- Engage in a balanced fitness program that includes walking, swimming, cycling, strength-building exercises, and stretching.

- Avoid exercises that put excessive stress on the joints, such as aerobic dancing, running, or competitive sports.

- Take acetaminophen, ibuprofen, or other mild pain medication 30 minutes before exercise to help prevent pain during activity.

- Consult an exercise specialist or a physical therapist to determine specific activities or exercises that are right for you.

- If a particular activity causes excessive or severe pain to a specific joint, avoid that activity or substitute another that uses different joints.

If You Have Low Back Pain

- Perform daily stretching exercises. Physical activity can prevent further episodes of pain and disability. Walking, swimming, and strength training with light weights are good preventive measures.

- Certain exercises and sports such as cycling, racquet sports, golf, and jogging may worsen back pain. Stop exercising but maintain normal daily activities during an episode of acute low back pain. Use mild pain medications. Bedrest for more than 1 day slows the healing process.

- Resume your regular physical activity program once the pain resolves.

If You Have Osteoporosis

- Weight-bearing exercises such as walking and strength-training exercises with weights can help slow the progression of osteoporosis. For women who are receiving estrogen replacement therapy, exercise is most beneficial when it is combined with a calcium supplement of at least 1,000 mg per day.

- Exercise and other forms of physical activity may hasten recovery and lessen pain due to osteoporotic fracture.

- Physical therapy programs strengthen specific muscle groups around a fracture site.

If You Have Diabetes Mellitus

- Exercise helps control blood sugar and aids in weight loss. A balanced fitness program is especially beneficial in controlling diabetes.

- Monitor your blood sugar closely to ensure that you don't become hypoglycemic after an exercise session.

- Do not fast for a prolonged period before or after exercise.

If You Have Cancer

- An exercise program can make you feel better physically and mentally.

- Special rehabilitation programs may help people with specific types of cancer. For example, women who have had mastectomies should participate in exercise programs to strengthen and stretch the arm and chest muscles to recover full function in the affected arm.

Follow These Guidelines

Physical activity, in particular the moderate-intensity activity we recommend here for sedentary individuals, is low risk. However, injuries and health problems, even catastrophic ones, do occur, and it is sensible to be aware of this possibility. If you are planning large increases in activity, including strenuous activities, at least give your physician a call about your plans. This becomes more important the older you are.

We urge you to follow the guidelines discussed in this chapter, and be alert to early warning signs of heart problems. The overall risk of remaining sedentary far outweighs the small risk associated with being physically active.

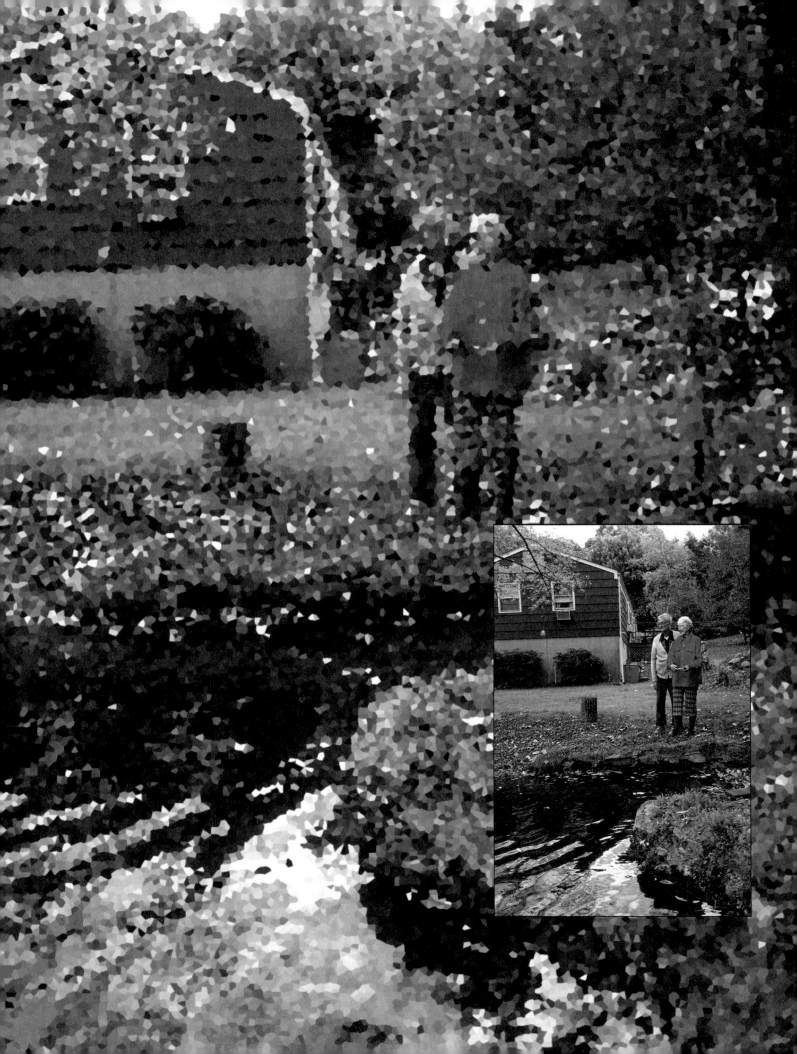

CHAPTER 5

How Physically Active Are You?

It is important to assess your current level of physical activity before you begin your fitness program. If you want to change and maintain a health habit, self-assessment is crucial for three reasons:

- You need a clear view of your current level of activity so that you can set appropriate and realistic goals.

- Ongoing assessment of your activity will help you to monitor your progress over time. There's nothing like success to keep you motivated!

- Research studies have shown that people who regularly assess and monitor their activity, especially when they are getting started, are more likely to succeed than people who don't monitor their progress.

This chapter contains several tools for assessing and monitoring your physical activity. Some are more complex than others. Choose the ones that will work best for you.

Energy Expenditure—Past and Present

The average daily energy expenditure of people in the United States has progressively declined over the past century. This trend accelerated after World War II with the explosion of technology and labor-saving devices at home and on the job. It is now possible for most people to go through the day without expending much energy.

Life-style and Physical Activity—1900 versus 1990

Compare the daily life of a white-collar worker today with the daily life of a similar professional at the turn of the 20th century. In 1900, the hypothetical worker might have walked to work, or at least to a trolley stop. Several more minutes of walking would have taken him or her from the trolley stop to the office building. There might have been three or four flights of stairs to climb to reach the office itself, where the absence of numerous labor-saving devices would have required a slightly higher energy expenditure over the course of 1 day.

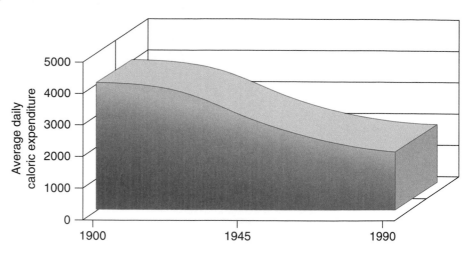

In the late afternoon, our worker would have returned home where, perhaps, the furnace needed stoking or the lawn needed mowing with a manual mower. Shopping or visiting friends and relatives might have required a horse for transportation. Hitching the horse to a carriage, driving, and reversing the process at the end of the journey required a lot more effort than getting in the family car and driving to a parking spot closest to the mall.

Leisure time was undoubtedly more active. Our ancestors did not have television, video games, stereophonic equipment, and other distractions that are available to us and that encourage us to be sedentary.

Energy expenditure requirements for most Americans have gradually declined since 1900. Current estimates are that Americans' average daily energy expenditure is about 500 calories less per day than it was 100 years ago. This difference amounts to a decline in average energy expenditure of only 5 calories per day each year from 1900 to the present—a trivial amount, you might think, equaling the difference in energy cost between sitting and standing, or reclining and sitting in a chair for less than an hour. Nonetheless, over the past 100 years, this small daily difference adds up to a net decline of 500 calories per day—or more than 180,000 calories per year. And this many calories is the energy equivalent of 50 pounds of fat.

Tip

To become more physically active, begin by decreasing, as much as possible, the number and amount of your sedentary activities.

It is unrealistic for all of us to revert to a turn-of-the-century life-style, but we need to be aware that the sedentary habits of contemporary life are new and not natural to us. The sedentary life-style that characterizes our lives today explains, at least in part, the rapidly increasing rates of obesity and the higher rates of heart attack, stroke, adult diabetes, and some cancers.

Self-Assessment Tools

How Much Time Do You Spend Sitting?

One way to assess your current physical activity level is to determine how much time you spend in sedentary activities, such as sit-

Hours Spent in Sedentary Activities

	Sunday	Monday	Tuesday	Wednesday	Thursday	Friday	Saturday
Sleep							
Sitting in a car							
Sitting at work							
Sitting at home							
Sitting—other							
Total hours							

ting. You may be surprised at the results. Make a chart like the one on this page. Complete it faithfully for 1 week. Divide your day into 4-hour blocks, and at the end of each block, note what you did for that time. Before you go to bed, complete the chart for that day.

How Often Do You Take the Elevator or Escalator?

The energy cost of waiting for and riding an elevator is approximately 1.5 calories per minute for a 175-pound person. The energy cost of climbing stairs depends on the rate at which you climb, but it is relatively easy for the average individual to expend 8 to 9 calories per minute in this activity.

To monitor your use of elevators or escalators for 1 week, keep a tally card in your pocket like the one at the foot of this page or make a note on your personal calendar of the number of floors for which you used an elevator or escalator. After a week, find the stairs and climb to the floor, especially if you are going up fewer than three or four flights. If your destination is above the fourth or fifth floor, get off a few floors early and climb the stairs the rest of the way. Keep another tally like the one on the next page to monitor the number of floors you climbed during 1 week.

Take the Stairs—Burn Calories and Save Time!

Waiting for or riding the elevator	1.5 calories per minute
Climbing stairs	8 or 9 calories per minute

Number of Times You Used an Elevator/Escalator

	Sunday	Monday	Tuesday	Wednesday	Thursday	Friday	Saturday
Per day							

Number of Flights of Stairs Climbed

	Sunday	Monday	Tuesday	Wednesday	Thursday	Friday	Saturday
At home							
At work							
During leisure time							
Total number							

After establishing this new habit over a few weeks, monitor the number of floors for which you used an elevator or escalator over 7 days. Were you able to reduce the number? Perhaps you completely shunned the use of electrical power in favor of stair climbing?

How Much Time Do You Spend Walking?

In addition to monitoring your sedentary activities, it also is useful to measure how much energy you expend in routine daily activities. Use your calendar or a chart like the one below to record how many flights of stairs you climb or how much time you spend walking.

There are several ways you can use the chart to record your time spent walking. You can wait until the end of day and try to recall the time walking for each of the categories. This method is

Minutes Spent Walking

	Sunday	Monday	Tuesday	Wednesday	Thursday	Friday	Saturday
Walking to work							
Walking on the job							
Walking at home							
Walking during work breaks							
Walking during leisure time							
Walking for exercise							
Total minutes							

convenient, but it may be more accurate to pause periodically throughout the day to complete the chart. You might do this at lunchtime, before going home at the end of the day, and before going to bed. Or, you can stop every hour on the hour and record your walking.

Some people find it easier to count 2- or 5-minute blocks of time spent walking. For example, you might decide to tally only blocks of 5 minutes of continuous walking for each category in the chart. Thus, if you went for a 20-minute walk at lunchtime, you would enter four tally marks in the category "walking during work breaks."

It really doesn't matter what technique you use to record your walking time. Simply select the approach that will work for you, the one that fits your life-style and personality. Tally your walking time for a week and monitor your progress as you become more active.

How Many Steps Do You Take Each Day?

Counting the number of steps you take each day is another helpful way to monitor your physical activity level. And, it's one of the easiest tallies to take if you use a pedometer. These devices are about the size of a large wristwatch and can be worn on your belt or waistband. They are available in nearly all sporting goods stores for less than $20 and automatically record every step you take in 1 day. The pedometer will not measure the distance you walk, but it will accurately record the number of steps you take.

Use a pedometer to establish a baseline number of steps. Wear the pedometer for 1 week while following your normal routine and record the number of steps per day on your calendar or on a chart like the one below. At the end of the week, calculate the average steps per day. This is your baseline. Your goal is to find ways to increase this number by building more activity into your daily routine. The average number of steps most people take during a routine work day ranges from 2,500 to 5,000. An unusually sedentary day will result in 1,500 to 2,000 steps. If the day involves more walking than usual, perhaps traveling and walking in

Examples of Sedentary Activities

- Taking naps
- Watching television
- Reading
- Writing
- Sitting at a desk
- Lying on a couch
- Riding in a car or bus
- Flying in an airplane
- Playing board games or cards
- Sewing
- Writing letters
- Sitting while talking on the phone
- Working at a computer

Number of Steps per Day

	Sunday	Monday	Tuesday	Wednesday	Thursday	Friday	Saturday
Number of steps							

Average steps per day _____

MET Values of Various Activities

MET refers to metabolic equivalent, or the amount of energy your body expends during rest or activity.

Activity	MET Value
Sitting	1
Standing	1.8
Walking (2 mph)	2
Walking (3 mph)	3
Walking (4 mph)	4
Low-impact aerobics	5
Doubles tennis	6
Racquetball	7
Bicycling (12–14 mph)	8
Jogging (5 mph)	9

airports or sightseeing while on vacation, the number of steps you take may be as high as 15,000 to 20,000.

How Is Physical Activity Measured?

Most health behaviors are difficult to measure accurately, and physical activity is no exception. The basic measure of physical activity is also a measure of energy expenditure. The human body is a machine that converts calories from food into energy which fuels the body's metabolism (all the involuntary processes that sustain cellular life) and the body's voluntary movements. The minimal level of energy expenditure necessary to sustain life is called the "basal" or "resting" metabolic rate. The basal metabolic rate is the amount of energy that cells in various body organs and systems expend to maintain cellular integrity and function. The average basal metabolic rate is 1 calorie per kilogram of body weight per hour.

Basal metabolic rate is calculated in a laboratory by measuring the rate of oxygen use. The resting metabolic rate that expends 1 calorie/kg of body weight per hour requires approximately 3.5 ml of oxygen/kg of body weight per minute.

In addition to measuring the resting metabolic rate, scientists can also measure the metabolic rate of different physical activities. For example, walking at 3 mph on a level surface requires about 10.5 ml of oxygen/kg of body weight per minute. Walking at 3 mph expends three times as much energy as quiet rest (10.5 ml/3.5 ml = 3).

Physiologists refer to the energy expenditure at rest as 1 metabolic equivalent, or MET. Energy expenditure for all activities can be expressed as multiples of this resting rate. Walking at 3 mph is a 3 MET activity, for example.

To determine your metabolic rate, multiply the MET value of your activity by your weight in kilograms.

Example:

- Person weighs 176 pounds = 80 kg (176/2.22 = 79.28)

- Walking at 2 mph burns 160 calories per hour (2 METs X 80 kg)

- Walking at 3 mph burns 240 calories per hour (3 METs X 80 kg)

- Walking at 4 mph burns 320 calories per hour (4 METs X 80 kg)

The MET value of walking will be higher if you are:

- Walking on a soft surface soft (sandy beach)

- Walking uphill

- Carrying a load such as groceries

Estimate Your Energy Expenditure

Energy expenditure can be measured accurately in the laboratory, but these methods are not feasible or necessary for your purposes. You can estimate your average daily energy expenditure from a record of your physical activity habits and a few simple calculations.

How Intense Is the Activity?

An important factor in calculating energy expenditure is assessing the intensity of your activities. Most sedentary adults spend very little time in *moderate-* or *high-intensity activities*. These relatively few episodes of intense activity stand out in the daily routine. Most people spend most of their time in *low-intensity activities*.

Use the chart on this page to categorize the intensity of your activities. This list is not exhaustive. Many of your common activities may not be included. However, a few guidelines may help you correctly classify any activity.

- If an activity seems *less intense than moderate to brisk walking* (3 to 4 mph), it is probably a *light-intensity activity* and need not be recorded.

- If the activity seems *about as intense as moderate to brisk walking*, classify it as *moderate*.

Moderate, Hard, and Very Hard Physical Activities

	Moderate Intensity (3 to 5 METs)	*Hard Intensity (5.1 to 7 METs)*	*Very Hard Intensity (More than 7 METs)*
Transportation	Walking at 3 to 4 mph (15 to 20 minutes per mile)	Walking faster than 4.5 mph	Jogging at any speed
Household activities	Housework such as vacuuming, mopping, scrubbing, lifting and carrying laundry	Raking, light digging or hoeing, lifting and carrying heavy boxes, moving furniture	Shoveling heavy snow, carrying heavy loads upstairs, heavy carpentry, sawing hardwood
Occupational activities	Operating machine tools, assembly line work (standing, lifting loads less than 50 pounds)	Using heavy power tools (like jackhammers), lifting and carrying 50 to 75 pounds, moving heavy objects	Trimming trees, carrying bricks or stones, leveling concrete, heavy digging
Sports and recreational activities	Shooting baskets, curling, golf, social badminton or frisbee, horseback riding, table tennis	Doubles tennis, casual racquetball, fencing, water skiing, moderate downhill skiing	Basketball, soccer, competitive singles tennis, cross-country skiing, skin or scuba diving, squash

- If an activity seems *harder than moderate to brisk walking, but not as hard as jogging*, classify it as a *hard activity*.

- *Jogging* at any speed is a *very hard activity*. Sports that involve *continuous running* (soccer or basketball) are *very hard activities*.

The chart shows you that you can get the same benefits from cleaning your house or going for a walk. You burn the same number of calories or earn the same METs in either activity. So don't feel guilty if you don't take a walk because you had to clean the house.

Use Common Sense to Classify the Intensity of Your Activities

- *Give your honest, subjective estimate* about the intensity of an activity when compared with some of the benchmarks discussed above.

- *Be reasonable.* It is possible to play basketball and not move very much. If you play basketball, soccer, or other typically strenuous sports but spend much of the time standing or moving at a walking pace, the sport probably requires moderately intense, rather than very hard, activity.

- *Be consistent.* You may wonder how short an interval to include in your daily total. This is partly a matter of personal preference. The shorter the interval you try to remember, the more complicated the procedure. We recommend that you not record intervals shorter than 5 minutes. If you prefer to record only activities that you did for at least 15 minutes, that's okay. Just be consistent in your approach from day to day.

How to Calculate Your Total Daily Energy Expenditure

Once you have assessed the intensity of your activities you are ready to estimate your total daily energy expenditure. Using the chart at the bottom of the following page, take these steps:

- Know your weight in kilograms. *(See the "Weight Conversion Table" at the top of the following page.)*

- In the second column, record the hours you slept and include any naps you took during the day.

- Then, think back over your day and record the number of hours you spent in moderate-, hard-, and very-hard-intensity activities.

- Next, total the hours spent in sleep, moderate-, hard-, and very-hard-intensity activities.

Weight Conversion Table

To convert pounds to kilograms
(your weight in pounds ÷ 2.22 = your weight in kilograms)

To convert kilograms to pounds
(your weight in kilograms X 2.22 = your weight in pounds)

Your Weight (lbs)	Your Weight (kg)	Your Weight (lbs)	Your Weight (kg)
100	45	180	82
105	48	185	84
110	50	190	86
115	52	195	88
120	54	200	91
125	57	205	93
130	59	210	95
135	61	215	98
140	64	220	100
145	66	225	102
150	68	230	104
155	70	235	107
160	73	240	109
165	75	245	111
170	77	250	113
175	79	255	116

Estimating Your Total Daily Energy Expenditure

Activity	Hours	MET Value	Hours X METs
Sleep		1	
Moderate		4	
Hard		6	
Very hard		10	
Total hours			
Light (24 minus total hours)		1.5	
		Total MET hours or calories/kg/day	

Total daily caloric expenditure: MET hours X your weight in kilograms = _____
(weight in pounds/2.22 = weight in kilograms)

- Subtract that number from 24 hours to get the time spent in light-intensity activities.

- Multiply the hours in each category by the MET value in the third column and enter the figures in the last column.

- Add the figures in the last column to get MET hours. This is your total daily energy expenditure in calories per kilogram of your body weight.

- To get the total calories you spent for the day, multiply this figure by your body weight in kilograms at the bottom of the chart.

- An example of calculating daily energy expenditure is shown below.

An Example: Pamela

Pamela works in an office, so she has a sedentary job.

- On this particular day she slept 8 hours.

- She walked from her apartment to the bus stop to take a bus to work. This walk took 15 minutes.

- The bus stopped in front of her office, and she took the elevator to the 20th floor where she works, so she did not have to walk more than a couple of minutes to get to her desk.

- She spent most of the morning working at her desk and moving around her office to the fax machine, copier, and filing cabinets. Although she made several trips to a coworker's office that was two floors above her own, she took the stairs for these trips.

- At noon she ate her lunch in a snack bar on the first floor of her office building. She normally takes an aerobics class at noon, but she did not have time today.

- To get some vigorous exercise, she decided to climb the stairs going back to her office, and it took her 8 minutes of steady climbing to reach the 20th floor.

- During the afternoon, she again made several trips to another department, which is three floors above her office. She always took the stairs.

- A friend gave her a ride home after work and dropped her at her door.

- Because she missed her aerobics class and her usual walk from the bus stop to her apartment, she thought she should get some additional physical activity before dinner. She changed into casual clothes and went across the street to a large park, where she took a brisk 30-minute hike on a soft, sandy trail that included a number of rather steep hills.

- Before going to bed, she completed her daily energy expenditure chart:

  0.25 hour @ moderate intensity. (Remember that she had a 15-minute walk to the bus stop, which was a moderate-intensity activity.)

  0.50 hour @ hard intensity. (She judged that her hike before dinner was more vigorous than a walk along the street because of the soft path and hills. She did not think that the hike was as strenuous as jogging, so she rated it as 30 minutes of hard-intensity activity.)

  0.25 hour @ very hard intensity. (She spent 8 minutes climbing stairs after lunch, and she estimated that over the course of the day she spent another 7 minutes climbing stairs. Therefore, she spent a total of 0.25 hour in the very-hard-intensity activity of stair climbing.)

Pamela's score of 37 calories/kg/day *(see chart below)* qualifies her as a moderately active person. A person who slept for 8 hours and spent the rest of the day in light-intensity physical activity would have an energy expenditure score of 32 calories/kg/day.

For Pamela, the difference between 32 and 37 calories/kg/day is 300 calories. This difference over 1 month is equivalent to the energy stored in about 2.5 pounds of fat, or 30 pounds per year. Small differences in daily energy expenditure do add up.

Here is Pamela's completed daily energy expenditure chart.

Activity	Hours	MET Value	Hours X METs
Sleep	8	1	8 X 1.0 = 8
Moderate	0.25	4	0.25 X 4 = 1
Hard	0.50	6	0.50 X 6 = 3
Very hard	0.25	10	0.25 X 10 = 2.5
Total hours	9		
Light (24 minus total hours)	15	1.5	15 X 1.5 = 22.5
Total MET hours or calories/kg/day			37

Total daily caloric expenditure: MET hours X your weight in kilograms = <u>37 X 60 = 2,220 calories</u> (Pamela weighs 133 pounds or 60 kilograms [133/2.22])

How Do You Rate?	
Score	*Life-style*
32-35	Too sedentary
36-42	Moderately active
42+	Very active

Note that Pamela did not go to a health club or take part in traditional forms of exercise, but she managed to maintain an acceptable level of physical activity by looking for opportunities to increase her activity level. The amount of activity she did on this day is consistent with the activity recommended by the American College of Sports Medicine (ACSM) and the Centers for Disease Control and Prevention (CDC). This amount of activity provides you with many of the known health benefits of an active way of life. It also helps you control your weight.

How Much Time Did You Spend on the Activity?

An important factor in accurately estimating energy expenditure is to provide an accurate time interval. For example, if you go the beach for 8 hours, do not record that as 8 hours of swimming at a hard or very hard level. Perhaps you spent 30 minutes actually swimming, 1 hour walking on the beach, and the rest of the time sitting and reading. In this example, you would record 1 hour of moderate-intensity activity and one-half hour of either hard or very hard activity, depending on how strenuously you swam.

Don't Be Surprised

You may have very few or even no hours in the moderate-, hard-, and very-hard-intensity activities. Perhaps as many as 40 to 50 million adult Americans spend virtually no time in moderate- or high-intensity activities.

What Does Your Activity Score Mean?

To put your energy expenditure in perspective, consider these examples:

- The person who stays in bed all day has a score of 24.

- The person who does not do any moderate-, hard-, or very-hard-intensity activity has a score of 32.

- The person who does 2 hours of moderate-intensity activity (such as housework and walking), 1 hour of hard yard work, and 1 hour of jogging has a score of 50.

Monitor Your Activity Level

Carefully monitoring your physical activity patterns is an important first step in making permanent changes to your activity habits. Self-monitoring helps you focus your attention on the behavior you are trying to change and also allows you to track your progress. We suggest that you try some of the relatively simple tools described in this chapter to measure how active you are. Find one or two tools that work for you, assess your activity at regular intervals, track your progress, and enjoy your success as you move toward permanent activity habits!

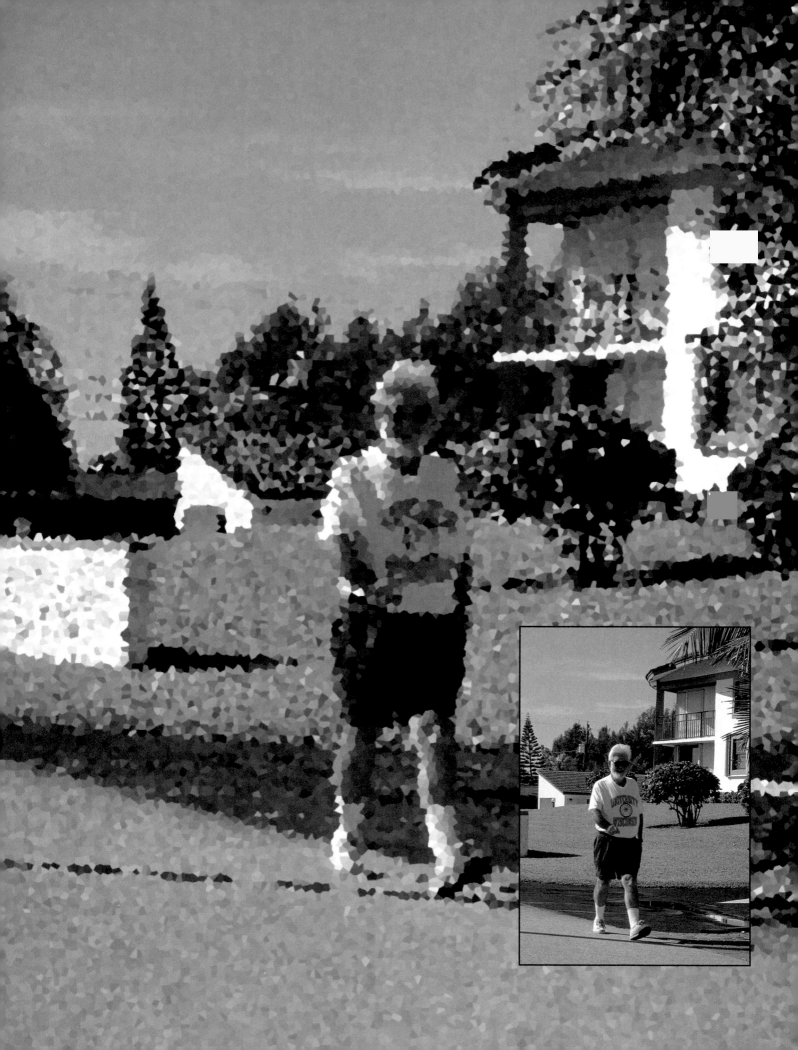

CHAPTER 6

Looking at Past Attempts to Be Active

The Challenge of Change

We have all tried to change our habits at one time or another—how we eat, how we spend money, and maybe even how much we exercise. We know that change is difficult. We are creatures of habit, and making adjustments in our routines usually requires thought, planning, and several tries before we succeed permanently. Although difficult, change is possible. And don't believe the old adage, "You can't teach an old dog new tricks." It's never too late to change. We've seen many elderly people who have successfully started and stayed with regular programs of physical activity.

As much as we've studied and learned about behavioral change, people, by their very nature, defeat our understanding of the exact process that's involved. We're all so different. What works for one person may not work for another. We've known people who can decide to change and can act on their decisions immediately. Most of us, however, find that gradually reshaping our habits, slowly building on success, and returning to an activity after we stop is a better way to adopt a new behavior.

It's appealing to think that we should be able to "type" individuals and match behavior-change strategies to individual differences. Unfortunately, such diagnostic tools either are not available or have had limited success. Our best plan is to understand some principles of behavior change and carefully analyze our preferences and dislikes using a try-and-try-again method, evaluating our success, and formulating new plans.

→EVALUATE → TRY → EVALUATE → TRY → EVALUATE → TRY

There are many theories about why and how we make substantial changes in our life-styles. Many health professionals promote behavior-change programs that focus on immediate and dramatic results. This approach, known as the action-oriented approach, assumes that when individuals decide they need to change their health behavior, they immediately and overtly take steps to make the change. The expectation is as about as dramatic (and realistic) as anticipating that a person who has pursued minimal exercise since childhood will embark on a training course for a marathon.

Many people find this action-oriented approach appealing, because they are hoping for a "quick fix." Thousands of people flock to weight-loss programs that promise 10 pounds off in the first week, or to health clubs that suggest you'll look like a bodybuilder after 6 weeks of training. Even though we all know better, many of us fall for it, and unfortunately most of us who attempt such programs are disappointed and ultimately give them up.

Many of us who have more realistic expectations and follow carefully supervised programs nevertheless fail to stick to our plans to change. Dropout and relapse rates are high, and we become disillusioned. Some of us feel we shouldn't have attempted to change at all.

Why didn't the programs work? Who's at fault? Usually, we blame ourselves. We figure we didn't have enough willpower or determination. But perhaps the problem is not with the individual but with the approach. It's unrealistic to expect overnight change in lifelong health behaviors. Change is a complex process that takes time!

One problem we face is considering a health behavior as an "either/or" event—for example, I am either sedentary or active, but nothing in between. In reality, health behaviors can be measured on a continuum, and although many questionnaires box us into a couple of categories at one or the other end of the continuum, most of us fall between the two extremes of sedentary and highly active. Try to view your physical activity as a fluid concept. You can move up and down the continuum. Where would you place yourself right now? Your overall objective should be to progress gradually along the continuum so that you consistently lead a more active life.

Behavior Change Is Not an "Either/Or" Event

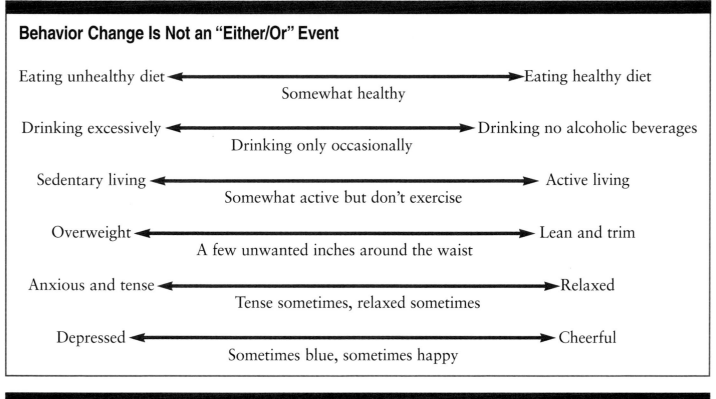

Eating unhealthy diet ⟷ Eating healthy diet
Somewhat healthy

Drinking excessively ⟷ Drinking no alcoholic beverages
Drinking only occasionally

Sedentary living ⟷ Active living
Somewhat active but don't exercise

Overweight ⟷ Lean and trim
A few unwanted inches around the waist

Anxious and tense ⟷ Relaxed
Tense sometimes, relaxed sometimes

Depressed ⟷ Cheerful
Sometimes blue, sometimes happy

Physical Activity Is a Continuum—Where Are You?

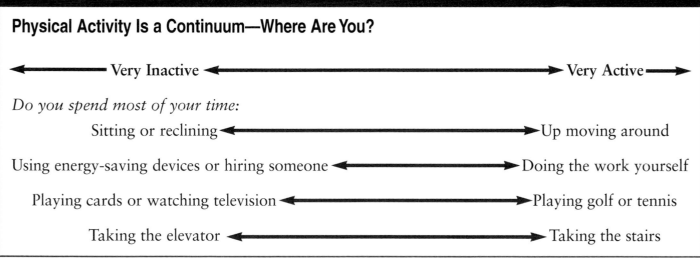

⟵ Very Inactive ⟷ Very Active ⟶

Do you spend most of your time:

Sitting or reclining ⟷ Up moving around

Using energy-saving devices or hiring someone ⟷ Doing the work yourself

Playing cards or watching television ⟷ Playing golf or tennis

Taking the elevator ⟷ Taking the stairs

What Health Behaviors Have You Successfully Changed in the Past?

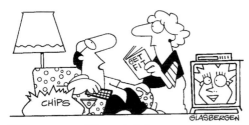

"Change my life-style? At my age, I get tired changing my socks!"

Virtually everyone has succeeded in changing a health behavior. Perhaps you implemented daily flossing as part of your dental-health program. Maybe you quit smoking 10 years ago. Perhaps you get a regular flu shot or limit the fat in your diet. You may have lost weight or learned how to manage stress more effectively. In any event, you probably can identify some positive health behaviors that you have incorporated in your daily routine.

As a first step, list your successes at changing health behaviors in Action Box 1 on the following page. By analyzing and identify-

ACTION BOX 1

Analysis of Past Behavior Change Attempts

Current positive health habit	Why did you change?	How did you change?	What makes you continue the health habit?
Example: Don't smoke	Tired of smell	Just stopped	Got rid of the smell
	Concern about health		Feel healthier
	Bad example for kids		Stopped coughing, breathe easier

Your positive habits:

1.			
2.			
3.			

ing factors related to those successes, you can develop strategies that apply some of the same tried-and-true methods to increase your physical activity.

What Have You Tried That Did Not Work?

Just as everyone can point to some successes in health behavior change, you can also identify attempts that didn't work for you. It's helpful to review unsuccessful attempts to change your health behavior so you can learn from them. (Complete Action Box 2 on the next page.)

By completing these two action-box worksheets, you've taken an important step in planning a behavior change. Analyzing your experiences can help you develop a strategy for future changes. For example, if you tried to lose weight by not eating dessert while your family ate dessert in front of you, you may now try to get your family's support by having everyone forego dessert. Or, you may simply leave the table before dessert is served. This type of careful preparation increases your likelihood of success in future efforts to improve your health and life-style.

We will occasionally refer you back to these two worksheets. Later, you may be able to elaborate on your responses on the

ACTION BOX 2

Analysis of Unsuccessful Behavior Change Attempts

Unsuccessful attempts to change a health behavior	Why did you want to change?	What were your reasons for not changing?	What resistance did you face, from yourself or others?
Example: Eating dessert	To lose weight	Couldn't resist eating	Family always had dessert with meals
	To look better		Craved it
	To feel better		
	What techniques did you use to try to change?	**Were you successful for a short period?**	**What made you stop trying?**
	Left the table when dessert was served	Yes, about 1 week	Didn't want to miss the conversation during dessert
			Tired of trying to resist it
	Why did you want to change?	**What were your reasons for not changing?**	**What resistance did you face, from yourself or others?**
Your attempts: 1.			
	What techniques did you use to try to change?	**Were you successful for a short period?**	**What made you stop trying?**
	Why did you want to change?	**What were your reasons for not changing?**	**What resistance did you face, from yourself or others?**
Your attempts: 2.			
	What techniques did you use to try to change?	**Were you successful for a short period?**	**What made you stop trying?**

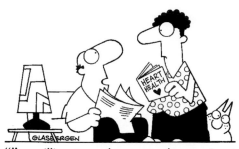

"I'm willing to make some changes in my life-style, as long as I don't have to do anything different."

worksheets and further analyze and understand the factors affecting your success in changing health habits.

Resisting and Embracing Change

When you consider the word *change*, what thoughts enter your mind? Do you think of terms like *difficult* or *easy*, *important* or *unimportant*, *slow* or *fast*, *later* or *now*, or do you have other thoughts? Write your thoughts about change in Action Box 3 below.

Look for a pattern in your responses. The pattern will allow you to better understand how you feel about change so you can deal with it. Although we don't know what you've written in this space, we do know that your thoughts are unique. If we were to pose the same questions to a large group of people and collect their responses, the list would be quite long and varied because change is multifaceted.

Do you think of change as a threat? Some of your thoughts about change may center around avoidance. Resisting change is natural, and everyone does it. Use Action Box 4 on the following page to list ways you have resisted change, especially change related to becoming physically active. Take some time to go over all your responses on the worksheets and look for patterns so that you understand how you think.

Most people tend to alternate between resisting change and embracing it. It's even possible to pursue your goal to be active and simultaneously embrace your sedentary life-style. Many people ignore or underestimate the consequences of a negative be-

---

ACTION BOX 3

Your Thoughts About Change

Circle the words that most appropriately describe your thoughts:

Difficult	*or*	Easy
Important	*or*	Unimportant
Slow	*or*	Fast
Later	*or*	Now
Threat	*or*	Opportunity

Write your other thoughts about change.

_____

_____

_____

_____

_____

havior or situation. This is partly why it's so difficult to make and sustain a change. Just as the payoffs of becoming more active will pull you toward your goal, unforeseen forces will pull you back to your old sedentary patterns. Recognize that you rarely embrace a change once and for all. Evaluate the positive and negative forces that pull you toward and push you away from your goal. See if you can add others to the lists in Action Box 5 below.

ACTION BOX 4

Ways You Have Resisted Change

Did you deny that the problem existed? _____

Did you procrastinate or drag your feet? _____

Was complaining about the change part of your response? _____

Were you impatient with your progress? _____

Write other ways you have resisted change.

_____

_____

ACTION BOX 5

Evaluate Your Positive and Negative Forces

Disadvantages to Remaining Sedentary	*Disadvantages to Being Active*
Poor health	Possibility of injury
Low fitness	No television
Feeling tired	Cost of shoes and clothing
_____	_____
_____	_____

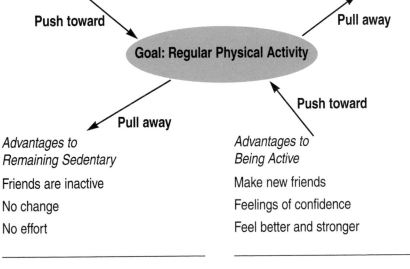

Push toward   **Pull away**

Goal: Regular Physical Activity

Pull away   **Push toward**

Advantages to Remaining Sedentary	*Advantages to Being Active*
Friends are inactive	Make new friends
No change	Feelings of confidence
No effort	Feel better and stronger
_____	_____
_____	_____

In your efforts to become more physically active, how can you tell when you are moving into a phase of resistance? When you become aware of resisting change, what can you do to start embracing this challenge? Complete Action Box 6 below to help prepare you to move through periods of resistance toward positive health habits.

ACTION BOX 6

Resisting and Embracing Change

	Resisting Change	Embracing Change
Thoughts	What are your thoughts? _____ _____ Are you thinking you can't do it? _____ Are you thinking it's not worth the effort? _____ _____	Believe that you can do it if you start slowly. Think about how being active will improve your health. _____ _____ _____
Feelings	What are your feelings? _____ _____ _____ Are you feeling discouraged about your progress? _____ Are you too tired to exercise? _____	Focus on feeling good. Enjoy the satisfaction of accomplishing your goal. _____ _____ _____
Behaviors	What are your behaviors? _____ _____ _____ Are you having to force yourself to be active? _____ Is it difficult to find time to be active? _____	Commit to being active, even if you don't want to. Schedule a time for physical activity and mark it on your calendar, just like any other important appointment. _____ _____
Social Relationships	How are others responding to your life-style change? _____ _____ Are your inactive friends trying to sabotage your efforts to be active? _____	Acknowledge the compliments you get from others who notice you are active. Enjoy the camaraderie of others who are active. _____ _____

Empower Yourself

If you become physically active, your body and health will change. Have you thought about how a stronger body and better health will positively affect how you feel, how you behave with others, and what you think and believe? One of the most exciting things about making a change in one aspect of your life is that it will spill into other areas of your life and into the lives of others around you. Can you recall how this has happened before?

When you open your mind to the potential benefits of being active, when you choose to embrace physical activity as a challenge for growth, you empower yourself. You'll begin to see options and alternatives where before you saw only obstacles and frustrations.

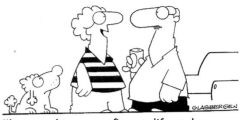

"I started my new fitness life-style today. From now on, I expect to look younger and feel younger. I'm even planning to get pimples again!"

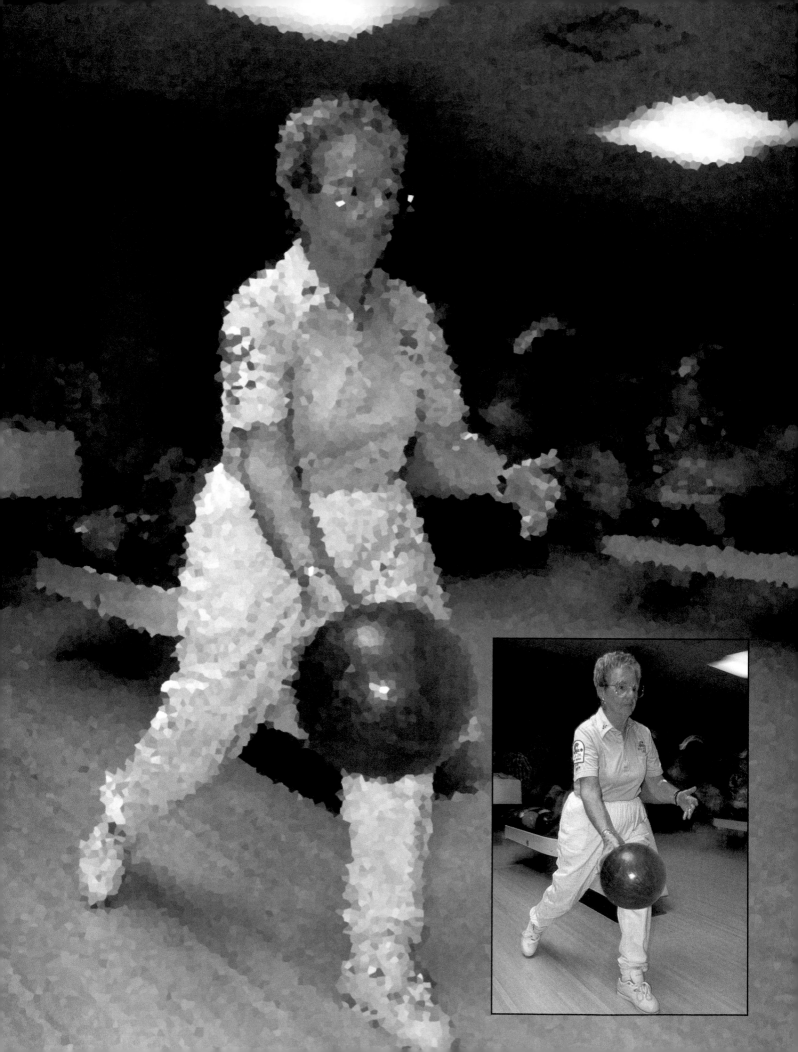

A New Approach to Change

Nobody else can do it for you. As you attempt to change your activity habits, you must become your own health counselor. Our plan is to help you develop the skills necessary to change old behaviors so that you become more physically active and fit.

How People Change

We believe that change occurs in stages. Dr. James Prochaska and his colleagues at the University of Rhode Island have followed thousands of people struggling to overcome their negative health habits and have observed that people change their behaviors gradually, progressing through a series of stages. They have identified five stages of change.

Dr. Bess Marcus of Brown University applied the Stages of Change model to analyze how people change their physical activity habits. The major premise of the model is that people are at varying degrees of readiness to change. Each stage in the process of change begins with a mindset. In Stage 1, you may not be thinking about exercise at all. In Stage 2, you may be thinking about it but not ready to do it. If you're in Stage 3, you are ready, willing, and planning to change but still not putting on your walking shoes. In Stage 4 you are ready and have taken action; you're off and running (or walking or swimming). In Stage 5, exercise has become a habit; you don't even think about not doing it, although you still have to negotiate obstacles in your life that might interfere with your new health regimen.

Stages of Health Behavior Change

Stage 1 Not thinking about change

Stage 2 Thinking about change

Stage 3 Developing plans to change

Stage 4 Implementing the change

Stage 5 Maintaining the new habit

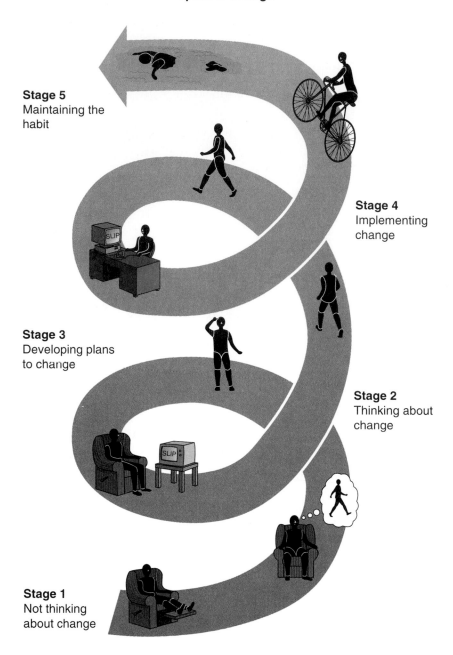

Spiral of Change

Stage 5
Maintaining the habit

Stage 4
Implementing change

Stage 3
Developing plans to change

Stage 2
Thinking about change

Stage 1
Not thinking about change

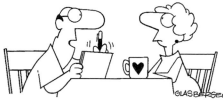

"I'm making a list of everything I can possibly do to get back in shape. For starters, I'm using a fountain pen because it's heavier than a regular pen!"

We believe that you will not permanently give up your sedentary habits until you have passed through Stage 5 and are committed to staying active for a lifetime. The key strategy for becoming ready is to structure your efforts around these Stages of Change. The chapters following this one (chapters 8 through 12) provide you with that structure. Each chapter begins with a brief self-assessment that helps you to measure your readiness for change. Depending on where you are on the spiral *(see above)* between not wanting to exercise and wanting to, the chapters ask you to participate actively in a series of tasks that are designed to move you along the path to greater readiness and greater activity. Many of the tasks ask you to consider your thoughts and behaviors so that you can identify obstacles to becoming active and find ways to overcome them.

There are quantities of white space in the pages of these chapters where we want you to write your responses. Take a pencil or pen and write in the book! Use it as a workbook. There is no greater force than action itself for changing how you think. Our principal objective is to engage you actively in a process of change that positively influences how you think about your behavior (your readiness to change) and provides you with the skills for putting thought into action.

Each stage represents a period of time as well as a set of tasks that you must master before moving to the next stage. You will use a variety of skills as you progress. A skill that you learn in one stage will be used again in a later stage, but in a different way. For example, "increasing knowledge" in Stage 2 may mean that you are learning the benefits of physical activity and the hazards of inactivity. In Stage 3, "increasing knowledge" means learning about different physical activities and exercise options. You will learn to apply previously learned skills to future stages of change, building on what you already know and increasing your likelihood of long-term success.

We believe that having completed the tasks for one chapter, you will be ready to move to the next stage and toward the ultimate goal—being active every day or nearly every day just as you do other activities, like eating and sleeping, that are natural to you.

The first step in the behavior change process is to determine "where you are"—how ready you are to change your physical activity habits. Later in this chapter you will complete a Stages of Change questionnaire that helps you assess your readiness for change. Once you have identified where you are in this process, you will begin to build new skills that move you toward permanent exercise habits. The short-term goal is to move to the next stage. For example, if you've just starting to think about becoming active, your goal is to develop a plan to increase your physical activity. It's too early at this stage to think very much about your ultimate goal—being active for the rest of your life.

How long does it take to progress through the five stages? There is no universal answer to this question. Some people may progress very rapidly, while others may take years to move from Stage 2—thinking about change—to Stage 3—making firm plans to change. In general, however, if you are thinking about changing and are willing to make a serious attempt, you will probably spend a few months at each successive stage. Many people spend about 6 months in each stage between Stage 2—thinking about change—and Stage 4—implementing change. Truly maintaining a habit (Stage 5) may take several years, even a lifetime. It's important to give yourself ample time to progress through each stage.

A few people move from thinking about change to deciding to change to acting on their decisions without a hitch, but they are the exception rather than the rule. Slips and setbacks are a natural and predictable part of the process and will occur at every stage of change. Nearly everyone attempting change experiences them.

Behavioral change is not a linear progression. You move ahead and backtrack, then go forward a little farther. For this reason, a spiral rather than a straight line is the better way to illustrate normal behavior change. *(See p. 112.)*

Fortunately, most people who get off track don't go all the way back to "square one." They learn from their experiences and, after some time, try new approaches and start making progress again. Managing slips and preventing setbacks are critical aspects of the behavior change process. You will learn how to manage slips and get back on track to sustainable physical activity habits.

We believe that your chances of success with this staged approach to change are greater than with any other approach you may have tried. In fact, the Stages of Change model is somewhat eclectic—it incorporates many of the best concepts from other behavior change models. The strategies you will use have been applied successfully to change a variety of health habits.

Setting Goals

Learning new skills and setting realistic goals are the foundations on which change is built. Your goals will vary depending on your readiness for change. We'll help you set goals that are realistic and appropriate at each stage. In the early stages, your only responsibility is to commit to working toward specified goals that are set for you. As you progress through the Stages of Change, you will assume more responsibility for setting your own goals.

Goals and Responsibilities

	We Will	You Will
Stage 1	Assume responsibility for identifying specific tasks for you.	Work on the tasks we suggest and evaluate your success.
Stage 2	Continue to identify tasks for you.	Monitor your progress in accomplishing your tasks.
Stage 3	Identify a few new tasks and teach you to set goals for yourself.	Monitor your progress in accomplishing tasks and meeting goals.
Stage 4	Suggest a limited number of tasks.	Assume responsibility for setting and monitoring your goals.
Stage 5	Suggest a limited number of tasks.	Assume responsibility for setting and monitoring your goals.

Factors Related to Health Behavior Change

A number of factors are instrumental in the behavior change process. Individual differences in how people approach and implement behavior change complicate the process considerably. Early attempts to understand how individuals change their behaviors were overly simplistic and not very predictive of success. Some factors that consistently play a role in the change process have, however, been identified.

Knowledge

Knowing is not believing or doing. If we all did what we knew was good for us, no one would smoke cigarettes, eat fat, or sit for 6 hours watching television. You need knowledge to know what is or isn't good for you, but knowledge by itself is no guarantee that you will behave in an enlightened way. You need only to look around you to see that knowledge alone cannot persuade people to change their habits or shift their behaviors to more active lifestyles. So why is the learning model of behavior change the one most used by teachers, physicians, and other health care professionals who ply you with information about the benefits of exercise? Because it's easy to lecture about the facts and physiology of exercise. Teachers are comfortable giving you information, and it's assumed that if you understand what is good for you, you will do it. But this approach is overly simplistic. Many other factors influence your behavior and affect your decision to exercise or not.

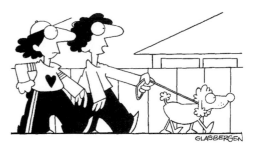

"The doctor told my husband to double his physical activity, so now he changes channels with both hands."

Attitude

If you don't want to do something, you won't, and nobody can make you. You must believe that physical activity is good for you. A positive attitude is essential if exercise is to be an important part of your life. Most adults believe they should maintain normal weight, exercise regularly, and manage stress effectively. However, positive attitudes are not always strong enough to make these difficult changes.

Affirmations—positive statements you make to yourself about changing a health habit—can effectively improve your attitude. Affirmations can refer to any aspect of the behavior change process. For example, you might tell yourself, "I will begin to think about the benefits of being active" or "I know I can give up watching television for 3 hours for a few nights each week." These positive statements will bolster your confidence that you can make changes. Later, we will suggest other affirmations that will help you to take a strong, positive attitude to your physical activity program.

"I will drink eight glasses of water every day, I will exercise for 30 minutes each morning, I will take the stairs instead of the elevator, I will bicycle instead of driving, I will flap my arms instead of using the airlines...."

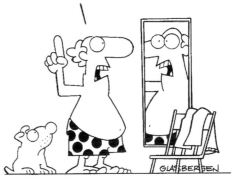

Motivation

A common misconception is that one person can "motivate" another to do something. Only you can motivate yourself. The primary motivation to make health habit changes comes from within the individual. *Motive*, after all, means "a need or desire that causes or 'moves' a person to act." Needs and desires come from within. "External" motivation—wanting something because

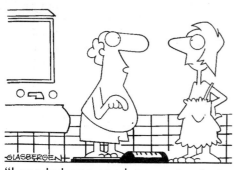

"I needed one good reason to start exercising. I think I just found 235 good reasons!"

someone else tells you you should—may help you develop the "internal" motivation to act, but the internal motivation is the key. Therefore, we do not believe that this book will "motivate" you to increase your physical activity (only you can do that), but we hope that it will influence you to make changes in your health habits.

Knowledge, attitude, and motivation are important components of the health behavior change process. Furthermore, most readers of this book probably already possess these characteristics to some, perhaps considerable, degree. If you didn't, you probably would not have obtained this book or at least have read this much of it. The information presented here should increase your knowledge, promote more positive attitudes toward physical activity, and enhance your motivation to become more physically active. However, other factors are crucial to your success in behavior change.

Maybe you're feeling content with the way you are. You have no apparent health problems and no complaints. Then some crisis or dramatic event captures your attention. You experience chest pain while jogging across the lawn to pick up the newspaper. A favorite uncle who has been a lifelong smoker dies of a massive heart attack. Your spouse says, "I want a divorce."

You begin to think about the future. You have expectations and unfulfilled dreams. Maybe your kids are in college, or you have other financial responsibilities. Poor health is not what you want in your future.

Intense emotional experiences and life-changing events can get your attention and may be a powerful stimulus to change. Suddenly, health and life-style are on your personal agenda. You begin to look seriously at the advantages of exercising. If your motivation to change comes primarily from fear or from a wish to please someone else, you may lose your desire to change. A life-crisis can jump-start the process of behavior change, but it may also be the underlying reason you slip back to your old routines. It's important at this stage to broaden your knowledge and understanding of the benefits of change and to determine which benefits are likely to mean the most to you.

Self-Confidence

Many individuals have long histories of failed attempts to change health habits. If you are one of these, you may be discouraged about the likelihood of succeeding in making permanent, lifelong changes to your health habits. Behaviorists have recently identified self-confidence as vital to the process of change. Several studies have shown that individuals who are confident they can change are more likely to do so than those who downrate their chances for success.

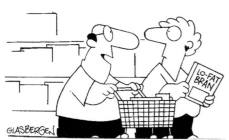

"I'm always losing my car keys, my temper, my memory, and my patience... so losing weight should be a breeze!"

Behavioral Analysis

An effective way to improve the chances of successful change is to thoroughly analyze the targeted behavior. Research shows that self-monitoring your behavior, exploring your motives, tracking your progress, and assessing your attitudes along the way are often helpful in making a change. Understanding the stimuli or cues that prompt a behavior may help you to control it. We will teach you the skills of behavior change, but you must become your own health counselor.

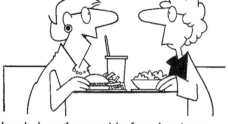

"I've noticed that I only overeat when I'm depressed. So I taped jokes and cartoons on the refrigerator door to cheer me up before I get to the food!"

Persistence

A pessimistic view is that failure breeds failure, and that a person who repeatedly fails learns a pattern of behavior and cannot break it. If you keep trying techniques that fail, then you will fail too. But new methods of change can break old patterns. Moreover, research in behavior change indicates that one of the best predictors of success is the number of previous attempts to change. Contrary to the belief that failures breed more failures, the persistent person demonstrates a high degree of determination to succeed and a willingness to learn from problems and mistakes. This person is more likely to succeed with the next attempt.

Skill Building

After analyzing the behavior you want to change, you need specific skills to facilitate changes. Skills that are helpful in a behavioral change program include developing a personal plan, solving problems, setting goals, rethinking old behaviors, identifying barriers, and planning for high-risk situations. For example, if you want support from your family and friends, you will need to develop

"I only lost 1 pound before I quit my diet. But if I can do that 50 times, I could lose 50 pounds!"

Behavioral Skills and Strategies

Setting goals. Targeting a specific habit for change

Affirmations. Making positive statements about yourself and the change process

Thinking differently. Reviewing and challenging your thoughts and beliefs

Becoming more knowledgeable. Learning new information about the habit you want to change

Monitoring your progress. Assessing your habits and progress

Planning systematically. Developing a careful plan for change

Recognizing cues. Looking for things in yourself and your surroundings that stimulate a behavior

Building relationships. Identifying and developing support of others for your attempt to change

Building self-confidence. Believing that you can make and sustain a change

Managing time. Allowing time to practice your new habit

Managing stress. Coping with stresses associated with changing a habit

Rewarding yourself. Recognizing the progress you make

Dealing with slips. Anticipating problems and getting back on track if you lose some of your gains

skills to identify and mobilize people to get the kind of support you want.

In Which Stage Are You?

The first step in applying the Stages of Change approach to changing your physical activity is to determine your current stage. The following questionnaire *(Action Box 1)*, developed by Dr. Bess Marcus, acknowledges that different individuals require different intervention strategies based on their stages of readiness for

ACTION BOX 1

Stages of Change Questionnaire

Physical activity means walking briskly, vacuuming, jogging, gardening, climbing stairs, or any other similar physical activity.

Regular physical activity or exercise means accumulating 30 minutes or more in the above activities on most days of the week. For example, you could take one 30-minute walk; three 10-minute walks; or 5 minutes of vacuuming, 10 minutes of walking, 10 minutes of gardening, and 5 minutes of stair climbing. You also are considered regularly physically active if you play vigorous sports, jog, or participate in other vigorous activities for at least 30 minutes for at least 3 days a week.

Please check "Yes" or "No" for each statement listed below.

	Yes	No
1. I am currently physically active.		
2. I intend to become more physically active in the next 6 months.		
3. I currently engage in regular physical activity.		
4. I have been physically active regularly for the past 6 months.		

Scoring

If you answered "No" to questions 1 to 4, you are in Stage 1. Read chapters 8 to 12.

If you answered "Yes" to Question 2 and "No" to questions 1, 3, and 4, you are in Stage 2. Read chapters 9 to 12.

If you answered "Yes" to questions 1 and 2 and "No" to questions 3 and 4, you are in Stage 3. Read chapters 10 to 12.

If you answered "Yes" to questions 1, 2, and 3 and "No" to Question 4, you are in Stage 4. Read chapters 11 and 12.

If you answered "Yes" to questions 1, 3, and 4, you are in Stage 5. Read Chapter 12 and the rest of the book to find out how to enjoy staying active for the rest of your life.

Key to Chapters

Chapter 8: If You Haven't Thought Much About Exercise (Stage 1)

Chapter 9: Thinking About Starting to Exercise (Stage 2)

Chapter 10: Developing Your Exercise Plan (Stage 3)

Chapter 11: Developing Regular Exercise Habits (Stage 4)

Chapter 12: Staying Active for a Lifetime (Stage 5)

Adapted from "The Stages and Processes of Exercise Adoption and Maintenance in a Worksite Sample," by B.H. Marcus, J.S. Rossi, V.C. Selby, R.S. Niaura, and D.B. Abrams, 1992, *Health Psychology, 11*, pp. 386–395. Copyright © 1992 LEA Publishers.

change. After you learn where you are in the change process, you will be directed to specific activities suited to your stage of readiness. Matching specific strategies and techniques with your current stage of readiness enhances your chances of long-term success.

You will begin with small changes that are relatively easy to implement. Your success in maintaining these changes will give you a good foundation from which to move to more extensive changes. This approach, which builds on successes, can help you to increase your self-confidence and raise the odds for future success.

Take a moment to answer these questions honestly. There are no right or wrong answers. The questionnaire will help you determine how ready you are to change your physical activity habits so that you can start at a place that will work for you.

After you have determined your stage of readiness, go to the appropriate chapter to find specific strategies to help you progress to the next stage. Move to a more advanced stage when you are ready. After Stage 5, physical activity will have become a regular part of your life, and you will be ready to maintain your new active habits indefinitely.

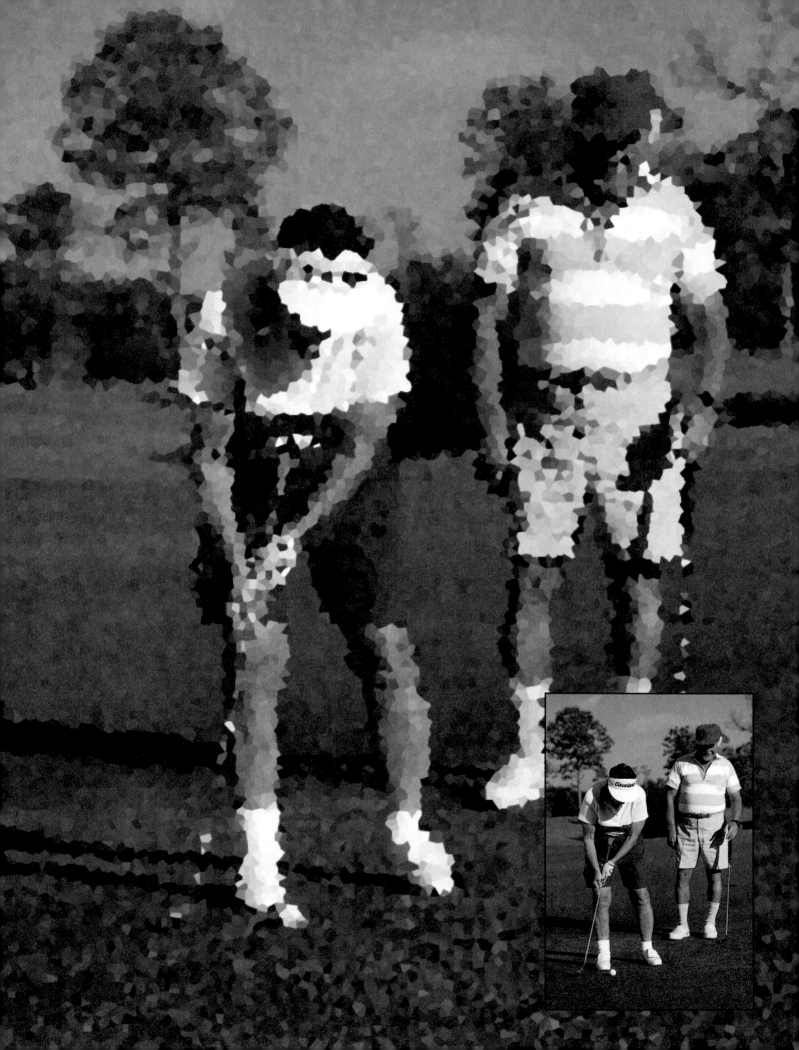

CHAPTER 8

If You Haven't Thought Much About Exercise (Stage 1)

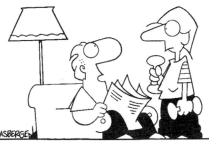

"I got plenty of exercise today! I ran up a phone bill, jumped to a conclusion, stretched my patience, and pushed my luck!"

Your responses to the readiness quiz in Chapter 7 *(see p. 118)* indicate that you are not currently physically active and have not been regularly active in the past 6 months. You say you do not intend to become more physically active in the next 6 months. Even if you were regularly active at some time in the past, perhaps when you were in high school or college, but have been inactive for the last 6 months and are not intending to become active any time soon, then you are also in Stage 1.

ACTION BOX 1

Self-Assessment

Do any of these statements apply to you?

	Yes	No
I don't need to be more active.		
I don't think being more active would be beneficial.		
I'm not really that inactive.		
I can't think of any reason to be active.		
I can give a long list of reasons *not* to become active and very few, if any, for being active.		
I become anxious or defensive if someone suggests that I should be more active.		
I have given up on the idea of becoming physically active.		
I don't want to think, talk, listen, or read about being active.		
I am definitely not ready to get started on an activity program.		

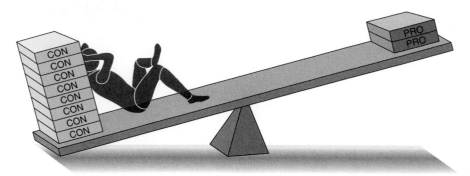

People in Stage 1 typically see more "cons" (reasons for not being active) than they see "pros" (reasons for changing). A few of the most common reasons given by people who aren't thinking of being active are listed below in Action Box 2. Are any of these true for you?

Those of you in Stage 1 are hardly alone. There are probably 15 million inactive American adults. Many of those who are currently sedentary aren't thinking of becoming active within the next 6 months. (Six months seem to be about as far into the future as people seriously plan to make changes in their physical activity.)

In Stage 1, an important task is to begin thinking about your reasons for and against ("pros" and "cons") becoming active. List all your "cons" on the Action Box 2 worksheet below. Be honest with yourself. Be aware of what's holding you back, but also try to identify a few "pros"—reasons why being physically active might add something positive to your life.

ACTION BOX 2

Weigh the "Pros" and "Cons" of Change

Date _____

Check the "pros" and "cons" below that apply to you and add others.

Pros	Cons
Advantages to Being Active	**Disadvantages to Being Active**
I might feel better.	*I'm too old.*
I might enjoy it.	*It would take too much time.*
I might have more energy.	*I don't know anyone who is active.*
	I could get hurt.
	I wouldn't enjoy it.
Disadvantages to Staying Sedentary	**Advantages to Staying Sedentary**
I might lose the ability to live independently.	*I wouldn't have to change.*
I might have to take medicine.	

Program for Change

Tasks

We believe the tasks listed below will help you move to the next stage of change. Try to accomplish all the tasks listed for this stage.

☐ Read Chapter 3 of this book to learn about the many benefits of physical activity.

☐ Collect newspaper and magazine articles about the benefits of physical activity from reliable sources.

☐ Identify at least five new advantages ("pros") of being physically active *(Action Box 2)*.

☐ Identify at least five new disadvantages ("cons") to staying sedentary *(Action Box 2)*.

☐ Repeat affirmations about physical activity every morning and night for at least 1 week when you brush your teeth.

Evaluate Your Success

As you accomplish the tasks for Stage 1, answer the questions below and score your success. Aim for a score of at least 12. If your score falls below 10, perhaps you should rethink your motivation and keep working before moving forward. When you have accomplished the tasks for Stage 1 and feel you are ready, move to Stage 2.

	Score
How committed were you to accomplishing these tasks? (3) = very committed, (2) = somewhat committed, (1) = not very committed	
How difficult were these tasks to accomplish? (3) = very easy, (2) = somewhat easy, (1) = very difficult	
How much did you learn from working to accomplish these tasks? (3) = a great deal, (2) = some, (1) = not very much	
How much motivation, help, or support did you need from others to accomplish these tasks? (3) = not very much, (2) = some, (1) = a great deal	
Are you thinking seriously about becoming more active? (3) = yes, definitely, (2) = yes, I am beginning to, (1) = no, I'm not ready yet	
Total Score	

Affirmations

Affirmations are positive statements you can repeat regularly to motivate you to become active. You can say affirmations out loud or silently. You should repeat them often and with real commitment. Begin each affirmation with "I am," "I can," or "I will" rather than with "I am not." Schedule a time in your day, such as when brushing your teeth, to say affirmations. Some people believe it is helpful to say affirmations while looking in the mirror. Begin with the affirmations listed below. Add one of your own.

☐ I can be more active than I am now.

☐ I'll enjoy being more active.

☐ I'll be healthier when I'm active.

Stage 1 continues on the following page

Program for Change

☐ I'll feel better when I'm active.

☐ I'll look better when I'm active.

☐ I'll stay independent if I'm active.

☐ _____

Tips for Success

☐ If you can move from not thinking about being active to thinking seriously about being active in 1 month, you double your chances of starting an activity program within the next 6 months.

☐ Be sure you're changing because *you* want to.

☐ Lack of internal motivation is likely the reason for slips in people who attempt changes when they aren't ready. They probably never intended to change in the first place.

Dealing with Slips

If you start to slip back to not thinking about being active, try these strategies to get back on track:

☐ Review the benefits ("pros") of physical activity.

☐ Read something new about physical activity.

☐ Think about how inactivity affects your health.

☐ Consider how your inactivity affects the people closest to you.

☐ Talk to people like yourself who are physically active.

Reward Yourself

_____ will be my reward for starting to think about being active.

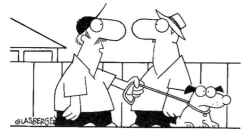

"I started exercising because I had a close brush with death—my wife threatened to kill me if I didn't get off the couch!"

How to Approach Change

Don't Wait for a Crisis to Happen to You

Some people consider changing their health habits only after personal crises. They may have a heart attack after years of sedentary living and may recognize the need for life-style changes. Or, their doctors may tell them that their blood pressure, blood sugar, or blood cholesterol levels are too high and that physical activity will help control these factors. Sometimes the crises strike relatives or close friends. A person might think, "That could happen to me. Perhaps I should think about making a change before it's too late." We hope there won't be a crisis in your life to cause you to think seriously about physical activity.

Learn About the Benefits of Activity

It's important to know as much as possible about physical activity as you think about making a change. This book will help answer many of your questions. Chapters 3 and 4 discuss the proven benefits and risks of physical activity that have been documented by research.

Seek information from other sources. Read and collect articles about activities you think you might enjoy. But, be cautious. The media are full of information and products that provide seemingly simple answers and quick fixes. Unfortunately, not all the information or products you see in print or hear about on television or radio are valid and reliable. Chapter 14 of this book gives you guidelines to help evaluate health and fitness information, products, and services. Don't be vulnerable to products and services that are scientifically unproved and unsound.

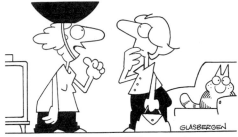

"I ordered it from TV! You use it to stand on your head for 20 minutes a day so gravity can change your big belly into a big chest!"

Become More Aware of Your Habits and Health

Obtaining personal feedback about your physical activity habits and your current level of fitness may motivate you to begin thinking about a change. This book contains several self-assessment and self-monitoring tools. Review Chapter 5 to learn how you can assess your current level of physical activity. This chapter will help you better understand how physical activity is measured and how it relates to calories and metabolism, a topic that will interest you if weight management is on your "pro" list for being physically active.

You can also participate in health screenings. Health fairs that offer blood pressure checks, cholesterol screenings, and fitness and health risk assessments are fairly common events in many communities. Hospitals and other health care providers often sponsor these events in shopping malls on weekends to increase awareness about their services. Some worksites offer health promotion or wellness programs for their employees, and screenings and educational resources may be included in these programs.

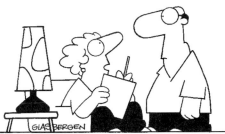

"Today I walked 2 miles and burned 200 calories. But I deducted 50 calories for breathing the air outside of Nickerson's Bakery on Third Street."

Take advantage of these benefits and services if they are available. Screenings are low cost, and it's usually easy and convenient to participate. The test results are confidential and you're under no obligation to participate in any further program or service.

Although screenings are educational and motivational, they are not intended as medical diagnoses. If your assessment indicates that you are at risk for a medical condition, see a physician to confirm the results and receive medical advice or treatment.

Take a Look Around You

Sometimes your surroundings can help to motivate you to change a health habit. As positive health practices become more socially acceptable in our culture, more people will consider adopting them. Perhaps the desire to be part of the "norm" motivates us.

Do you think you might like to participate in, rather than observe, the trend toward a more active life-style? More people are physically active than 30 years ago. It's not unusual to see people walking, jogging, cycling, or skating on streets and roads in cities, suburbs, and rural areas. More people are taking the stairs or walking instead of waiting for the elevator, escalator, or moving sidewalk. Almost any fall or spring weekend, you can participate in a "fun run" or walk with hundreds of other active people.

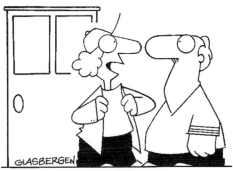

"It seems like everyone is into fitness these days! This morning the park was full of walkers and joggers, the squirrels were bench-pressing stones, and the goldfish in the pond were swimming laps!"

Whatever it takes to inspire you to start thinking seriously about being more active, it's the change in your thinking that counts.

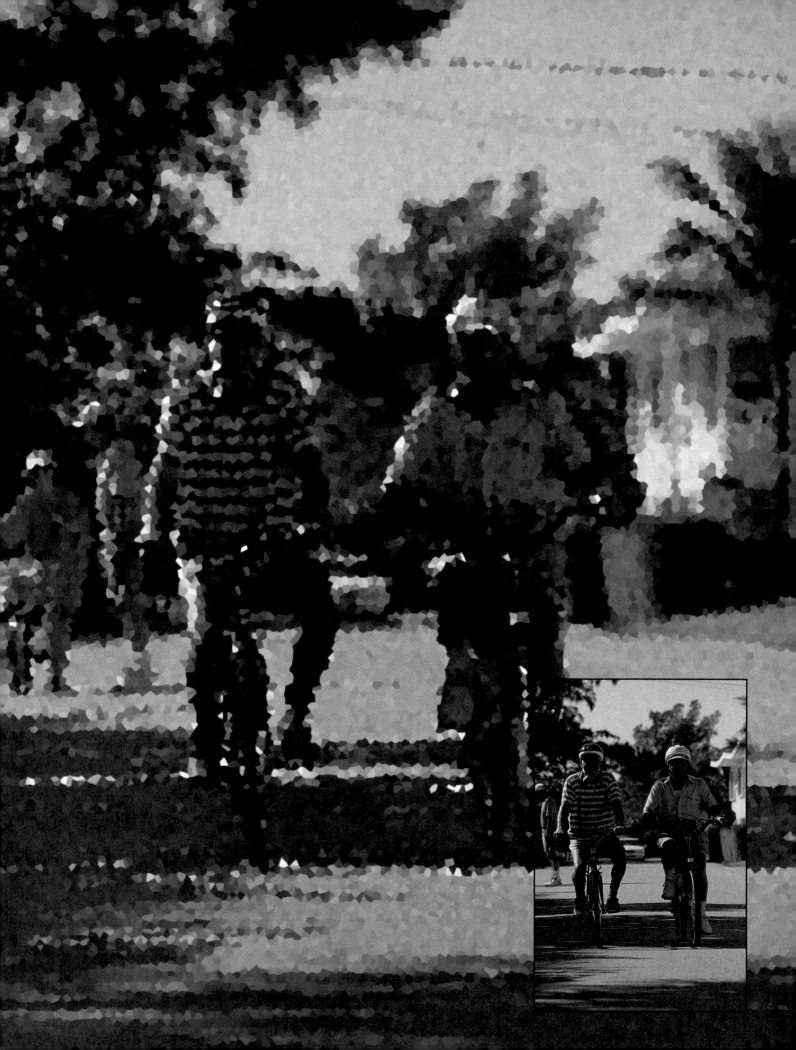

Thinking About Starting to Exercise (Stage 2)

Your response to the readiness questionnaire in Chapter 7 *(see p. 118)* indicates that you are not currently physically active but that you intend to start exercising in the next 6 months. If you are reading this book, you are probably at least in Stage 2—thinking that you will start exercising soon, but not quite ready to start.

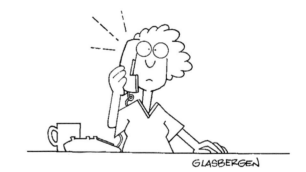

GLASBERGEN

"Thank you for calling the Weight Loss Hotline. If you'd like to lose 1/2 pound right now, press 1 18,000 times."

ACTION BOX 1

Self-Assessment

How many of these statements apply to you?	Yes	No
I know I need to or should be more active.		
I know some of the benefits or "pros" of physical activity, but the "cons" still win.		
I feel ambivalent about physical activity. I don't care one way or the other.		
I don't believe I can become active or stay active once I start.		
I've been thinking about becoming more active for years, but I've never done anything to get started.		

ACTION BOX 2

Weigh the "Pros" and "Cons" of Change   Date _____

If you are beginning the process of change at Stage 2, fill in your specific "pros" and "cons" for changing your physical activity below.

Pros	**Cons**
Advantages to Being Active	Disadvantages to Being Active
Disadvantages to Staying Sedentary	Advantages to Staying Sedentary

Weighing the "pros" and "cons" for activity and deciding in favor of activity is one of the best predictors of success for becoming and staying active. Why? Because the hardest part of changing a behavior is changing your thinking. Once you have abandoned an old habit of thinking, you've taken your first step toward changing your behavior. From inertia, you have begun to advance along the spiral of change. *(See p. 112 in Chapter 7.)*

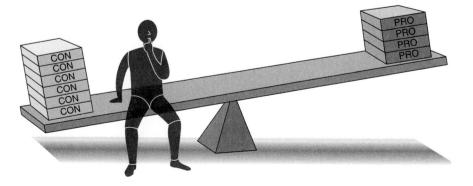

People in Stage 2 still find more reasons for staying sedentary than for exercising, but the list of "pros" and "cons" is more balanced.

Program for Change

Tasks

The tasks for Stage 2 will encourage you to think seriously about becoming physically active. The information you gain by completing these tasks will be very useful as you start to develop your plan for increasing your physical activity in the next few weeks. You may want to start a notebook or filing system for the information you collect. Try to accomplish all of the tasks. Check your success. When you're ready, proceed to Stage 3.

- [ ] Identify at least two new advantages of being physically active *(Action Box 2)*.
- [ ] Identify at least two new disadvantages of staying sedentary *(Action Box 2)*.
- [ ] Give up at least one of your advantages for staying sedentary *(Action Box 2)*.
- [ ] Give up at least one of your disadvantages for being physically inactive *(Action Box 2)*.
- [ ] Spend at least 5 minutes each day thinking about yourself as an active person.
- [ ] Repeat affirmations about physical activity every morning and night for at least 1 week when you brush your teeth.
- [ ] Talk to someone who has recently started to be physically active to learn why and how he or she is active.
- [ ] Read newspaper and magazine articles from reliable sources about the benefits of physical activity.
- [ ] Practice visualizing yourself as an active person at least once each day.
- [ ] Evaluate your thoughts, feelings, and behaviors regarding exercise *(Action Box 3)*.
- [ ] Recognize your excuses for being inactive *(Action Box 4)*.

Evaluate Your Success

As you accomplish the tasks for Stage 2, answer the questions below and score your success. Aim for a score of at least 12. If your score falls below 10, perhaps you should rethink your motivation and keep working before moving forward. When you have accomplished the tasks for Stage 2 and feel you are ready, move to Stage 3.

	Score
How committed were you to accomplishing these tasks? (3) = very committed, (2) = somewhat committed, (1) = not very committed	
How difficult were these tasks to accomplish? (3) = very easy, (2) = somewhat easy, (1) = very difficult	
How much did you learn from working to accomplish these tasks? (3) = a great deal, (2) = some, (1) = not very much	
How much motivation, help, or support did you need from others to accomplish these tasks? (3) = not very much, (2) = some, (1) = a great deal	
Are you ready to start developing a plan to become more active? (3) = yes, definitely, (2) = yes, I am beginning to, (1) = no, I'm not ready yet	
Total Score	

Stage 2 continues on the following page

Program for Change

Affirmations

These positive statements will help you get ready to develop your plan for physical activity. Write these affirmations on index cards and carry them with you or post them on your bathroom mirror. One of the most important affirmations for you at this stage is repeating the date for developing a plan. Give yourself at least 1 month to accomplish your goals for Stage 2. As the date approaches, you should feel confident about your ability to move forward. Add some of your own affirmations to the list below.

- [ ] I can be more active than I am now.
- [ ] I will enjoy being more active.
- [ ] I will be healthier when I'm active.
- [ ] I will feel better when I'm active.
- [ ] I will look better when I'm active.
- [ ] I will start to develop a plan to begin to be active on (date)_____.
- [ ] _____
- [ ] _____

Tips for Success

Many people spend years thinking and talking about being more active. You may fool your spouse, friends, or even your doctor with well-intended thoughts and promises, but don't fool yourself. Don't just think about being active, develop a systematic plan now. Here are some tips:

- [ ] Imagine a new you. Create in your mind the image of yourself engaged in physical activity. How do you look? How do you feel? Visualize your success with physical activity.

- [ ] Describe specific situations related to being inactive that are bothering you. Consider the effects that becoming more active will have on you. What will you do differently? How will you feel? What else in your life will be different as a result of increasing your physical activity?

- [ ] Focus on working toward the next stage of change rather than attaining the ultimate goal of becoming and staying physically active.

- [ ] Congratulate and reward yourself for thinking about being physically active.

- [ ] Keep your list of advantages and benefits of being active in front of you each day. Try to add something to the list each day.

- [ ] Make a list of positive statements (affirmations) about yourself and physical activity. Read and review them often and add to them regularly.

- [ ] Recognize when you're having irrational or self-defeating thoughts. Analyze and challenge your thinking. Your behaviors will reflect and reinforce your thoughts.

Dealing with Slips

If you start to slip back to the early stages of change, try these strategies to get back on track:

- [ ] Review the benefits ("pros") of physical activity.
- [ ] Read something new about physical activity.
- [ ] Think about the health hazards of inactivity.

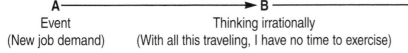

Program for Change

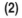   Consider how your inactivity affects the people closest to you.

Talk to people like yourself who are physically active.

Reward Yourself

Choose a reward that is meaningful to you. You'll find some suggestions in Chapter 12.

_____ will be my reward for starting to develop my physical activity plan.

How to Start Thinking Differently

Consider Your Thoughts, Feelings, and Behaviors

Because you have not thought much about exercising, you must work on changing some of your thoughts and beliefs. More than likely, you've had at least some negative thoughts that have sabotaged your intentions to become physically active. The A-B-C model for thinking rationally developed by Dr. Albert Ellis will help you understand the relationship between your thoughts, feelings, and behaviors and will suggest ways you can change them to help you become active.

Most people believe that a particular event or situation causes their feelings and behaviors. For example, assume you have a new assignment (Point 1A) that requires you to travel frequently over the next several months. You feel depressed about your job demands, so you remain sedentary (Point 1C). However,

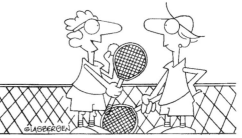

"I used to think exercise was just for kids, and I was right. If you want to be a kid again, you've got to exercise!"

(1)

A ◄————————————————————————————————► C
Event   Feelings and behaviors
(New job demand)   (Feel depressed, remain sedentary)

between Point A and Point C, something else happens—you think. These thoughts are called "inner dialogues." The thinking you do at Point B can be rational or irrational. Most people think irrationally at least some of the time (Point 2B). Irrational thinking is illogical, inaccurate, self-defeating, and catastrophic. It prevents goal attainment. In contrast, rational thinking is reasonable and realistic and does not automatically reject negative thoughts or simply substitute positive thinking. A negative thought may be

(2)

A ——————————————► B ——————————————————► C
Event   Thinking irrationally   Feelings and behaviors
(New job demand)   (With all this traveling, I have no time to exercise)   (Feel depressed, remain sedentary)

accurate, and a positive thought may be inaccurate. Thinking rationally means looking at what is accurate and accepting it as accurate. It challenges negative irrational thoughts and replaces them with rational responses.

You *can* change your thoughts. At Point B ask, "Is this an accurate assessment of the situation?" It's true the travel may be unavoidable, but it's not true you can't be physically active. A rational thought may be that activity could help relieve the stress of your new job demands. Changing your thoughts (Point 3B) will change how you feel and behave (Point 3C).

(3)

A ────────────────► B ────────────────► C

Event   Thinking rationally   Feelings and behaviors

(New job demand)   (Exercise will relieve the stress of all this traveling)   (Feel motivated, find ways to exercise while traveling)

Evaluate Your Thoughts

Irrational beliefs about physical activity may pop into your head from time to time. To substitute more accurate and rational beliefs, stop, analyze your thoughts (inner dialogues), and change your thoughts (if necessary) before you act. *(See Action Box 3 below.)*

ACTION BOX 3

Substitute Positive or Rational Thoughts for Negative or Irrational Thoughts

Example

1. Identify the thought:	(Exercise is for athletes.)
2. Ask yourself if it's accurate and reasonable:	(No, I know several people just like me who aren't athletes but who are physically active. They participate in noncompetitive activities and seem to enjoy them.)
3. Restructure the thought as a more rational belief:	(I may not be an athlete, but I can participate in physical activity and have fun.)

Transform each inaccurate, irrational, or negative thought in the left-hand column below to an accurate, rational, or positive thought in the right-hand column.

Inaccurate, Irrational, Negative Thoughts	Accurate, Rational, Positive Thoughts
Exercise is only for athletes.	*I may not be an athlete, but I can participate and have fun.*
I'm too old to be active.	
I'm too out of shape to be active.	
I'm just too lazy to be active.	
I can't be active because I have to take care of my mother.	

You can interrupt the process of automatic thinking and change your feelings and actions. Ask someone to help you come up with a rational response if you have difficulty thinking of one on your own.

Recognize Your Excuses

Excuses are a type of automatic, irrational thought that can be unconsciously believed and accepted. Excuses can blind you to options and prevent problem solving. Others' excuses are easier to see than your own. One way to learn to be aware of your own excuses is to listen for "If only…" statements and "Yes, but…" responses. *(Complete Action Box 4 below.)*

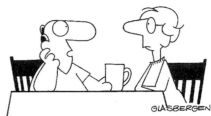

"Before I start an exercise program, I should talk to my doctor. I think I may have an overactive 'excuse gland.'"

ACTION BOX 4

What's Your Excuse?

Create three "If only…" statements that you or someone else might use to avoid being active. Then give a viable, constructive response to each statement.

Example

Excuse: *"If only…I weren't so tired at the end of the day, I'd feel like exercising."*

Constructive Response: *"Regular physical activity can make me feel more energetic."*

Excuse:	Constructive Response:
"If only…	
"If only…	
"If only…	

Below are several viable solutions to common problems in getting started with physical activity. Play the devil's advocate. Write a "Yes, but…" response for each.

Example

Solution: *If you go for a walk first thing in the morning, nothing else can prevent you from being active that day.*

Excuse: *"Yes, but I must prepare breakfast for my husband in the morning and I wouldn't have time to walk."*

Solution: An easy way to increase your physical activity is to park your car farther from the building and walk the extra distance.

Excuse: "Yes, but… _____

_____

Solution: If you work out to an exercise video at home, you can save money by not paying for a fitness club membership.

Excuse: "Yes, but… _____

_____

Solution: If you walk to lunch you can get an extra 15 minutes of physical activity 5 days a week.

Excuse: "Yes, but… _____

_____

Are you learning to recognize your excuses for inactivity?

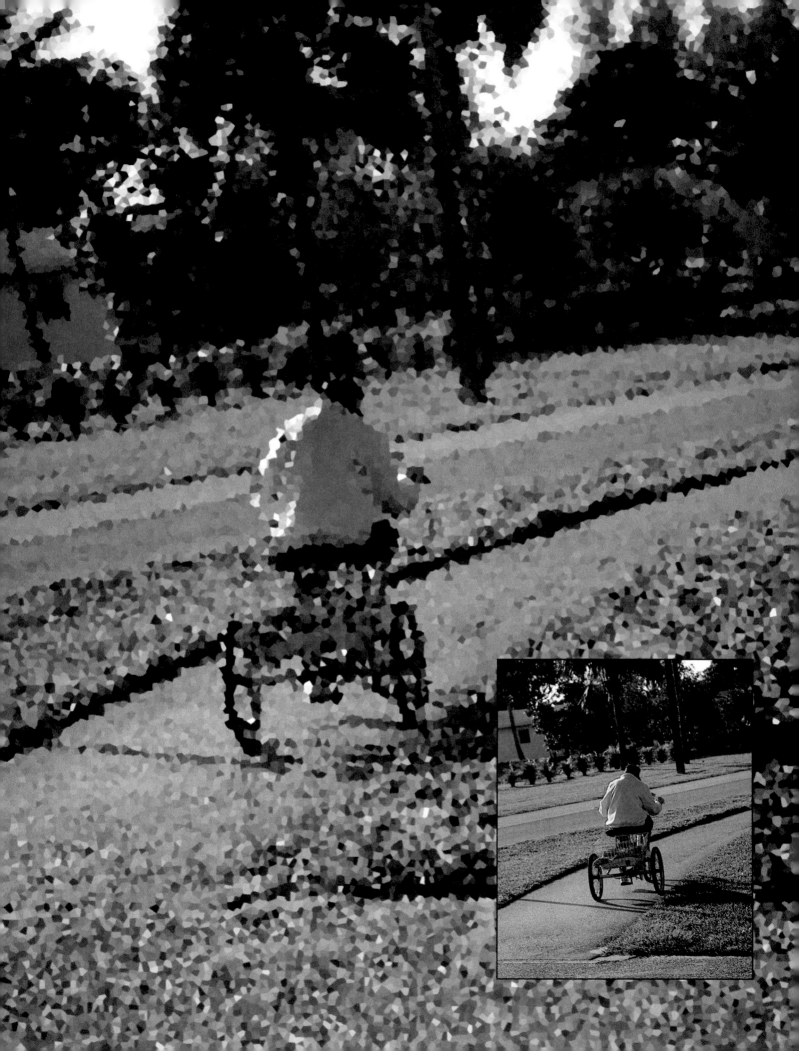

CHAPTER 10

Developing Your Exercise Plan (Stage 3)

I f you have progressed to Stage 3 from an earlier stage, congratulations! Keep up the good work! Remember that research in behavior change indicates that people who systematically progress through the Stages of Change by completing tasks appropriate to each stage are much likelier to make and sustain permanent changes.

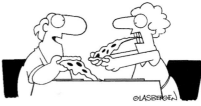

"It has the same chewy texture as mozzarella cheese, but it won't clog your arteries or make you gain weight. It's sugarless bubble gum!"

ACTION BOX 1

Self-Assessment

How many of these statements apply to you?	Yes	No
I know there are health benefits to being active.		
I have made at least one serious attempt to become active within the past few months.		
I have made a conscious choice and commitment to become more active.		
I believe I can be active.		
I have developed an individual plan for becoming active.		
I have sought help or support from my doctor in becoming more active.		
I have considered joining a group led by a health professional at a fitness center.		
I have considered joining a peer support group or club.		
I have purchased exercise clothes or equipment.		

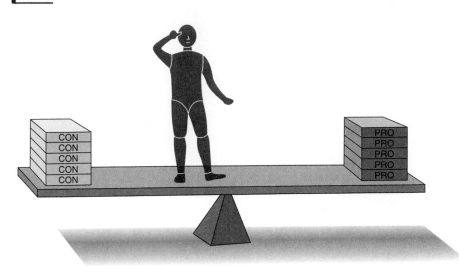

People in Stage 3 find at least as many reasons for being physically active as for remaining sedentary. The "pros" begin to weigh against the "cons," and people make serious plans to stay active.

Whether you have progressed from Stage 2 or you're beginning in Stage 3 based on your responses to the readiness questionnaire in Chapter 7 *(see p. 118)*, this is a very important stage for you. You have indicated that you intend to become more physically active in the next 6 months and that you are currently physically active.

People in Stage 3 have started practicing new behaviors. They are the most likely to enroll in action-oriented programs.

ACTION BOX 2

Weigh the "Pros" and "Cons" of Change   Date _____

If you are beginning the process of change at Stage 3, fill in the "pros" and "cons" for changing your physical activity habits below.

Pros	Cons
Advantages to Being Active	Disadvantages to Being Active
Disadvantages to Staying Sedentary	Advantages to Staying Sedentary

Program for Change

Tasks

The tasks for Stage 3 will be useful as you start to develop your plan for increasing your physical activity. You may want to start a notebook or filing system for the information you collect. Try to accomplish all of the tasks. Check your success. When you're ready, proceed to Stage 4.

- Before you set out to exercise, we recommend that you complete the PAR-Q in Chapter 4 (*see p. 75*) to determine that exercise is safe for you. If you answer "yes" to any questions, call your doctor before starting to increase your physical activity.

- Monitor your current activity level for 1 week *(Action Box 3)*.

- Identify 15 ways in which you can be more active in each of these areas: home, work, and recreation *(Action Box 4)*.

- Identify three places in your community where you could exercise *(Action Box 5)*.

- Establish at least one visual cue or prompt to remind you to be active at home, at work, and during leisure time *(Action Box 6)*.

- Evaluate your social support. Ask someone to help you to be active *(Action Box 7)*.

- Make a personal contract to be active *(Action Box 8)*.

- Set a few short-term goals to be physically active *(Action Box 9)*.

Evaluate Your Success

As you accomplish the tasks for Stage 3, answer the questions below and score your success. Aim for a score of at least 12. If your score falls below 10, perhaps you should rethink your motivation and keep working before moving forward. When you have accomplished the tasks for Stage 3 and feel you are ready, move to Stage 4.

	Score
How committed were you to accomplishing these tasks? (3) = very committed, (2) = somewhat committed, (1) = not very committed	
How difficult were these tasks to accomplish? (3) = very easy, (2) = somewhat easy, (1) = very difficult	
How much did you learn from working to accomplish these tasks? (3) = a great deal, (2) = some, (1) = not very much	
How much motivation, help, or support did you need from others to accomplish these tasks? (3) = not very much, (2) = some, (1) = a great deal	
Are you ready to start increasing your physical activity? (3) = yes, definitely, (2) = yes, I am beginning to, (1) = no, I'm not ready yet	
Total Score	

Affirmations

Having a positive attitude will help you to develop your plans and carry out your physical activity goals. Read your affirmations frequently, especially when you are feeling uncertain or negative about your activity efforts.

- I can be active.
- I enjoy being active.

Stage 3 continues on the following page

Program for Change

- [ ] I'm healthier when I'm active.
- [ ] I feel better when I'm active.
- [ ] I look better when I'm active.
- [ ] I'll make time every day to be active.
- [ ] Being active every day will be a priority for me.
- [ ] _____ will support me in my efforts to be active.

Tips for Success

- [ ] Be sure your goals are realistic. Disappointments that come from unrealistic goals can cause you to quit trying.
- [ ] As you set your goals, choose a balance between internal and external target areas. Internal target areas include adjusting beliefs and attitudes related to physical activity. External target areas include altering your environment or performing specific activities such as going for a walk or raking leaves.
- [ ] Set short-term goals in the beginning. You will probably find it easier to set goals for a day or a week at a time.
- [ ] If you are not willing to do what is needed to attain a specific goal, don't berate yourself. Rather, select another goal that is more realistic.
- [ ] Shift your focus from attaining the goal to simply working toward the goal.
- [ ] Congratulate and reward yourself for working toward, as well as completing, a goal.
- [ ] Establish your reward in advance. Repeat your reward as a part of your daily affirmations. It helps to have something special to celebrate when you accomplish each goal.
- [ ] Share your goals with people who care about you and who will support your efforts to be physically active.

Dealing with Slips

If you are making a new start, these strategies can help you to get back on track:

- [ ] Think about the type of person you will be if you keep exercising.
- [ ] Consider that you will feel more confident if you exercise regularly.
- [ ] Tell yourself that you are able to keep exercising if you want to.
- [ ] Tell yourself that if you try hard enough you can keep exercising.
- [ ] Make a new commitment to exercise.
- [ ] Remind yourself that you are the only one who is responsible for your health and well-being.
- [ ] Believe that regular exercise will make you a healthier, happier person.
- [ ] Remind yourself that only you can decide whether you will exercise.

Reward Yourself

_____ will be my reward for starting to develop my physical activity plan.

How to Develop an Activity Plan

Consider Your Current Activity Level

Now that you are ready to become more active, you should consider collecting some data on your activity level so that you can monitor your progress. You may decide to record how long you walk or how many flights of stairs you take, or you may use a pedometer to count the number of steps you take each day. The technique you select is not critical. What is important is that you systematically record your activity and document your success. Use the Action Box 3 activity record below or keep a similar record on your personal calendar. Research shows that individuals who monitor their activity do better in the long term than people who don't monitor their activity. See Chapter 5 for other tools to help you assess and monitor your activity level.

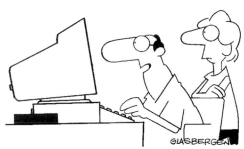

"I'm keeping track of the total amount of time I spend exercising. Does computer golf count?"

ACTION BOX 3

ACTIVITY RECORD

	Sun	Mon	Tues	Wed	Thurs	Fri	Sat
Walking	Minutes						
At home							
At work							
During work breaks							
For recreation							
During leisure time							
Total							
Climbing Flights of Stairs	Number of Flights						
At home							
At work							
During leisure time							
Total							
Steps	Number of Steps/Day						
Steps							
Weekly average steps per day							

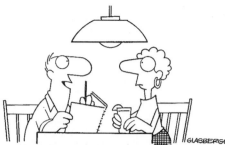

"Today I increased my daily walk by one-half mile, parked my car a little farther away from work, and gave my coffee an extra 25 stirs!"

Look for Small Ways to Increase Your Activity

There are numerous ways to incorporate small increments of activity into your daily life. Brainstorm at least 15 ways to incorporate moderate physical activity into your daily routine. *(Complete Action Box 4 below.)* Moderate activities are those equivalent to brisk walking or walking approximately 4 miles per hour.

Look for Places to Be Active

Where can you do various activities? Although you certainly don't need special facilities or equipment to be active, you have options.

ACTION BOX 4

List 15 ways to incorporate moderate activity into your daily routine. Rank them from the most vigorous to the least vigorous (most vigorous = 3; moderately vigorous = 2; least vigorous = 1). This will help you to become conscious of small increments in physical activity.

Place an asterisk (*) by the activities you currently do.

Ways to Be Active at Home

Hints: Labor-saving devices can encourage a sedentary life-style. Doing your own housework and yardwork can save you money while increasing your activity level.

Rate the Intensity (1–3)

Ways to Be Active at Work

Hints: If you supervise others, manage by walking around. Take the stairs instead of the elevator.

Ways to Be Active Through Recreation

Hints: Learn to dance. Walk when playing golf instead of using a cart.

Community

Your community is likely to have numerous outdoor areas or facilities where you can exercise. Investigate recreational and physical activity resources in your area. *(See Action Box 5 below.)* Many groups welcome newcomers and provide opportunities for novices to learn new skills. Start by considering activities you know you can do or in which you participated in the past. Look for places that are close to your work or home (within a 10-mile radius). You'll be more likely to use the resource frequently and regularly if it is within convenient traveling distance.

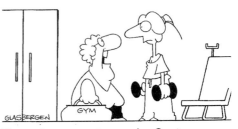

"I used to exercise at the Senior Center Fitness Room, but I switched to the Uptown Gym because that's where all the buff hunks are!"

ACTION BOX 5

Identify Community Resources for Physical Activity

Use this worksheet to identify resources in your community. Ask about the requirements for using these resources.

- What programs and activities are offered?
- What are the days and hours of operation?
- Are there fees for programs or services?
- What equipment is available?
- Are staff available for instruction and supervision?
- Is the setting safe?
- What, if any, amenities are available?
- Would you enjoy participating?

Locations	Notes
Parks/Recreation Centers	
Schools	
Clubs/Leagues	
Other	

Home

Although the social aspects of exercising at recreational facilities can be motivating, don't forget the advantages of exercising at home:

- You save travel time to another location.

- You may save money.

- You can use your own shower.

- You can wear whatever you want, even your underwear.

- You can do short bouts of activity rather than one extended activity session.

- You can be a positive role model for your family.

- You can do household chores (gardening, vacuuming, painting) that must be done anyway.

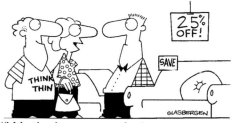

"We don't want a sofa that converts into a bed. We want a sofa that converts into a home gym."

Arrange Your Surroundings to Support Activity

When you are planning to increase your physical activity, it helps to arrange your surroundings to support your good intentions and make activity more convenient. Provide yourself with visible cues that will stimulate you to be active at home, work, and during leisure time. *(See Action Box 6 on the following page.)* Remove things from your environment that may encourage you to be inactive.

Involve Others in Your Efforts to Be Active

It's very important that you have the support of your spouse, family, or people you live with to sustain your interest in being more active. How can you involve your spouse or partner in your efforts to be active? Identify the type of support you want. Some people want praise and encouragement as they make changes, while others prefer to be ignored whether they are progressing or slipping.

Below are some ways in which a partner, spouse, or family member might help you:

- Ignoring your physical activity habits completely

- Reinforcing your successes, ignoring your setbacks

- Monitoring your physical activity with verbal reminders

- Offering to join you in physical activity

- Offering to assume your tasks or duties so you can be active

- Asking how you're doing with your activity

- Asking you how he or she can help

- Encouraging you to be active

- Other (you define)_____

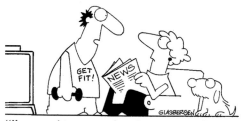

"I'm working very hard to get in shape and I need all the encouragement I can get. Does your old cheerleader uniform still fit you?"

Think about the people around you who can be supportive. What types of support do you need, and who can provide it?

ACTION BOX 6

List Cues and Prompts for Physical Activity

Make a list of cues to remind yourself to be active.

At Work

Schedule exercise or stretch breaks during meetings at work.

Have pictures of active people in view.

_____

_____

At Home

Lay out exercise clothes the night before.

Wear exercise clothes around the house.

Turn off the television for 1 hour after supper and go for a walk.

_____

_____

During Leisure Time

Spend time with others who are active.

Always carry exercise clothes, especially shoes, in the car.

_____

_____

Can you rely on more than one person? How broad and how deep is your support system? *Breadth of support* means that various types of support are available to you. *Depth of support* means that if someone who offers you a special type of support were no longer available, others would be available to provide that support.

If you lack one type of support, you may want to try to build support in that area. *(See Action Box 7 on the following page.)* If you cannot list more than one name for one type of support, you might consider strategies to increase the depth of your support system in that area. You might also consider expanding your support system if you depend on only one or two people for most of your support.

ACTION BOX 7

Evaluate Your Support

Name three people who could give you each type of support listed below:

Emotional support—people with whom you could share a very personal worry or concern

_____

Affection—people who show their affection and tell you they appreciate you

_____

Emotional challenge—people who challenge you to attain your goals

_____

Listening support—people who listen to your concerns, problems, and disappointments in your efforts to be active without being judgmental

_____

Feedback and appraisal—people who tell you how you're doing and who acknowledge your efforts and accomplishments

_____

Role models/partners—people who share similar experiences, priorities, values, and views related to physical activity

_____

Experts/information support—people who know more about physical activity than you do and whose opinions you can trust

_____

Ask for Support

Identify a person who could support you as you start your physical activity program. Write down what you would say to this person to ask for help. Asking for support may be easier if you remember what others have done to help you or what you have done to help others.

Types of Support Needed	From Whom	How You Will Ask

Increasing Your Social Support System

How do you expand a support system? Here are some tips:

- Call or write letters to long-distance friends and family members.

- Join organizations, clubs, or religious groups and get involved.

- Develop good listening skills. The most valued friends are those who are good listeners.

- Be an interesting person to know. Develop interests beyond your work and your family. Keep up to date on current events and develop interests you can share with others.

- Let others get to know the real you. Be willing to share personal experience.

- Question others to learn about their interests and needs rather than talking about yourself.

- Be a "taker" as well as a "giver." Some people are comfortable only when caretaking or helping others, while others reach out only when they need something. Look for mutually supportive relationships.

Make Time for Physical Activity

Your ultimate goal should be to engage in at least 30 minutes of moderate physical activity every day or nearly every day. Examples of moderate physical activity include walking briskly, vacuuming, gardening, climbing stairs, or any other similar physical activity.

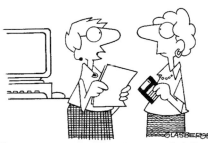

"I'm trying to fit 30 minutes of daily exercise into my busy schedule. Today I took 120 15-second walks."

You can plan 30 minutes of physical activity all at once, or you can break the 30 minutes into smaller time segments. Some people find it easier to plan extended activity time, perhaps first thing in the morning before breakfast or right after work. People who exercise first thing in the morning stay active most consistently, because it's unlikely that other responsibilities will interrupt an early-morning routine. Exercising at the end of the day can help to relieve stress that has built up over the day and boosts energy for the evening. If you plan to exercise in one extended session, you may need to allow extra time for travel, changing clothes, and showering.

Many people prefer to accumulate the time spent exercising over the day. If you have had difficulty finding time for regularly scheduled activity, consider shorter bouts of exercise. Three 10-minute brisk walks are equivalent to one 30-minute walk at the same pace. If time for 10-minute walks is hard to find, could you manage six 5-minute walks? You could even begin with 2-minute walks if that fits your needs. Use any approach, but make time for activity, and make it a priority.

Write a Personal Contract to Be Active

Use the information you've gained in this section to write a contract to be active for at least 15 minutes each day. *(See Action Box 8 on the following page.)* Sign the contract to show your commitment to the plan. Involve another person in your plan by asking for his or her support and signature.

ACTION BOX 8

Write a Personal Contract to Exercise

For the week of _____

I, (your name)_____ , will perform the following activities for a total of at least

_____ minutes over the course of at least _____ days this week.

Day	Activities	Minutes

When I complete the activities listed above, I will reward myself as follows: _____

Signed _____   Date _____

Witness _____   Date _____

Each week reevaluate your progress and rewrite your contract. Your goal should be to increase your physical activity to at least 30 minutes for every day.

Set Realistic Goals

We will continue to suggest tasks for each Stage of Change, but we will also help you to set and monitor your own goals. *(See Action Box 9 on the following page.)* Ask yourself these questions to help determine if your goals are realistic:

- Is the goal one that I've been able to attain in the past? The sedentary businessman who has decided to take up tennis at retirement with the goal of quickly climbing the competitive ladder at the tennis club has failed to consider that he will need skill as well as endurance. If he has played competitive tennis before, however, then he is likely to regain the skills and attain this goal.

- Could someone else, someone a lot like you, reach the goal you're setting for yourself? If you don't believe someone else can achieve it, then perhaps it's not an appropriate goal for you. People sometimes get stuck here. Be completely honest with yourself. Wanting and wishing don't make something happen. If you find yourself saying "I should do...," then you may need to rethink your degree of commitment.

- Is the timing right? Waiting until after the holidays or until the first of the month is appropriate only if the waiting period is necessary. For example, if you don't have a pair of comfortable walking shoes and can't go shopping until next week, then postponing walking until next week is appropriate. Begin as soon as possible to work on your goal. Unless you have good reason to wait, start now.

ACTION BOX 9

Set Physical Activity Goals

Use this worksheet as you begin to assume more responsibility for setting your own physical activity goals.

What do you want to accomplish?

Be as specific as possible. Break your general goal into smaller, short-term goals.

_____

_____

_____

By when do you want to accomplish your goal? Set a date.

_____

_____

_____

How will you know when you have reached your goal?

Identify the criteria to determine that you have achieved your stated goal to your satisfaction.

_____

_____

_____

What are you willing to do (or give up) to attain your goal?

Be honest with yourself. Timing, motivation level, and other factors will affect your ability to attain your goal.

_____

_____

_____

What's stopping you from reaching your goal?

Commit to increasing your awareness of your motivators, limitations, expectations, and barriers. Reassess your goals regularly.

_____

_____

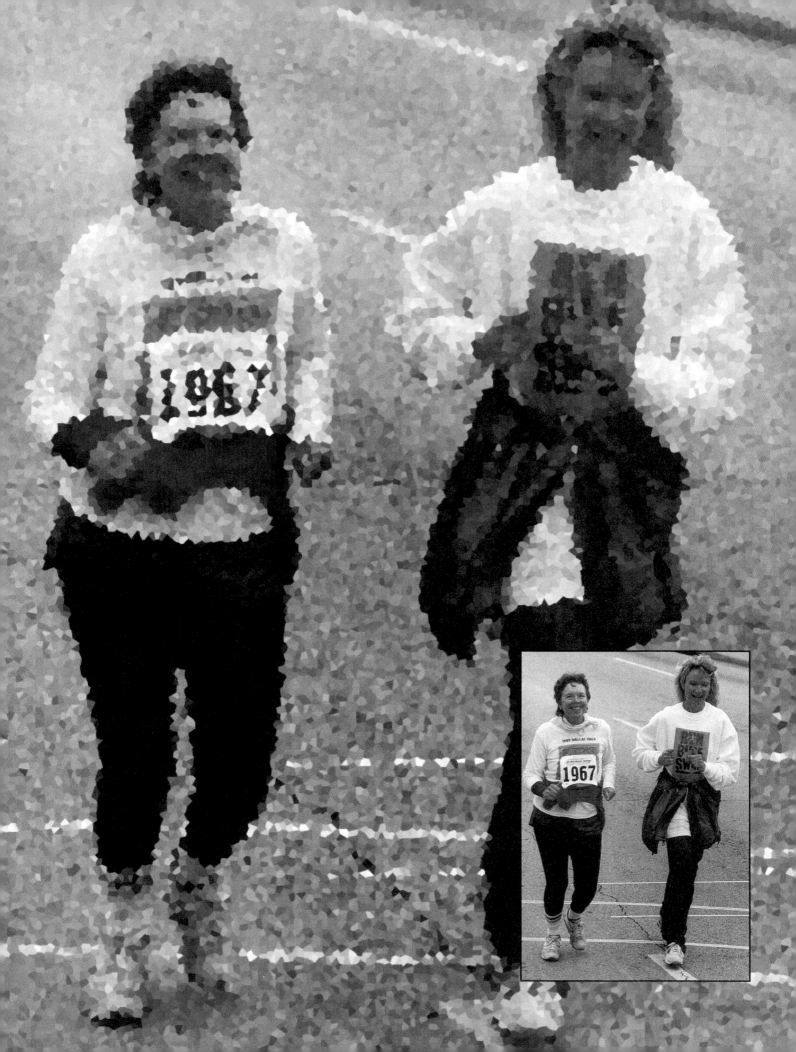

CHAPTER 11

Developing Regular Exercise Habits (Stage 4)

I f you have progressed to Stage 4 after carefully working through previous stages, you're well on your way to success in your goal to be active and stay active.

If you are starting Stage 4 based on your responses to the readiness questionnaire in Chapter 7 *(see p. 118)*, you are currently active but haven't been active regularly for at least 6 months. You can expect to spend approximately 6 months in Stage 4. Moving too quickly through this stage can precipitate slips and setbacks. Research shows that people who haven't taken adequate

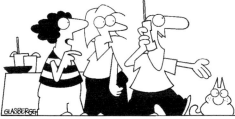

"Larry is exercising for 35 minutes a day now. Plus he probably burns an extra 500 calories a day raving to everyone about how great he feels."

ACTION BOX 1

Self-Assessment

How many of these statements apply to you?	Yes	No
I see more "pros" than "cons" for being active.		
I am keeping a daily record of my minutes of activity.		
I accumulate at least 30 minutes of moderate activity nearly every day.		
I have made others aware of my intent to be active.		
I seek support from others like my spouse, family members, coworkers, and friends.		
I try to avoid people and places that could sabotage my efforts to be active.		
I substitute physical activity for sedentary activities, such as turning off the television and going for a walk.		
I reward myself for being active.		

ACTION BOX 2

Weigh the "Pros" and "Cons" of Change   **Date** _____

If you are beginning the process of change at Stage 4, fill in your "pros" and "cons" for becoming physically active below.

Pros	Cons
Advantages to Being Active	Disadvantages to Being Active
Disadvantages to Staying Sedentary	Advantages to Staying Sedentary

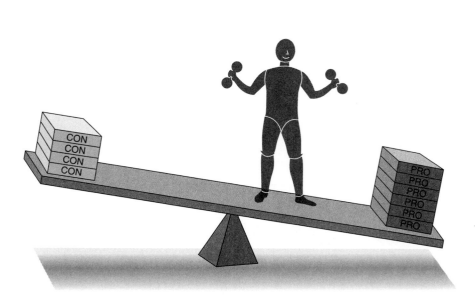

People in Stage 4 see more benefit to being active than to staying sedentary. For the first time since they have started to think about change, the "pros" of becoming physically active truly outweigh the "cons."

time to progress through the previous stages and master the critical tasks are candidates for early slips. It requires time to practice new behaviors before they become habits.

People in Stage 4 who have become active have made the greatest and most visible commitment. They are actually doing something different, not just thinking or talking about it.

Even though you realize and enjoy the benefits of physical activity, you should keep your list of "pros" in mind. Continue to review your list regularly and add more "pros" as you become ever more committed to an active lifestyle. You might even want to look back at your lists from previous stages. Which "cons" were easiest to give up? Do any "cons" remain challenges?

Program for Change

Tasks

The tasks for Stage 4 will help you to stay with your activity plan. Try to accomplish all of the tasks. Check your success. When you're ready, proceed to Stage 5.

- ☐ Try at least one new type of physical activity that you have not done recently.
- ☐ Engage in physical activity for at least 30 minutes each day and record it on your calendar or log.
- ☐ Identify and evaluate at least one high-risk situation *(Action Box 3)*.
- ☐ Practice assertive communication *(Action Box 4)*.
- ☐ Ask someone to support your efforts to be active *(Action Box 5)*.
- ☐ Evaluate your level of confidence that you'll stay active *(Action Box 6)*.

Evaluate Your Success

As you accomplish the tasks for Stage 4, answer these questions and score your success. Aim for a score of at least 12. If your score falls below 10, perhaps you should rethink your motivation and keep working before moving forward. When you have accomplished the tasks for Stage 4 and feel you are ready, move to Stage 5.

	Score
How committed were you to accomplishing these tasks? (3) = very committed, (2) = somewhat committed, (1) = not very committed	_____
How difficult were these tasks to accomplish? (3) = very easy, (2) = somewhat easy, (1) = very difficult	_____
How much did you learn from working to accomplish these tasks? (3) = a great deal, (2) = some, (1) = not very much	_____
How much motivation, help, or support did you need from others to accomplish these tasks? (3) = not very much, (2) = some, (1) = a great deal	_____
Are you able to maintain your activity on a regular basis? (3) = yes, definitely, (2) = yes, I am beginning to, (1) = no, I'm not there yet	_____
Total Score	_____

Affirmations

Read your affirmations frequently to help you maintain your exercise habits.

- ☐ I enjoy being an active person.
- ☐ I feel and look better since I've started being active.
- ☐ I feel more relaxed and less tired.
- ☐ My health has improved since I've started being active.
- ☐ I feel more confident about my ability to stay active.
- ☐ It's getting easier to perform activities, such as climbing stairs.
- ☐ Physical activity is becoming a habit for me.

Stage 4 continues on the following page

Tips for Success

- ☐ Recognize that you are a unique and worthy individual. Fulfill your needs first.
- ☐ Don't use taking care of others first as an excuse not to take care of yourself. If you take care of yourself, you will be in better shape to take care of others.
- ☐ Become self-reliant. Depend on others only when necessary.
- ☐ Know and accept yourself and take responsibility for your thoughts, feelings, and actions.
- ☐ Stop fighting change—embrace it! Look for opportunities to change for the better.
- ☐ Keep company with positive people.
- ☐ Concentrate on your assets and qualities. Give yourself a pep talk.
- ☐ Imagine an ideal you. Think of yourself as an attractive person.
- ☐ Take care of your appearance.
- ☐ Be good to yourself. Treat yourself as you treat your best friend.
- ☐ Stand tall and smile. Your body language tells a lot about how confident you are.

Dealing with Slips

If you are making a new start, these strategies can help you to increase your physical activity.

- ☐ Keep thinking about the type of person you will be if you keep exercising.
- ☐ Remind yourself that you will feel more confident if you exercise regularly.
- ☐ Review the strategies that have helped you to be active in the past.
- ☐ Remind yourself that you have been active before and that you can be active again.
- ☐ Remember that you are the only one responsible for your health and well-being.
- ☐ Remember that regular exercise will make you a healthier, happier person.
- ☐ Remember that only you can decide whether you will exercise.

Reward Yourself

_____ will be my reward for starting to develop my physical activity plan.

How to Develop Regular Exercise Habits

Reward Yourself

You've heard it before, but it's true: Small steps build success. The staged approach that you have used thus far has helped you to progress at a realistic pace. You haven't tried to accomplish too much too fast. Remember, you're in this for the long haul. Your ultimate goal is to make physical activity a permanent part of your life-style. You're getting closer to making that goal a reality every day. Each day that you are active should strengthen your resolve. Recognize, reinforce, and reward yourself at each small success, no matter how trivial it may seem. There are many easy ways you can reward yourself:

- Check off small goals on your "to-do list" each day.

- Practice positive affirmations.

- Write a positive statement in your journal.

- Buy yourself a gift when you've reached a preset milestone. Put aside a small amount of money on each day that you follow your activity plan. At the end of the week or at a preset time, use the money to buy something you would like. The reward doesn't have to be associated with physical activity. It could be a plant for your office, a long-distance phone call to a friend or family member, or a new pair of jeans. Don't buy something that could sabotage your efforts—a fudge sundae or a lounger.

- Instead of something tangible, give yourself the gift of time. Put aside 10 minutes for each day that you accomplish your activity goal. At the end of the week you'll have at least an hour you can spend doing something just for you, such as browsing at a flea market or museum, building something in your workshop, or volunteering for a community project.

Others can be a part of your reinforcement plan, too:

- Listen for and accept compliments from other people as you progress toward your activity goals.

- Agree to share a reward with another person who is being supportive. For example, take dance lessons, stay overnight at a bed and breakfast, go fishing or hiking—anything that you both enjoy and that doesn't undermine your efforts by putting you in a situation in which you might be tempted to slip back into your old sedentary habits.

- Ask someone to give you positive feedback on a regular basis. Remember that support from others is essential when you are trying to stay active.

Establish Supportive Relationships

- Learn to ask for the type of support you need. Be specific when you ask for support. Don't wait for others to read your mind. Tell them what would and would not be helpful.

- Don't be afraid to set limits on any behaviors or situations that could sabotage your efforts.

- Effective communication is important. Let others know your goals and expectations.

- Know that some people may have difficulty accepting or adjusting to your new life-style practices. Be prepared to modify previous relationships, at least temporarily, if someone sabotages your efforts.

- Actively avoid the naysayers who put down or otherwise diminish your efforts.

- Seek people with similar values and habits who can be supportive. Identifying good role models helps you to picture yourself as an active person. Ask how they successfully maintain their active life-styles.

Control Cues for Inactivity

As you begin to become more active, you will notice that you are gaining control over situations that were previously uncomfortable or problematic. You are learning to manage the cues that trigger sedentary habits. You may not even be conscious of your cues; nevertheless, they are real and can damage your best attempts at staying active. Learning to manage cues is a very personal skill because not everyone has the same reaction to a particular cue. You must learn to identify factors in your life that act as cues for inactivity. You can then develop strategies to adjust or adapt your responses when you encounter bothersome cues.

There are two major types of cues: internal cues (thoughts and feelings) and external cues (events and objects in your environment). If you believe that external events are always responsible for your actions, your focus is outside yourself. Psychologists call this an "external locus of control." When your sense of responsibility and control over your actions is within you, this is called an "internal locus of control." It is associated with a sense of personal responsibility and empowerment. Your thoughts, beliefs, and feelings are major sources of your internal cues.

Learn to identify situations in your environment (external cues) that put you at high risk for being inactive, such as:

- Traveling on business

- Going on vacation

- Seeing other people engaging in sedentary activities

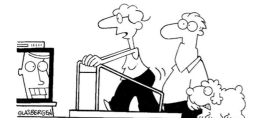

"I used to miss a lot of exercise whenever I was too busy. Mostly I was too busy looking for reasons not to exercise!"

- Statements from others encouraging you to give up your physical activity

Manage High-Risk Situations

- Try to predict specific times when you'll be faced with situations that encourage inactivity. Mark these times on your calendar so they don't sneak up on you.

- Assess the cues that lead to high-risk situations and determine how well you handled them. *(See Action Box 3 below.)*

- Plan strategies for breaking the typical behavior pattern or response associated with your cues for inactivity.

- Think of appropriate substitutes and alternatives. Have a long list of acceptable alternatives available to help ensure success in a variety of high-risk situations.

ACTION BOX 3

Assess High-Risk Situations

Describe what happened in one high-risk situation within the last week.

Before the situation? _____

_____

During the situation? _____

_____

After the situation? _____

_____

Overall, how well did you handle the situation? Rate your success on this scale:

Not very well   **Very well**

  1   2   3   4   5

If you believe you were generally successful (rating of 3 or higher), what was the key to your success?

Describe it. _____

_____

If you believe you were generally unsuccessful (rating below 3), what could you do differently next time?

Before the situation? _____

_____

During the situation? _____

_____

After the situation? _____

- Practice your responses through role playing or imagery to help you feel confident that you won't slide back into old sedentary habits.

Communicate Assertively

Assertiveness is a behavioral style that helps you reach your personal goals. It is highly unlikely that someone can be both personally responsible and nonassertive at the same time. When you affirm your rights, you are less likely to feel irritated or manipulated by others. Learning to communicate in an assertive and direct manner can help you stay active when people or situations obstruct you.

Characteristics of Assertive People

Assertive people do:

- Ask for what they need or want.
- Make clear and forthright statements.
- Say "no" to unreasonable requests.
- Take responsibility for their feelings and behaviors.
- Recognize and respect the boundaries of others.
- Protect their rights and interests without abusing others.
- Attempt to negotiate when conflicts arise.
- Know they won't always get what they want.
- Take risks.

Assertive people don't:

- Expect others to read their minds or interpret what their needs or limits are.
- Expect others to meet their needs.
- Get angry, make demands, or behave rudely toward others to get what they want.
- Passively allow others to make decisions.
- Feel mistreated or blame others for their problems.
- Rely on hints, sarcasm, or emotional manipulation to meet their needs.

Learn to Negotiate

As you begin to become more physically active, there will be times when you must say "no" to requests. Learn to negotiate by considering the other person's requests while not sacrificing your need to exercise. Be direct instead of making excuses. Learn to use "I" statements instead of "You" statements when responding to requests. *(See Action Box 4 on the following page.)* Consider these responses to a request to change your physical activity plans:

> "I can understand that you would like me to stay home, but I really want to go for a walk" (emphatic statement).

> "Part of me would like to go to the movies with you, but the other part is saying that I really need to exercise and that's the part I need to listen to" (mixed-feelings statement).

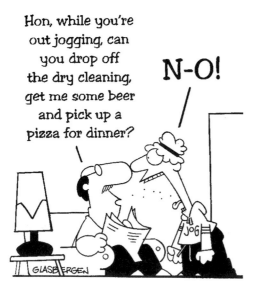

Hon, while you're out jogging, can you drop off the dry cleaning, get me some beer and pick up a pizza for dinner?

N-O!

I don't want to give up my morning workout to meet early every day this week, but I can come in early 2 days and stay late 2 days" (agree with certain conditions).

Ask for Help

There will also be times when you'll want to request assistance from others. Part of taking care of yourself is asking for help when you need it. *(See Action Box 5 on the following page.)* Most people are happy to help if the request gives them a choice to say "yes" or "no" and if it considers their needs and feelings.

ACTION BOX 4

How Would You Respond?

Write assertive responses to these comments or actions by others. Considering your responses in advance will help you feel prepared and confident to deal with these situations if they happen.

Example:

Comment: *"Why should I stay home while you're out exercising?"*

Assertive Response: *"I want to spend time with you, but I'm also excited about participating in the walk/run. I would really appreciate it if you would go with me. I would enjoy your company, and I'd feel you are supporting my efforts to be active."*

Comment: *"Aren't you afraid you're going to hurt yourself by being active?"*

Assertive Response: _____

_____

Comment: *"What are you trying to prove by wearing those exercise clothes?"*

Assertive Response: _____

_____

Comment: *"Why don't you slow down and act your age? You know, you're not so young."*

Assertive Response: _____

Tips for Assertive Communication

- Avoid hints and sarcasm.
- Speak firmly and make eye contact.
- Use your voice and body language to communicate confidence.
- Remain calm and don't let your emotions interfere.
- Take time to think over your response. If necessary, indicate a specific time when you can respond so it doesn't appear you're avoiding the issue.

When making requests, give clear, specific information that will help others decide whether to say "yes" or "no." For example:

"Would you help do the dishes so that I can go for a walk after supper?"

"Would you consider a vacation this year that includes physical activity? Think about it, and we'll talk more later."

"Would you like to participate in the 'Fun Run' in 2 weeks? It's okay if you say 'no.'"

ACTION BOX 5

Make Requests

What requests might you need to make to gain support for your physical activity?

_____

_____

_____

_____

_____

Set Limits

Don't be afraid to set limits when other people's behaviors might sabotage your efforts to be active.

- Describe the specific behavior that is bothering you and how you're feeling.

- Specify what behavior you'd like the person to change and what the consequences of this change will be for you.

- Inform the person of what will happen if he or she is able or not able to do what you have requested.

Build Self-Confidence

Confidence will help you deal with difficult or high-risk situations. Having confidence means that you have a feeling of control. *(Test your confidence in Action Box 6 on the following page.)* Research has shown that a high level of confidence is a very good predictor of future performance, perhaps even better than past performance. In other words, if you think you can stay active, then it's very likely that you will!

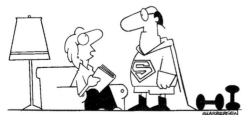

"You've come a long way, dear, and you're much more athletic than you used to be...but aren't you getting a little *too* confident?"

ACTION BOX 6

Test Your Confidence

Listed below are some situations in which you might be tempted to stop your physical activity. Add others that are likely to be problems for you to the list. For each situation, use the Confidence Scale to evaluate how confident you are that you can stay active.

Confidence Scale

Not confident at all				*Somewhat confident*				*Very confident*		
0	10	20	30	40	50	60	70	80	90	100

	Your Confidence Score
Your exercise partner didn't show up.	
Your spouse is sick.	
Your car is being repaired.	
You had too much to eat or drink the night before.	
It's cold outside.	
The pollen count is high, and you have allergies.	
It's raining.	
You've sprained your ankle and will be on crutches for 3 weeks.	
You must travel out of town on business.	
You're feeling blue.	
You stayed up too late and overslept.	
Your workout clothes are dirty.	
It's hot and humid.	
You had surgery.	
You're bored with the activity you are doing.	
You're not making much progress.	
You've been inactive for 5 days.	
You've been inactive for 2 weeks.	
You've gained a few pounds.	
You don't feel very motivated.	
You feel self-conscious.	
There's a miniseries on television you want to watch.	
You're going to lots of holiday parties.	
The piece of exercise equipment you use (treadmill, cycle) is broken.	

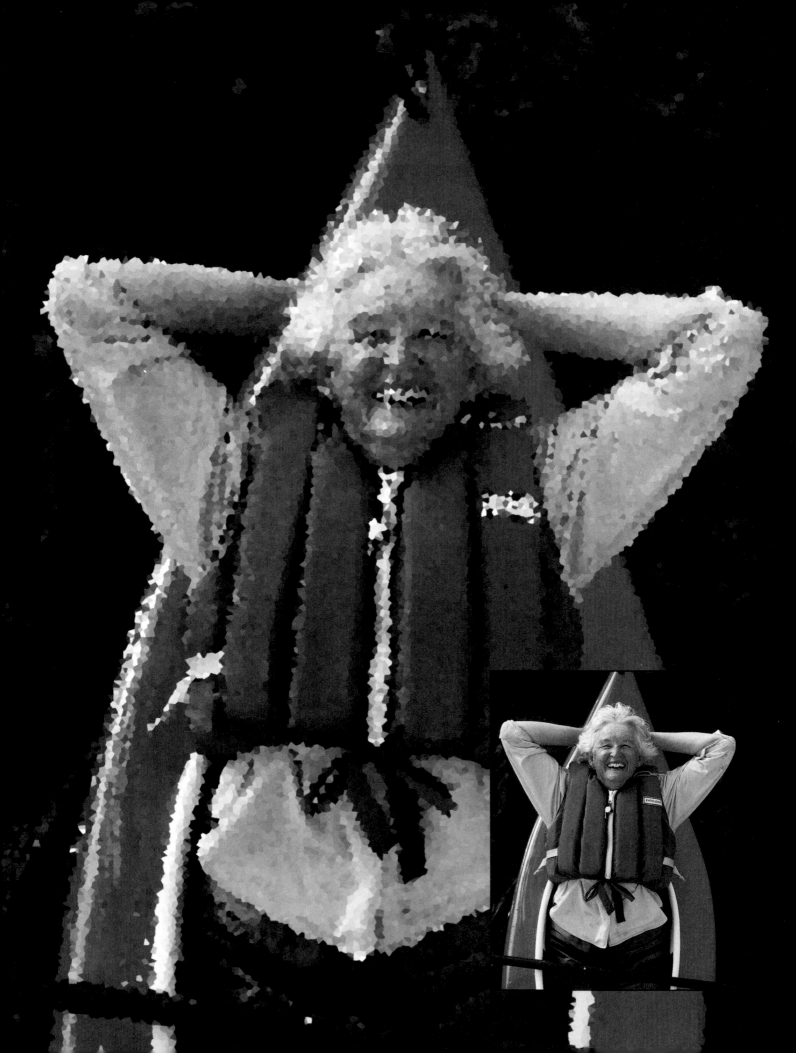

Staying Active for a Lifetime (Stage 5)

Congratulations on reaching Stage 5 in the behavior change process! You can now answer "yes" to all four questions on the readiness questionnaire. *(See p. 118 in Chapter 7.)* Your most important response is that you have been regularly active for the past 6 months. But the change process is not complete until you can say with confidence that you will never return to your sedentary life-style no matter what the obstacle.

How long does it takes to get to this high level of confidence? Every person is different, but it probably takes at least 6 months to 1 year of regular physical activity to begin to feel confident. Something unexpected can always happen.

ACTION BOX 1

Self-Assessment

How many of these statements apply to you?	Yes	No
I may be inactive from time to time, but I feel less and less tempted to return to my sedentary ways.		
I experience fewer and less frequent periods of inactivity.		
I learn and practice more and new ways to be active.		
I rely less on external rewards and more on internal rewards.		
I continue to increase the list of "pros" for physical activity. The "cons" decrease steadily.		
I feel more confident about my ability to maintain my current level of physical activity.		

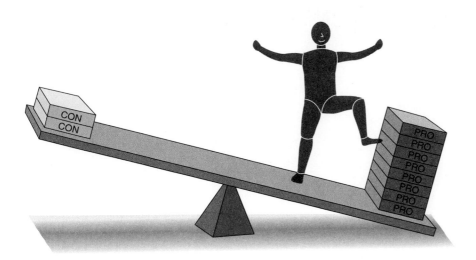

People in Stage 5 have made exercise a habit. Reasons to be sedentary ("cons") scarcely weigh in the decision to be physically active ("pros"). Daily exercise begins to come easily and naturally.

For behaviors such as physical activity and weight control, change is a lifelong pursuit. The end of the behavior change program for physical activity marks the beginning of a lifetime of maintenance.

As physical activity continues to become more and more a part of your life-style, you will notice that you discover new and different benefits to being active. You'll be surprised at how long your list of advantages is, and you'll enjoy looking back at your "pros" and "cons" from previous stages.

ACTION BOX 2

Weigh the "Pros" and "Cons" of Change

Date _____

Fill in the "pros" and "cons" for staying active for a lifetime below.

Pros	Cons
Advantages to Being Active	Disadvantages to Being Active
Disadvantages to Staying Sedentary	Advantages to Staying Sedentary

Program for Change

Tasks

The tasks for Stage 5 will help you stay active for a lifetime if you do them at regular intervals.

- ☐ Engage in physical activity for at least 30 minutes every day or nearly every day of the week.
- ☐ Repeat a self-assessment at least once every 3 months to monitor your fitness level.
- ☐ Review your advantages for staying physically active at least once each month *(Action Box 2)*.
- ☐ Repeat affirmations about physical activity regularly.
- ☐ Support another person who is attempting to become more active.

If increasing your physical activity level is a goal for you, focus on the following tasks in addition to the ones above. Add any other goals you have.

- ☐ Increase your physical activity by engaging in more vigorous activities.
- ☐ Increase your physical activity by extending the time of your activity.
- ☐ Learn to perform one new type of physical activity.
- ☐ Participate in a special event.
- ☐ Develop a cross-training plan to ensure a balanced workout *(Action Box 3)*.
- ☐ _____
- ☐ _____

Affirmations

- ☐ I'll always be an active person.
- ☐ I enjoy physical activity.
- ☐ Being an active person is very important to me.
- ☐ I'd really miss being active if I couldn't.
- ☐ I'm confident that I can continue to be active no matter what the situation.
- ☐ I'm confident that I can make other positive changes in my life.

It's still important to give yourself positive strokes about your new, active life-style. In fact, you can use your accomplishments in becoming physically active to support other positive changes you want to make. Perhaps you want to manage your finances more effectively or make some new social contacts. If you can make and sustain a change that is as difficult as becoming and staying active, you can use what you've learned to tackle other changes.

Dealing with Slips

If you are attempting to reestablish your physical activity patterns, try these strategies to help get back on track and stay active.

- ☐ Consider adjusting your exercise goals from your previous level. Be sure to set realistic goals for yourself rather than set yourself up for failure by expecting too much.

Stage 5 continues on the following page

Program for Change

- Tell yourself that you are being good to yourself by taking care of your body when you exercise.

- Do something nice for yourself for making an effort to exercise more.

- Identify people you can depend on when you have problems with exercising. Tell them how they can help.

- Put objects that serve as cues to exercise around your home and at work.

- Avoid spending time in environments that promote inactivity.

- Use exercise to relieve your worries when you're feeling tense.

- Engage in some physical activity instead of remaining inactive. Just do something!

Your Reward

You'll know when you've reached the stage where you're confident that you can remain physically active for the rest of your life. At this point you won't need tangible rewards to keep yourself motivated to stay active. Your active life-style and all the benefits that accrue from it will themselves be the reward.

How to Stay Active for a Lifetime

When you reach Stage 5, you are well on your way to making physical activity a permanent part of your life. You have experienced many successes along the way, and you should now view yourself as a new person as far as activity is concerned. You have learned from your experiences—what works and what doesn't. Through this process of developing, implementing, and evaluating your plans, you have acquired many strategies and alternatives to support your new, active life-style.

Consider Cross-Training

One strategy that will help to maintain your activity routine is cross-training. Cross-training means that you include a variety of activities in your fitness program. One example of cross-training is performing several different types of aerobic exercises. Triathletes train for events that include swimming, cycling, and running. But you don't have to participate in competitive events to cross-train. If you participate in an exercise class on Monday, Wednesday, and Friday; walk on Tuesday and Thursday; clean the house or work in the yard on Saturday; and play golf on Sunday, you are cross-training.

Another approach to cross-training emphasizes balanced fitness—including the three components of fitness (aerobic, strength, and flexibility). This approach is especially important to people who exercise primarily for health benefits. In addition to performing one or more types of aerobic activities, you would add strength training and flexibility (stretching) exercises to your routine. For strength

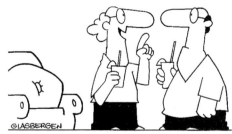

"On Monday I run, Tuesday I bicycle, Wednesday I lift weights, Thursday I power walk, Friday I row, Saturday I hike, and on Sunday I brag about it!"

ACTION BOX 3

Plan a Cross-Training Program Emphasizing Balanced Fitness

Monday	Tuesday	Wednesday	Thursday	Friday	Saturday	Sunday
Stationary cycling	Walking	Stationary cycling	Walking	Stationary cycling	Tennis	Tennis
Weight machines	Calisthenics	Weight machines	Calisthenics	Weight machines	Rest	Rest
Stretches	Stretches	Stretches	Stretches	Stretches	Stretches	Stretches

Use this worksheet to plan your own cross-training program.

Monday	Tuesday	Wednesday	Thursday	Friday	Saturday	Sunday

training, you could choose from calisthenics (exercises that use the body's weight as resistance, such as push-ups or sit-ups), weight training machines, handheld weights, or other resistance equipment such as rubber bands. *(See Action Box 3 above.)* Stretching is easily added as part of the warm-up and cool-down components of your routine. Cross-training has at least two distinct advantages:

- You are less likely to get bored with an exercise program that includes a variety of activities. Boredom is a common reason people give for quitting.

- You may avoid overuse injuries by exercising muscle groups in a more balanced way.

As you vary your activities through cross-training, your confidence will continue to improve. This technique will be useful when you are faced with staying active on business trips and vacations or when your routine is interrupted. See Chapter 1 for more information about establishing a balanced fitness program.

Have Fun

Some people say they don't like to exercise. It's just not fun for them. If they continue to think and feel this way, it will be difficult for them to stay with an exercise program. If this is likely to be a problem for you, try to think of ways to make exercise fun. Add your own ideas to this list:

- Wear bright socks
- Put on a funny hat
- Tie bells to your shoelaces

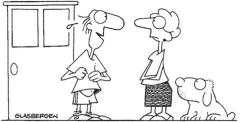

"I found a way to make exercise more fun. When I jog past the pizza parlor window, I lift my shirt and make everyone jealous!"

- Listen to music that you danced to as a teenager
- Tell jokes with your partner
- Make up chants or songs
- Say "hello" in a foreign language to everyone you see
- Wave to everyone you pass
- Play games
- Tell yourself you're having fun

  No one ever quit exercising because it was too much fun!

Reward Yourself

Children aren't the only ones who respond to rewards. Adults do too! Give yourself rewards as you establish and maintain your physical activity routine to help you stay with it. If at the end of the week you have achieved your goal—a given number of exercise sessions, a specific number of minutes of physical activity, or some other measurable outcome—reward yourself with something meaningful.

You are the only one who knows what reward is meaningful to you. These questions may help you determine which rewards are likely to work best for you:

- What would be a nice present to receive from a friend or family member?

- If you had an extra $10, $50, or $100, how would you spend it?

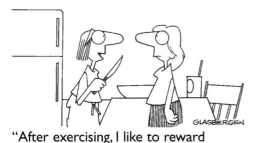

"After exercising, I like to reward myself with a pizza. But I use lettuce instead of crust, carrots instead of pepperoni, and fat-free dressing instead of mozzarella cheese."

Rewards

Tangible rewards do not have to be related to physical activity. The following rewards have worked for others. Do any of them appeal to you?

- Bubblebath
- Massage
- Pedicure or manicure
- Perfume or cologne
- Flowers
- Tree or shrub planted outdoors
- Trip
- Books
- Music
- Cowboy boots (and two-step lessons)
- Long-distance phone calls to friends or family

- Contributions to charity
- Movies or videos
- Plays or concerts
- Weekend in a local hotel or bed and breakfast
- Baby-sitting
- Detail shop for the car
- Birdhouse
- Wind chimes
- Jewelry
- Tools

- What do you like to do for fun?

- What are your hobbies or major interests?

- Whom do you like to be with?

- What makes you feel really good?

- What would you hate to lose?

- Whom would you like to tell about your success?

- Who would be proud of you for achieving your physical activity goals?

Your rewards will not always be tangible or externally motivated. As you become more confident about your physical activity, your greatest reward will be the internal satisfaction you get from accomplishing your goal. There will be a time—it may already have come—when the activity itself and the feelings that result will be all the reward you need to stay active.

Build Helping Relationships

Researchers studying the behavior change process have learned that people need social support to attain and maintain new habits. One study randomly assigned subjects to participate in an exercise program either as part of a team or as individuals. The people assigned to the team had not met before entering the study. During the study, the number of exercise sessions was observed. At the end of the study, the people who were part of the team approach had logged more exercise sessions than the people who exercised independently. Also, they had improved their fitness levels the most.

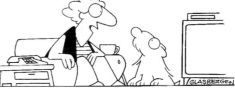

"I'm having trouble finding a good exercise partner. Paul Newman, Robert Redford, and Tom Cruise all have unlisted phone numbers!"

Many people report that joining another person or a group for physical activity makes exercise more fun and helps them stick with it. Having someone remind you to exercise or to let you know you were missed if you skip a session can be motivating. Some people say that they are more likely to show up for an exercise session if they know someone else depends on them to be there.

It is probably best and easiest to involve the people closest to you—family members, neighbors, and coworkers. Even if you don't involve a close friend or family member in your activity program, you can use physical activity to make new friends. You will meet some of the nicest people while participating in exercise or recreational fitness activities. For one thing, you automatically have something in common with people you meet while participating in physical activities. These people are likely to hold some of the same values as you.

Help Others Become Physically Active

As you become more confident about your ability to maintain your physical activity program, you may want to consider your influence on others. Just as you looked to others as positive role models when you were getting started, you can help someone else. Remember, though, not everyone is ready to take action right away.

Follow these tips to help a sedentary friend or family member become active:

- Ask the four readiness questions to determine where he or she is in the change process. *(See p. 118 in Chapter 7.)*

- Share information about the benefits of physical activity.

- Answer questions honestly about your experiences when getting started.

- Brainstorm ways to replace sedentary time with physical activities.

- Give specific examples of how you were able to overcome your barriers and problems.

- Help him or her develop a plan or contract for activity. *(See p. 146 in Chapter 10.)* Sign the contract as a supporter.

- Ask about specific ways you can help.

- When he or she is ready to take action, invite him or her to participate with you in an activity of his or her choice at his or her level of intensity.

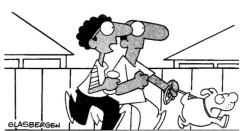

"Whenever I try to take a nap instead of exercising, I have this horrible nightmare where I'm being chased by 50 pounds of ugly fat!"

ACTION BOX 4

Conduct an Experiment in Self-Confidence

Date of experiment _____

Before

- What are your greatest fears about being inactive?

- Whom did you ask to support you, and what did you ask him or her to do?

During

- What are you doing at the times when you were normally active?

- Do you really miss physical activity?

- Do you still think of yourself as an active person, even though you're inactive?

- How does being inactive affect other aspects of your life (work, home, leisure, relationships)?

After

- What did you miss most about not being active?

- How did you start again, and how long did it take you to get back into your routine?

- How difficult was it to get started again?

- What did you learn from this experience, and how could you apply it in future situations?

- Give appropriate praise and reinforcement.

- Acknowledge that change is difficult.

Test Your Self-Confidence

After you have been active on a regular basis for at least 6 months, or whenever you feel very confident about your ability to stay active, you may want to try an experiment. You're the subject, and the test is this: You deliberately plan to be inactive for 1 week (a planned slip). At first, you may resist this idea, but you can learn some valuable lessons from this experience. Your confidence and will increase significantly when you know you can start again.

If you decide to try this experiment, keep a journal about your feelings before, during, and after your period of abstinence. Also, be sure to tell someone close to you what you are doing so he or she can monitor your experiment and support you when you resume your regular activity habits.

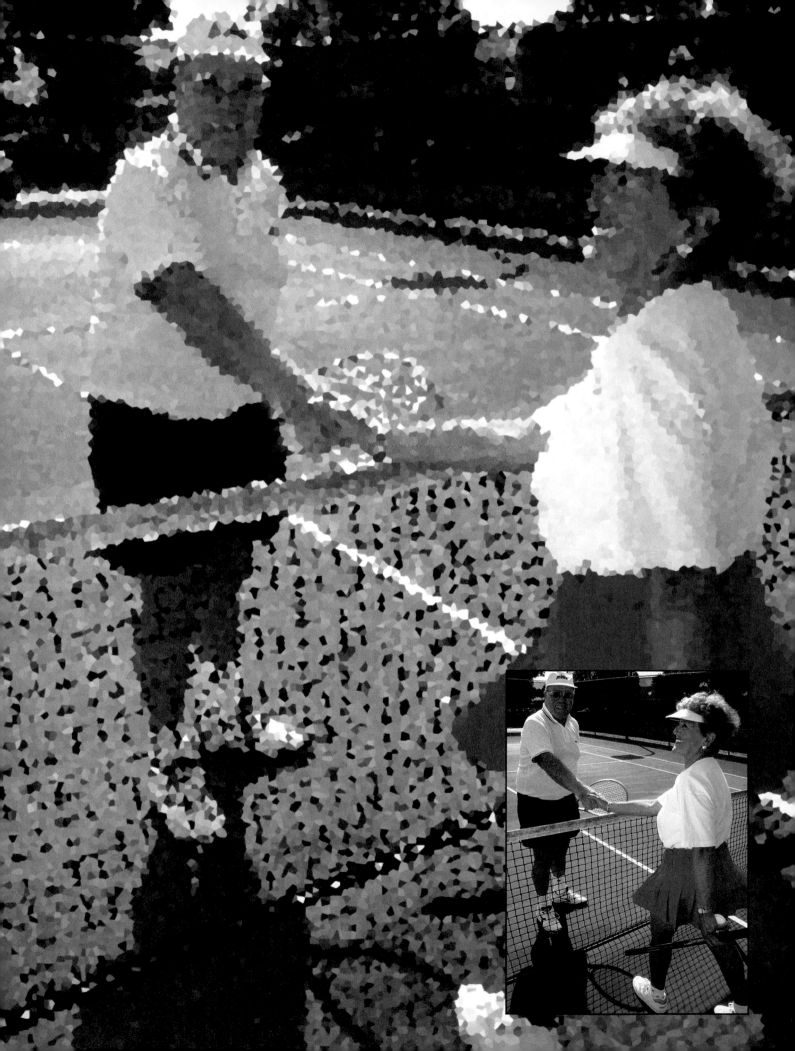

CHAPTER 13

Returning to Physical Activity After a Slip

Anyone who starts an activity program will have difficulty staying with it at some time or another. Many people will drop out or slip after only a brief period of increased physical activity. Others will experience setbacks after long periods, perhaps even years, of being active. Slips can occur at any stage of the behavior change process. Why do people slip out of activity habits?

Reasons for Slips

At Stage 1 (Not Thinking About Becoming Physically Active)

It's common for people who aren't even thinking about change to be unaware that they need to be active. Families, friends, and coworkers, however, may pressure them to change. Feeling coerced into starting to exercise, such people may be able to make and sustain a change as long as the pressure is on, but once the pressure is off, they quickly return to their old, sedentary ways. Lack of internal motivation is probably the most common reason people return to their sedentary habits. They may never have intended the changes to be permanent.

At Stage 2 (Thinking About Becoming More Active)

People who are thinking about change and wishing they could be more fit may not have made firm commitments to take action. They've weighed the "pros" and "cons" of physical activity but still aren't ready to change their habits. People can stay stuck in this stage for a long time. If they have not started to be more active after thinking about changing for several years, they may be no different from the people who are not thinking at all about changing.

At Stage 3 (Planning to Increase Physical Activity)

People who are getting ready to increase their activity levels are likely to begin exercising. They may buy exercise shoes and clothing and even invest in health club memberships or pieces of home exercise equipment. More than likely, they have attempted to start exercising several times within the past year but have not been able to maintain the new habit for very long.

It's easy for these people to get discouraged. Perhaps a fear of failing holds them back. They may not be confident they can maintain their new activity habits for very long, even if they start with the best intentions. Likewise, people sometimes fear success. Making a positive change, such as starting to exercise, requires them to address new issues. Change, even positive change, is stressful.

At Stage 4 (Developing Regular Activity Habits)

People who have taken action to change their activity habits have made the greatest and most visible commitment. They are actually doing something different, not just thinking or talking about it. But it takes time to develop regular habits you can sustain when events and obstacles throw you off track. Preparing well by progressing slowly but surely through the Stages of Change, and picking yourself up after each setback, will build confidence and eventually lead to activity habits that nothing can shake.

At Stage 5 (Maintaining an Active Way of Life)

People who have taken action and are sustaining new habits must also work hard at preventing slips. For most behaviors, including physical activity, this means staying with it for a lifetime. It's unrealistic to expect instant gratification. Establishing new patterns and avoiding setbacks are lifelong challenges.

Recycling Through the Stages of Change

Most people who work to become more active will not be successful on their first attempts. Slips, setbacks, and recycling through the Stages of Change are the rule rather than the exception. Many people make the same New Year's resolution 5 or more consecutive years before they actually stick to their goals.

Such patterns are normal. Change is not a linear progression. People don't march in a forward, stepwise fashion from one stage to the next. The expression "two steps forward and one step back" is an accurate description of how we make changes in our lives. A certain amount of regression is normal and natural. Yet, we often expect too much of ourselves, so that slipping back to a previous stage makes us feel like failures—embarrassed, disappointed, and guilty. Sometimes we regress more than one stage and slide back to a point at which we resist thinking about changing or exercising at all.

Fortunately, research in the area of behavior change indicates that most people who experience slips will recycle back to a point at which they contemplate exercising once more and make new plans to change. We can use the slip as a learning experience and begin to consider plans for our next attempts to change. Each time we recycle through the stages, we learn from our mistakes and try something different the next time around. We aren't revolving endlessly in circles, and we rarely go all the way back to where we started. We aim at progress, not perfection, and stay willing to give progress our best shot.

Dealing with Slips

Most of us lead busy lives, with family, job, community, and other responsibilities. Sometimes we have to compromise and adjust our schedules, and our exercise programs are frequently the things we cut. This is to be expected, and several days, or even a few weeks, without exercise is not a tragedy.

You lose some of the benefits of physical activity within a few days of stopping, but others persist for several weeks. The important thing is not to be surprised when your exercise program is disrupted. Be prepared with a plan to resume your activity. Numerous events can cause you to forego your regular physical activity. Some events you can anticipate and develop plans for; others are not within your control.

The remainder of this chapter will discuss each of these categories of events and will suggest how you can make adjustments after an event occurs or plan to avoid potential problems.

Events You Can't and Can Control

Events You Can't Control:
- Injury
- Illness
- Family responsibilities

Events You Can Plan For:
- Social activities
- Heavy workload on the job
- Travel

Substitute Activity Programs If You Are Injured

- Water aerobics
- Chair exercises
- Exercises using handheld weights
- Stationary cycling

If You Get Injured

- Apply the PRICE method (Protection, Rest, Ice, Compression, Elevation)
- Choose a substitute activity
- Continue to set aside time for exercise
- Plan to resume your chosen activity after the injury heals

"What If I Get Hurt?"

The only way to guarantee you will never have an exercise-related injury is never to exercise. Although you can't plan for injuries, expect occasional minor discomforts and injuries, such as sore muscles and blisters, as you become more physically active. The benefits of physical activity far outweigh the risks, so don't allow concern about injuries to deter you from increasing your activity. Fortunately, most injuries associated with physical activity are not serious and heal without medical care. This is especially true with the type and amount of moderate exercise that we recommend in this book.

Injuries are much more common with high-intensity exercises, such as skiing or roller blading, in which falls cause serious injury. Research studies have shown that 2 or 3 percent of individuals who run more than 20 miles a week will have injuries each year that necessitate medical care. Most injuries, even in this group, resolve within 1 or 2 weeks without medical intervention. There is a direct association between the risk of injury and how much you exercise, with injury rates increasing rapidly if you run more than 30 miles per week or play several hours of vigorous sports, such as racquetball or singles tennis. This amount and intensity of exercise is far more than you need for health benefits, and your risk of injury is relatively low with moderate amounts of exercise.

If you sustain a minor injury, see Chapter 4 for an easy self-treatment to prevent or reduce swelling and pain and speed recovery. Look for a substitute activity, and plan to resume your chosen activity after the injury heals. If you become injured, find another activity that does not put additional stress on the injured part. If, for example, you walk briskly in your activity program and sprain your ankle stepping off the curb, you might try a stationary cycle until your ankle heals. Or you might participate in water aerobics for a few weeks so that you don't put too much weight on the injured joint. If you do not have access to a stationary cycle or a pool, you might do some stretching or strength-building exercises using calisthenics or small handheld weights. *(See appendices 1 and 2 for stretching and strength-building exercises.)*

If your regular exercise is swimming and you develop shoulder bursitis which makes swimming painful, you could walk or climb stairs until your shoulder improves. If you still want to swim, use only your legs and feet for propulsion, perhaps using swim fins and a kickboard. If you cannot perform your golf swing because your back is sore, or your elbow gives you trouble when you play tennis, consider walking in your neighborhood or around a park.

Find a substitute activity to sustain your activity habits when your regular program is interrupted by injury. Even if you cannot exercise for as long or as vigorously as you normally would, you will find it easier to resume your regular program after your injury heals if you don't break your routine and continue to set aside time for exercise.

"What If I Get Sick?"

Illness can disrupt an activity program. Disruptive illness can be as minor as a sore throat or as major as a heart attack or stroke. How sick must you be before you stop your physical activity?

There are few hard-and-fast rules, but let common sense and some general principles be your guide.

Listen to your body. If you have a stuffy head from a cold and no fever, gentle physical activity may make you feel better. However, if you take a walk when you have a mild cold and feel very tired or much worse after you have walked a few minutes, stop and return home.

Never exercise when you have a fever or pain and symptoms below the neck, such as muscular pain from the flu. Strenuous exercise when you have a viral infection such as a bad cold or influenza can cause serious problems. You can damage your heart and muscles if you exercise during the course of a fever or an infection.

Never ignore pain, pressure, or a sense of fullness in your chest that is caused by physical activity. Be especially alert to pain or pressure that radiates to the jaw, shoulder, or arm. If you notice these symptoms when you are physically active, even when walking, especially if the symptoms go away when you rest, call your doctor immediately. Many people assume that this type of pain is due to indigestion, and they ignore it. It may well be a minor problem, but it is better to be cautious now than sorry later. If the pain is due to coronary artery disease, which disrupts blood flow to the heart, you may be having a heart attack, in which case, minutes count. The sooner you get appropriate medical attention, the smaller the amount of damage to your heart and the less serious the consequences.

Serious medical conditions such as heart attack, stroke, or severe arthritis require a medically supervised physical activity program. Even if you have these conditions, however, you can follow a physical activity program on your own, although you may need to follow your doctor's advice and heed more restrictions than usual. (*More specific advice on physical activity for individuals with serious chronic disease is presented in Chapter 4.*)

Recovery time differs depending on the illness, but the principles of getting back to your activity program are the same. Your objective is to repeat the same steps that helped you get started when you began your exercise program.

If your illness forced you to be inactive for several days or longer, you will have lost some fitness. Do not expect to go back immediately to doing the same amount of activity you were doing before the illness. The longer you were inactive, the more fitness you will have lost, and the more you will need to cut back on your activity program when you resume.

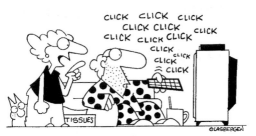

"The doctor said you're not supposed to exercise when you have the flu—and that includes aerobic channel changing!"

WARNING:
Stop Exercising Immediately If You Experience These Symptoms

- Chest pain, pain down your arm, heaviness in chest (angina)
- Persistent, uneven, rapid heartbeats
- Extreme breathlessness with light to moderate activity (not necessarily exercise)
- Wheezing, inability to catch breath
- Lightheadedness
- Nausea
- Extreme fatigue
- Numbness

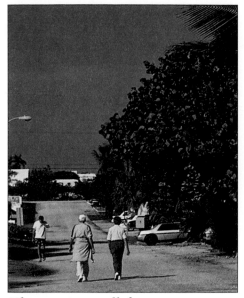

The evening walk becomes a doubles routine when your partner goes with you.

Keep a positive attitude, and don't despair. Expect illness to disrupt your activity program occasionally and plan for such eventualities. With good planning and dedication to your activity goals, you can start again.

"What If Family Responsibilities Interfere with My Activity?"

"What do I do *when* family responsibilities interfere with my activity plans?" is a more accurate question, because this will inevitably happen. Family responsibilities differ with life stage. Young couples with children sometimes have difficulty managing both childcare and exercise routines. Many parents find ways to exercise that include their children, such as canoeing, bike riding, walking, and even running with strollers. For most of you reading this book, the demands of childcare are no longer pressing problems, but professional responsibilities may absorb a great deal of your time. If you also spend much of your leisure time exercising, your partner may feel ignored and resentful.

If your partner feels neglected when you exercise, find opportunities for exercise that you both enjoy. Scheduled activities may offer one of your best times for communication. If you walk or bicycle together, you can listen without noise or distractions to your partner's news or daily concerns. In addition, each partner can help the other stay active. Some days, you may not feel like exercising and might be inclined to watch television. But if your partner says after dinner, "It's such a pleasant evening, let's go for a walk," you may be more likely to get up and go. It's certain that if you go for that walk, you'll feel better when you return.

"What If Social Activities Keep Me from My Activity Program?"

Most people have a limited amount of leisure time. There are only 168 hours in a week, and after sleeping, working, and taking care of basic personal needs, many people feel pressed for time. What leisure time you have, you may want to spend with friends. Perhaps you like to go with your friends to concerts or ball games. The time spent socializing is essential to your well-being. Friendships are an important part of life, and we certainly do not suggest that you ignore friends to be physically active. One alternative you might consider is to seek more active recreational opportunities that you and your friends can enjoy together. Dancing, hiking, bicycle riding, ice skating, bird watching, and traditional sports all offer good opportunities to combine social activities with exercise.

Let your friends know that you are concerned about being too sedentary and that you are trying to become more physically ac-

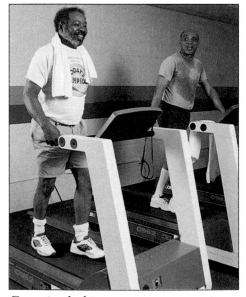

Exercise habits are easy to sustain when you have the support of a friend and training partner.

tive. You may be surprised how many of them will want to join you in your effort to be more more active.

"What If Job Pressures Interfere with My Activity?"

Your work may prevent you from being active. You may have new assignments, or your work may follow cycles when sometimes you are working much longer than usual. You probably should expect that work will sometimes interfere with your activity plans; when it does, you should have some alternatives in mind.

Perhaps you are putting in many additional hours on a special project and you do not have time to jog or go to your health club after work. In this situation, you may try to fit brief, unscheduled periods of activity into your daily routine. Try taking a 5-minute walk every 2 or 3 hours. Perhaps you can go around the block, climb several flights of stairs in your building, or simply take a brisk walk down the hall and back. Taking this short amount of time away from your work will not make you less productive; in fact, you will likely fell better and concentrate better after a brief break.

Relieve sedentary work habits by building activity into the job. If you meet with a colleague to discuss a project, build in some activity at the same time. A great deal of business is conducted on golf courses. If there is a park near your office, meet with coworkers while taking a brisk 15- or 20-minute walk through the park. If you manage projects or supervise employees, walk around to their offices and workstations.

"How Can I Be Active When I Travel So Much?"

Travel, either for business or pleasure, offers many possibilities for increasing your physical activity. When traveling on business, you might try walking from one appointment to another rather than taking a taxi. Take a vigorous walk in the morning before breakfast. There is nothing like some activity early in the day to make you feel invigorated and ready for the day's events.

Look for time during the day to build in a few minutes of physical activity. A short walk before or after lunch will heighten your senses and make you more productive the rest of the day. At the end of a day of sitting in meetings, you may be tempted to go to your hotel room to relax and watch the news or have a drink. Try some activity before doing either of these; you'll feel much better.

There is usually time for activity during the day, even on the busiest business trips. For example, if you carry your walking shoes with you, you can check your luggage or stow it in a locker and take a brisk walk through the airport terminal while waiting for a plane. If you take advantage of opportunities like this, you will get an immediate payoff in feeling better and being more

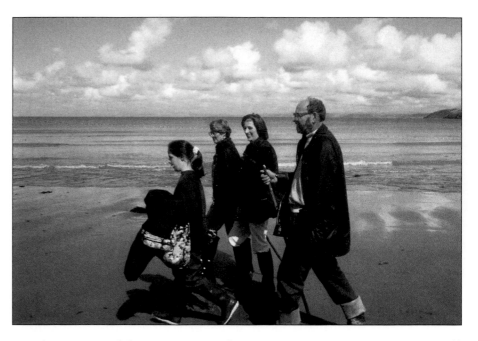

Vacations by lake and ocean shores offer irresistible opportunities for walking.

productive, and by staying with your activity program, you will continue to make positive contributions to your health.

"What Can I Do When I'm on Vacation?"

Vacations offer some of the best opportunities to increase your physical activity level. There is no better way to explore a new city than by walking. You see the sights and you experience the sounds, smells, and mood of the place more intensely than if you ride in a vehicle. In many cities, walking from one location to another is faster and more convenient.

Many of the world's largest, busiest cities have magnificent parks to be explored and enjoyed. Museums provide unique opportunities for combining activity with culture. You'd be surprised by the length of your walk through the museums of the Smithsonian Institution in Washington, DC. In many cities, like Washington, several museums are located in one area of the city. Tour buses can take you from one to another, but why ride when you can walk? The walk is part of the pleasure.

Many cities, like Boston, San Francisco, New Orleans, and Chicago, have waterfronts on rivers, oceans, or lakes where you can walk or even bike. Paved paths line the Charles River in Boston and the Mississippi in New Orleans. Pedestrian paths span the San Francisco Bridge. In Chicago, one of the United States' most handsome cities, you can walk along Lake Michigan then visit the Aquarium. Or you can walk down Michigan Avenue for some fine window shopping and hike a little farther to visit Chicago's Art Institute.

Foreign cities also are best seen on foot. In London, it may take you the greater part of a day to walk from the British Museum to the Victoria and Albert Museum. But what a walk it is! You pass through the West End, stop for tea at Fortnum and Masons on Piccadilly, stroll through Green Park and down Pall

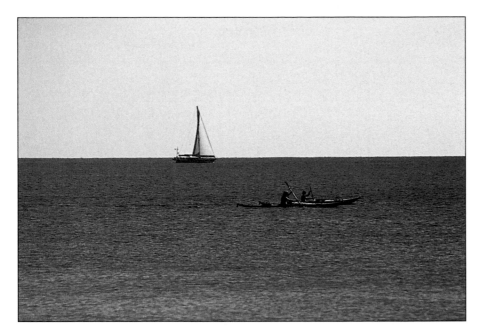

Salt air and warm seas are often best enjoyed in physical activities such as canoeing, sailing, swimming, or beachcombing.

Mall to view Buckingham Palace where you can watch the centuries-old ritual changing of the guard.

Vacations outside the city also offer many opportunities for active recreation. Hiking through the Appalachian Trail or in the Rocky Mountains will take you through uplifting scenery. Other vacations that take you fishing, hunting, bird watching, horseback riding, water skiing, canoeing, and bicycling keep you active while you take a break from your normal routine.

Slips as Learning Experiences

Most slips don't just happen. Slips occur along a continuum of change. What happens after the slip is more important than the slip itself. Use the slip as an opportunity to learn something new about yourself and the behaviors you need to change. Evaluate your efforts. There are likely to be numerous points along the way where you could have changed your behavior and prevented slips. Review the chain of events for the two scenarios described on the following page. Add at least one more preventive strategy for each event on the list.

Tips for Getting Back on Track

- Focus on the advantages of being physically active and the disadvantages of remaining sedentary.

- Revisit your tasks and goals from Chapter 10. Set new goals.

- Reward yourself for getting started again.

- Commit to being active for at least 15 minutes each day. This will usually get you started. Use the time to practice mental imagery.

- Think of yourself as an active person, enjoying being active.

Preventing Slips

Scenario #1

Chain of Events	Preventive Strategy
Monday—It rains so you can't walk outdoors.	• Climb stairs in your office building. • Vacuum the carpet at home, working as fast as you can to burn more calories.
Tuesday—The rain continues. You miss another day of activity.	• Drive to a shopping mall to walk. • Play an exercise tape and work out in your living room.
Wednesday—You must go out of town on a business trip. You spend most of your time in the airport.	• Make reservations at a hotel with a fitness center or swimming pool. • Take your walking shoes and other appropriate clothing for activity. • Store or check your luggage and walk in the airport while waiting for your flight.
Thursday—The meeting starts early and ends late.	• Use physical activity to relieve stress and relax. • Convince yourself that the trip will not cause you to stop your activity altogether.
Friday—When you return home, you feel too tired to do anything.	• Do something active even if you're tired. Physical activity is a great way to overcome fatigue and help you sleep better.
Saturday/Sunday—Because you've been out of town all week, you want to spend time with your family. You realize that it has been a week since you participated in any activity. You think you might as well quit for good.	• Get up early and go for a walk by yourself. Enjoy the quiet time. • Plan an activity the family can do together—biking, hiking, or skating. • Resolve to resume your regular program on Monday.

Scenario #2

Chain of Events	Preventive Strategy
Monday through Sunday—You've had a cold and a low-grade fever.	• Rest when you're sick or injured, especially with a fever. But don't let illness or an injury be an excuse to stop an activity permanently. • Set a date to resume your activity.
Monday though Sunday—Your fever is gone, but you don't feel 100% yet.	• When recovering from an illness, reduce your activity level for a few days, but strive to get back on your schedule.
Monday—You may return to exercise too intensely and experience minor muscle soreness on Tuesday, so you rest a few more days.	• Perform stretches to relieve and prevent soreness. • Choose a lower-intensity activity until the soreness diminishes.
Friday through Sunday—Relatives from out of town come to visit for the weekend.	• Show visitors the sites by taking a walking tour. • Enjoy recreational activities that include your visitors.
Monday through Friday—Your boss asks you to work overtime on a major project to meet a deadline on Friday. You agree to work late. You feel you must give up something, so you give up your time for activity at the end of the day. It's been 3 weeks since you were active.	• Get up early and exercise before going to work. • Emphasize to others that being active is a part of your life-style and that it is important to you. • Ask them to help you stay active. • Invite coworkers to join you in activities.

ACTION BOX 1

What Did You Learn from Your Slip?

What stage were you in when you started your program of change? _____

What stage of change were you in when you experienced your slip? _____

How many serious attempts have you made to be active? _____

What is the longest time you have remained consistently active? _____

What strategies were most helpful to you in your last attempt to return to activity? _____

Before the slip? _____

During the slip? _____

After the slip? _____

Anticipate Interruptions and Problems

Don't wait until a problem arises to look for a solution. Assume that there will be problems (because there will be), and plan ahead. Identify situations that are likely to be problems for you. Use the coping strategies that were introduced in this chapter. Ask someone to role play with you to work through some of the situations you are likely to encounter. Visualize the challenging situation and your positive response.

Strategies for Getting Back on Track

It's important to recognize that the more serious your previous attempts at change, the better your chance of long-term success with your next attempt. Also, the more quickly you can move into the action stage, the more likely you'll succeed at reestablishing and maintaining physical activity for a lifetime. In fact, most people will recycle through the Stages of Change several times before achieving long-term maintenance.

Those most likely to succeed in returning to physical activity are people who:

- Have made numerous serious attempts

- Begin in a later stage (action or maintenance)

- Are using the processes and strategies appropriate for their Stage of Change

- Can progress from one stage to the next within about 1 month

- Break large steps into smaller ones

For People in Stages 1 and 2

If you have slipped back to the early Stages of Change, try these strategies to get back on track:

- List the benefits ("pros") of physical activity.

- Read something new about physical activity.

- Think about the warnings of the health hazards of inactivity.

- Consider if you could be an active role model for others.

- Consider how your inactivity affects those closest to you.

- Talk to people like yourself who are physically active.

For People in Stages 3 and 4

If you are again beginning to make plans and trying to make a new start, these strategies can help you to increase your physical activity:

- Think about the type of person you will be if you keep exercising.

- Consider that you will feel more confident if you exercised regularly.

- Tell yourself that if you want to exercise, you will.

- Tell yourself that if you try hard enough you can keep exercising.

- Make a new commitment to exercise.

- Remind yourself that you are the only one who is responsible for your health and well-being.

- Believe that regular exercise will make you a healthier, happier person.

- Remind yourself that only you can decide whether you will exercise.

For People in Stage 5

If you are attempting to reestablish new patterns and behaviors, try these strategies to help you get back on track and stay active:

- Reward yourself when you exercise.

- Set realistic goals for yourself. Don't set yourself up for failure by expecting too much.

- Tell yourself that you are being good to yourself by taking care of your body when you exercise.

- Identify someone you can depend on when you have problems with exercising.

- Ask a healthy friend to encourage you to exercise when you don't feel up to it.

- Have someone provide feedback to you about your exercising.

- Keep objects around your home and at work that remind you to exercise.

- Remove obstacles in your environment that contribute to your inactivity.

- Avoid spending long periods in environments that promote inactivity.

- Engage in some physical activity instead of remaining inactive.

- Exercise even when you feel tired (you know you will feel better afterward).

- Use exercise to relieve your worries when you're feeling tense.

Try, Try Again

Always keep these points in mind as you move forward to try again:

- Try again as quickly as possible.

- Try again. This time you're probably at least one stage ahead of where you started last time.

- Try again, but do something differently. Learn from your experiences and mistakes.

- Try again. You can do it!

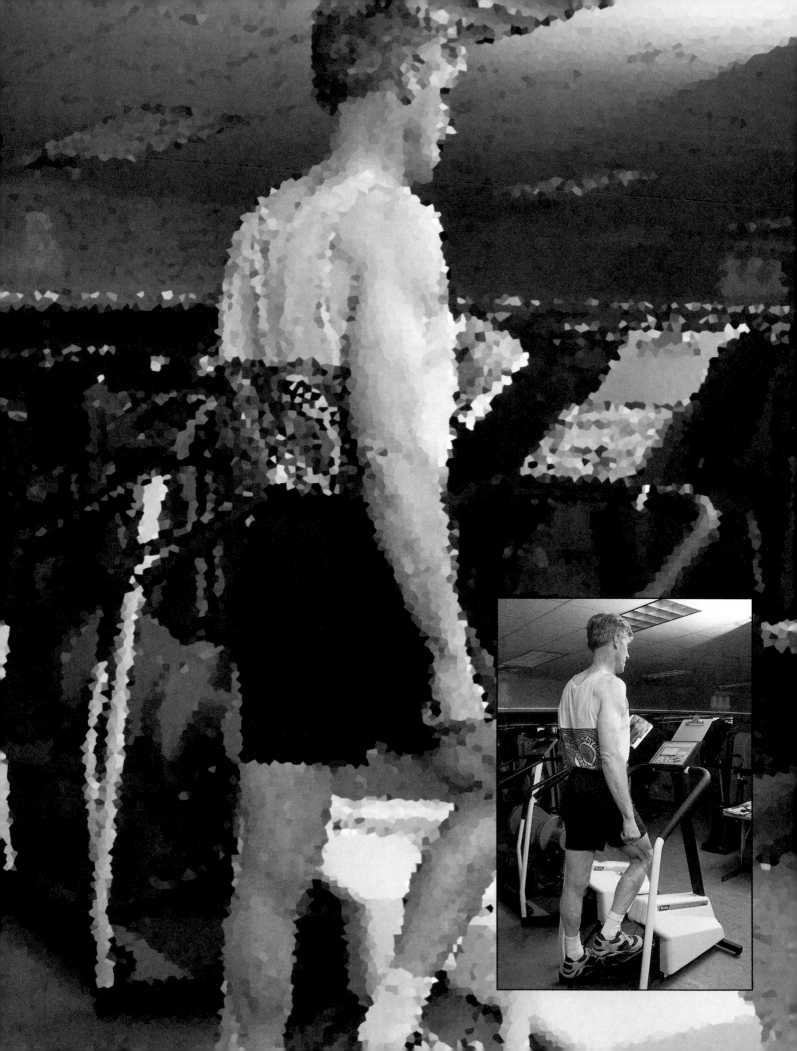

CHAPTER 14

Evaluating Exercise Resources, Equipment, and Facilities

You are now well on the road to healthy activity habits, exercising regularly, feeling good, and looking for opportunities to support your new life-style. At this point, you may be faced with some practical decisions and choices:

- How do you want to expand your exercise program?

- Where do you want to exercise? Do you want to exercise at home, perhaps purchasing weights or equipment, or do you want to join a health club?

Your personality and individual preferences, as well as practical considerations, such as where you live, how much money you want to spend, and your daily commitments, will influence your decision. It is important to choose the right setting for your exercise program because you are much more likely to stay with or expand your exercise routine if it is easy, convenient, and suits all your needs. Let's look at the two principal options: exercising at home and exercising at a health club or facility.

Should You Exercise at Home?

Like many other people, you may want to exercise at home, but you must first consider whether this choice is practical. Can you meet your exercise needs at home? For example, if you choose to walk or jog, do you have a safe, convenient place to do it, such as a quiet road, a park, mall, track, or community pathway? If none of these options is available, you may want to consider buying a treadmill, but you must put it where it's easy to use so that you'll use it regularly. If you want to bike, will bad weather prevent you from biking? If you live in a mild climate year-round, you're not likely to be frustrated by snow or ice, but in a northern state, winter weather may not permit outside biking for many months of the year. In this case, you might want to consider purchasing a stationary bike or a wind trainer, a device available at most bicycle stores that temporarily converts your bicycle to a stationary bike. Consider the following factors:

- What is your chosen exercise (indoor, outdoor)?

- If you exercise outside, do you have access to a safe and convenient exercise location?

- Is climate an obstacle to year-round outside exercise?

- If climate or weather is an obstacle, can you do alternative forms of exercise easily?

- Can you exercise at home easily? Do you have space for equipment?

Let's assume that you can exercise at home and there are no significant obstacles in your environment. You must now consider personal factors that still might influence your exercise routine:

- What exercise plan best suits your personality? Do you enjoy working out alone every day, or do you enjoy the support of training partners? What setting is most likely to help you stay with your exercise program?

- How social do you want to be? Do you prefer to exercise in privacy, or will your exercise routine thrive on the social contact a health club provides?

- How much money do you want to spend? If your funds are limited, or if you can't see spending money on equipment for the home, you may want to start by exercising without equipment. You can always decide later that you want to buy weights or an exercise machine.

Exercising at home has many advantages and a few disadvantages. Review the "pros" and "cons" in Action Box 1 on the following page to help you evaluate whether exercising at home is the right choice for you.

Overall, the home can be an excellent setting in which to establish unshakable exercise habits. Many people combine indoor and outdoor exercises at home, jogging and walking on weekends or in the early mornings when the weather permits and exercising quickly and easily on machines when the weather is bad or when they want to vary their schedules or work different muscle groups.

ACTION BOX 1

Weigh the "Pros" and "Cons" of Exercising at Home

Check which of the following is important or unimportant to you. If you check more boxes in the left-hand column than in the right, exercising at home may be a good decision. If you check more boxes in the right-hand column than the left, you probably would be happier joining a health club or exercising at a community recreation center.

	Important	Unimportant
Pros		
• You save time because you don't have to drive to another location.		
• You can enjoy the privacy, safety, and comfort of your home.		
• You can use your own shower.		
* You don't have to pack a workout bag.		
• You can exercise while you watch television or a video, listen to music, supervise your children, or talk to your child, spouse, or companion.		
• You can exercise at different times of the day and in brief intervals spread over the day rather than in one block of time.		
• You can save money (on club membership fees and clothes, if needed).		
• Once you buy a piece of exercise equipment, there are no additional ongoing costs.		
Cons	**Unimportant**	**Important**
• You don't have a variety of exercise equipment and activities from which to choose.		
• You need space to exercise or store exercise equipment.		
• You may not have the company or support of a training partner.		
• You may be easily distracted by other obligations built into the home setting, such as chores, child care, or (if you work at home) job-related work.		
• You may be interrupted by phone calls (even if you use the answering machine to screen your calls.)		

What Should You Know About Exercise Equipment?

Depending on your workout program, you may consider purchasing exercise equipment for your home. The marketplace has hundreds of products designed to appeal to people who want to improve their health and fitness. However, you must select the machine that fits your needs and use it correctly to benefit from your investment. Using the correct form is especially important to get the results you want. Many people compromise the effect of their workouts by supporting their weight on the handrails of treadmills or stair-climbers or gripping weight machines improperly. Poor posture and body alignment can cause injury and cancel the exercise's potential benefit. Read the instructions carefully to learn

Exercise Equipment for the Home

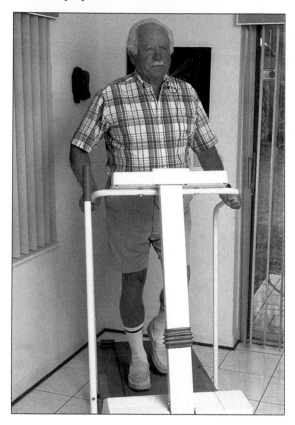

Motorized Treadmills

- *Fitness Benefits.* Improves cardiovascular fitness. Increasing the incline of the treadmill can increase the intensity of a 3-mph walk to an aerobic level equal to jogging. Walking and jogging improve lower-body muscle tone but do little for upper-body muscles. Some variations of treadmills now include poles that allow you to get a moderate upper-body workout while walking or jogging.

- *Special Features.* Select motors that permit speeds of at least 5 mph (required for jogging). Motor size varies from 1/2 horsepower to more than 1 1/2 horsepower. Monitors record your speed, distance covered, time elapsed, and sometimes heart rate and calories burned.

- *Ease of Use.* Most models let you adjust the incline to simulate hills and increase workout intensity. Choose a model that allows you to change the incline automatically (instead of using pins to change the slope). Select a treadmill that has a belt large enough to accommodate your full stride. A long, wide bed and full-length handrails make for easier use. Controls should be easy to reach.

- *Safety.* A slow minimum speed makes starting safer.

Straddle the treadmill to start. Gradually turn up the speed as you start to walk.

- *Durability.* Inexpensive treadmills are likely to be flimsy or have motors too weak to withstand heavy use or higher speeds. Most inexpensive treadmills are designed for walking, not jogging.

- *Cost.* Home-model treadmills generally range between $400 and $1,500. The higher-priced machines have larger motors, wider and longer belts, higher top speeds, and more special features and controls.

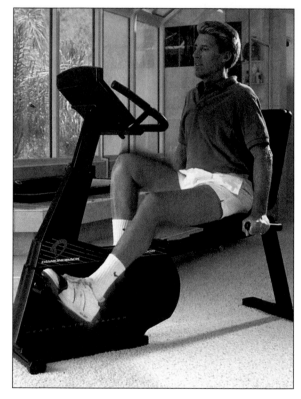

Stationary Cycles

- *Fitness Benefits.* Like walking and jogging, cycling is excellent aerobic exercise and has the added benefit of being a nonimpact exercise. Recumbent models work the hamstring muscles more than upright cycles and may be the preferred model for people with back problems. Dual-action models (ones in which you pump the handlebars as you pedal) can give you an upper- and lower-body workout. Stationary bicycles allow you to maintain a steadier activity level than outdoor bicycles.

- *Special Features.* Models vary according to how resistance is applied (belts around the wheel, air resistance, electromagnets) to regulate workout intensity.

Exercise Equipment for the Home (*continued*)

Recumbent models let you sit in a chair-like seat. Monitors record your speed, distance, and time, and, sometimes, heart rate and calories burned. Dual-action cycles may use a fan that cools you while you pedal. Pedal straps work your legs on the upstroke as well as the downstroke.

- *Ease of Use.* The seat should be adjustable, well padded, and comfortably shaped. You should be able to adjust the resistance easily by twisting a knob or by selecting a prescribed program.

- *Safety.* Stationary cycling is very safe.

- *Durability.* Inexpensive bikes may be flimsy and jerky.

- *Cost.* Most models cost between $100 and $1,200. If you already own a bike, you can purchase a training stand for less than $200 to convert it to a stationary model.

- *Special Features.* There are two types of stair climbers: steppers, which simulate climbing stairs, and ladders, which simulate climbing a ladder. Monitors display steps per minute, time, and calories burned. Some machines allow you to program changes in resistance at predetermined intervals.

- *Ease of Use.* Select climbers that have simplified monitors. Pedals and handles that ensure a comfortable and secure stance are also important. You should be able to adjust the resistance easily.

- *Safety.* With correct posture, using this type of equipment involves little risk for injury.

- *Durability.* Check the stability of the machine.

- *Cost.* Home-model stair climbers range from $200 to $700.

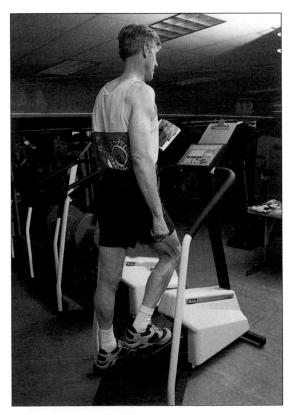

Stair-Climbing Machine

- *Fitness Benefits.* Stair climbing improves cardiovascular fitness and leg muscle strength. Because your feet stay on the levers, impact on the knees is less than when you go up and down a real flight of stairs. Models with independently moving steps give a better workout.

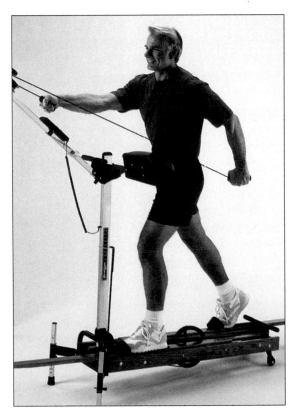

Cross-Country Ski Simulators

- *Fitness Benefits.* Ski machines offer the aerobic and muscle-toning benefits of cross-country skiing. They work the arms and legs so you get an upper- and lower-body workout.

Continues on following page

how to use a newly purchased machine. Better still, try to obtain access to a similar machine, perhaps at a club or a YMCA, and ask the instructors or supervisors about correct form.

Trying a piece of exercise equipment before you purchase it will also ensure that you don't buy a costly piece of equipment that—you discover too late—does not meet your needs. Using a machine for a few minutes in a store is not a sufficient trial to make a good decision. Many people purchase machines that they quickly discard, storing them in basements or attics because the machines do not live up to expectations, or they break. If you purchase exercise equipment for your home, shop carefully to get the most value for your dollar. Home exercise equipment can be expensive, and, as with most products, there is a wide range of features and levels of quality.

Use the worksheet in Action Box 2 on the following page to compare three different brands of exercise equipment. A thorough evaluation will help ensure that you get your money's worth.

Exercise Equipment for the Home (*continued*)

- *Special Features.* These machines have ski-like boards or sliding foot pads instead of skis and a rope-and-pulley device or ski poles. Leg motion can be linked to arm motion, or it can be done independently. Models that allow independent leg motion are more difficult to master but provide a more vigorous workout. Some models offer a variable incline that can increase the workout of your front thigh muscles. Monitors record heart rate. Some machines have indexed resistance settings.

- *Ease of Use.* Learning the correct technique can be challenging. Most machines fold compactly and can be stored in a closet or under the bed. Wheels let you move the machine easily.

- *Safety.* This is a safe, low-impact exercise machine. Expect a strenuous workout in the beginning if your fitness level is generally low.

- *Durability.* Check the machine's stability and make sure the electronic monitor is reliable.

- *Cost.* Basic ski machines begin at $300 and can cost much more.

Weight Machines (Home Gyms)

- *Fitness Benefits.* A typical home gym offers a variety of strength-building exercises—butterfly, triceps extension, pull down, shoulder press, leg extension, leg curl, chest press, and biceps curl. Home gyms can be effective in building strength, but so can handheld weights (which cost much less) and calisthenic exercises (which use the body's weight as resistance and cost nothing at all).

- *Special Features.* Home gyms use several methods to apply resistance: stacks of weight plates, thick rubber bands, flexible rods, hydraulic or pneumatic cylinders, and centrifugal brakes.

- *Ease of Use.* Minimal effort is required to set up and change weights, making it easy to use the various stations on the home gym. Select a gym that allows you to get in and out of the stations easily and quickly. Changing resistance is easiest on gyms with weight stacks or elastic bands. A wide range of resistance settings keeps you from outgrowing the gym too quickly. Comfort and fit are important features.

- *Safety.* On the whole, home gyms are very safe because you don't need a spotter to catch the weight if you lose the strength to support it.

- *Durability.* Home gyms made of heavier-gauge metal have more durable moving parts.

- *Cost.* Home gyms cost much less than the multistation gyms in health clubs. Prices range from $200 to $3,000. With home gyms, as with all exercise equipment, you get what you pay for. More money buys a better product.

ACTION BOX 2

Exercise Equipment Checklist

(Answer "Yes" or "No")

	Brand A	Brand B	Brand C
• Is the manufacturer reputable? Does the manufacturer provide strong customer support (toll-free telephone number)?			
• Does the equipment come with at least a year's warranty? Does the warranty cover replacement parts? For how long?			
• Is electricity required for operation (110 or 220 volt)?			
• Does the equipment appear sturdy? What is its life expectancy?			
• How much does the equipment cost? (More money usually buys better equipment.)			
• Is the equipment adjustable so that people of different sizes and fitness levels can use it? (This is especially important if several family members use the equipment).			
• Are training instructions, materials, and videos provided? Are they easy to follow?			
• Is the equipment safe and easy to operate? (Make sure you try it yourself.)			
• How much space is required to house and use the equipment? Can it fit into your living/exercise area?			
• Is it easy to move and store?			
• Does it come assembled or is it easy to assemble?			
• Is it noisy to operate?			

Arranging Exercise Equipment

Most exercise equipment is unwieldy and difficult to store. Banishing equipment to the farthest corner of the basement or garage may not be conducive to good exercise habits. If you want to get the most from the equipment you buy, place it where you know you will use it. Don't worry too much about how it looks. A pleasant upstairs study or bedroom will not be much pleasure to you if inactivity keeps you from climbing the stairs. Here are some tips for arranging equipment:

- Place your equipment in a pleasant, well-lit, well-ventilated area. You may want to keep it all in one room or distribute it throughout your home. Putting it all in one room has advantages. You can put your radio, stereo, and television in the same room and entertain yourself as you exercise. Or, if you have a porch or patio with a view, put a stationary bicycle or treadmill where you can enjoy the air and the view while you exercise. Wherever you put it, make sure you are not discouraged from using the equipment because you don't enjoy the setting.

- If you have limited space, purchase equipment that stores easily. Some treadmills fold easily to store under the bed. You can store free weights, especially those with plastic coatings, in closets or boxes that slide under a bed.

Would You Benefit from a Personal Trainer?

Certified personal trainers design and supervise individualized programs that monitor your progress and help you master skills and get results. Training sessions are performed in privacy at home (if space and equipment are available) or at a health/fitness center, where most trainers work as independent contractors, not as employees of the club. The trainer usually pays a portion of your fee to the club for use of space and equipment and for access to clients. Client fees range from $15 to $75 per hour depending on the trainer's experience and credentials.

Although personal trainers are useful for people in weight training programs, they are more a luxury than a necessity. You can design your own effective exercise program and be your own fitness counselor. We hope this book will help you learn the skills you need to fill this role.

Before hiring a personal trainer, ask yourself, "What's the added value to me? Will I exercise more regularly? Will I get better results?" If you decide to hire a personal trainer, decide whether you want a male or female trainer, then conduct face-to-face interviews with several trainers before making a final decision. More than likely, your choice will be influenced by whether you like the trainer and think you would enjoy working with him or her. Make sure you hire someone who is qualified and will help you get the most from your exercise program. Here are some questions for screening prospective trainers:

Questions for Personal Trainers

- What certifications do you have? (Ask the trainer to show proof, including CPR certification.)

- How much experience do you have as a personal trainer? (Ask for a list of previous and current clients.)

- Do you have professional liability insurance?

- Do you conduct medical screenings and fitness assessments before beginning an exercise program?

- What would the program include?

- What kind of improvement or upgrade can I expect after a specific time (such as 6 weeks)?

- When and where would the workouts take place?

- What is your relationship with the health/fitness club if the session is at a club?

- What is the cost per session? Must I sign a contract? Can I terminate it?

- Am I charged if I cancel an appointment?

Should You Join a Health Club?

You don't have to join a health club to be physically active, but you may want to consider it. The United States has a large number of well-equipped health clubs, and most major clubs have highly qualified staff. A number of inexpensive health clubs are also open to the public in local communities. Many YMCAs, YWCAs, JCCAs, schools, colleges and universities, public parks, and recreation centers charge small enrollment fees for the use of excellent exercise facilities. Some religious organizations providing fitness programs for their members emphasize the spiritual dimension of health as well as the emotional, mental, and social components of physical fitness. Churches and religious organizations are also unique in reaching out to promote health and fitness among the underserved, particularly families, minorities, and seniors.

ACTION BOX 3

Weigh the "Pros" and "Cons" of Exercising at a Health Club

Check which of the following is important or unimportant to you. If you checked more boxes in the left-hand column than in the right, joining a health/fitness club may be a good decision. If you checked more boxes in the right-hand column, you probably would be happier exercising at home.

	Important	Unimportant
Pros		
• You are motivated by seeing others exercise.		
• You enjoy regular social interaction.		
* You are less likely to be injured in a supervised setting.		
• You have access to emergency care if you are injured.		
• You have access to a wide range of equipment.		
• You don't have to invest in or maintain your own exercise equipment.		
• You have access to expert advice from staff and trainers.		
• You have access to information about nutrition and other health issues.		
• You have access to individualized assessments and programs.		
Cons	**Unimportant**	**Important**
• You must pay a membership fee.		
• You may have to sign a contract.		
• You're paying to use equipment that may not interest you.		
• You must commit at least 1 hour for each visit.		
• You may find the facility crowded, especially during peak times.		
• You can't exercise in private.		
• You must use public locker rooms.		
• You must travel to the facility.		
• You are restricted by the hours the facility operates.		

Special Facilities and Equipment

Exercise facilities

- Tennis courts
- Racquetball/handball courts
- Squash courts
- Basketball court, gymnasium
- Swimming pool
- Indoor track
- Outdoor track
- Aerobic dance studio

Locker room facilities

- Whirlpool
- Dry sauna
- Wet sauna
- Lockers
- Amenities (soap, shampoo, lotion, hair dryers, irons)

Equipment

- Weight machines
- Free weights
- Treadmills
- Stationary cycles
- Stair climbers
- Rowing machines
- Cross-country ski machines

Other

- Pro shop
- Food service
- Child care
- Well-lighted parking

Some corporations provide their employees with health and fitness programs and facilities at the worksite. Corporations know that fitness is good business. In addition to helping to attract and retain the best employees, health and fitness programs reduce absenteeism and health care costs.

From the employees' perspective, worksite health and fitness programs offer a convenient place to work out. If there is a fee, it is usually below market value and can often be paid through a payroll deduction plan. Some employers allow flexible work schedules to encourage workouts throughout the day. In companies that operate around the clock, it's not unusual to see employees going to the fitness center at 7 AM as they get off the night shift. If you're fortunate enough to work in a company that provides an onsite fitness facility, we strongly encourage you to take advantage of this valuable benefit.

Even if you don't have these options, you don't have to join a health club to be active. We don't discourage you from pursuing this option, but we do advise that before you join a health club or fitness center you make sure the club will meet your exercise needs.

Review the "pros" and "cons" in Action Box 3 on the previous page to help you evaluate whether exercising at a health/fitness club is the right choice for you.

What Should You Look for in a Health Fitness Club?

To evaluate health and fitness clubs in your area, begin by making a few phone calls. Ask about:

- Fees (read the contract and waivers and check the fees against the published price list)

- Brochures and applications to review

- Current membership and capacity

- An appointment to speak with a staff member and look at the facility

Select no more than three facilities to visit initially. Schedule your visit at the time of day you would use the facility, especially if this is during a busy period, such as after work or on the weekend. Don't be pressured to decide on the spot. Some businesses insist that you sign a contract immediately to get a special discounted price. Be suspicious of high-pressured marketing strategies; reputable health clubs do not use them. If you are still uncertain about which club to choose, call the Better Business Bureau in your area and ask if it has information on health clubs in your area.

Use the checklist in Action Box 4 on the following page as a guide during your evaluation. Add to this list if you are looking for special requirements in a health club.

ACTION BOX 4

Checklist for Evaluating Facilities

(Answer "Yes" or "No")

	Facility A	Facility B	Facility C
• *Convenience.* Is the facility convenient? Is it near home or work?			
• *Hours.* Do its hours of operation fit your needs?			
• *Parking.* Is there adequate parking?			
• *Facilities/equipment.* Does the club have the facilities or equipment you want to use?			
• *Space.* Is there ample space in the showers, locker rooms, and exercise rooms, and on the courts and tracks?			
• *Availability.* Is equipment available at the time you would visit?			
• *Physical plant.* Are the facility and equipment clean, neat, well-maintained, and in good working order?			
• *Air quality.* Are the temperature, humidity, and ventilation controlled and comfortable at peak times?			
• *Programs.* Does the facility provide comprehensive fitness programming (cardiovascular, strength, and flexibility training) as well as sports activities?			
• *Special services.* Does the facility provide comprehensive health/fitness services (fitness assessments, exercise prescriptions, physical therapy, arthritis therapy, cardiac rehabilitation, hypertensive exercise therapy, weight loss programs, nutrition counseling)?			
• *Staff.* Are staff experienced, well-qualified, and certified by recognized agencies like the American Red Cross (CPR and first aid), the American College of Sports Medicine (ACSM), the American Council on Exercise, and the Aerobics and Fitness Association? Are staff healthy role models? Are they friendly and supportive?			
• *Supportive systems.* Are activities available to encourage adherence (recognition programs, challenges and contests, monitoring systems, recreational leagues)?			
• *Safety and security.* Are safety and security practices emphasized (written policies and procedures)?			

What Will Help You Stay Active?

Regardless of where you decide to exercise, the principles outlined in the earlier chapters of this book will help you adhere to your program:

- Know the many benefits of exercise, especially moderate activity.

- Evaluate your current activity and fitness.

- Set realistic goals and expectations.

- Check your progress regularly.

- Develop a balanced fitness program.

- Find a convenient place to exercise.

- Make activity a priority.

- Get support from others.

- Make activity fun.

What About Other Health and Fitness Resources?

Unfortunately, not all the information about health and fitness you hear on television and radio or read in best-selling books is reliable. Our desire for the "quick fix" makes us vulnerable to products and services that are scientifically unproved and unsound. Be cautious! Don't believe what you read just because it is published in a popular magazine or book that makes the best-seller list. "Consumer beware" is good advice. To assess the reliability of any health resource, ask these questions:

- Who is saying it? What credentials, training, or experience qualifies the individual to make the claims? Even people who claim to have advanced educational degrees might provide misleading information. In addition, not all educational institutions are credible; some grant diplomas through the mail. Celebrities with no specific training or expertise in a given field often endorse products that are worthless. But remember, they get paid well for promoting products! Beware of paid endorsements.

- Does what is being claimed seem too good to be true? Does it promise to be "quick and easy"?

- Where is it being said? Some media are more careful than others in checking their sources before publishing information. You can probably trust peer-reviewed scientific journals, but most people don't read these journals. Scientific sources are frequently quoted, but sometimes research findings are misinterpreted or taken out of context. It's easy to be confused by "infomercials" and "advertorials," which are quickly becoming a common source of new information. Often complex issues are reduced to sound bytes that make good copy for the evening news but may fail to given an accurate overall picture.

Whom can you trust for accurate and reliable information? Your physician and other health care professionals are excellent sources for health and medical information. Write down your questions or collect pieces of information and take them with you to your next visit. Some health plans provide toll-free numbers you can call to have your questions answered.

You can also trust information from voluntary health organizations. The American College of Sports Medicine (ACSM) has a Fit Society program to provide information to consumers. Contact the program at (317) 637-9200. Nonprofit groups like the American Heart Association (AHA), the American Cancer Society, and the American Lung Association provide reliable information for consumers about important health topics. These organizations use rigorous scientific review processes before taking positions or releasing information on particular topics. Information from voluntary health organizations is generally written in an easy-to-understand format and is usually available free or for a nominal fee.

Other good sources of information are government health agencies. The Department of Health and Human Services provides numerous resources for consumers. Improving the health status of our nation is part of the mission of agencies like the Centers for Disease Control and Prevention (CDC), the National Institutes of Health, and the Public Health Service.

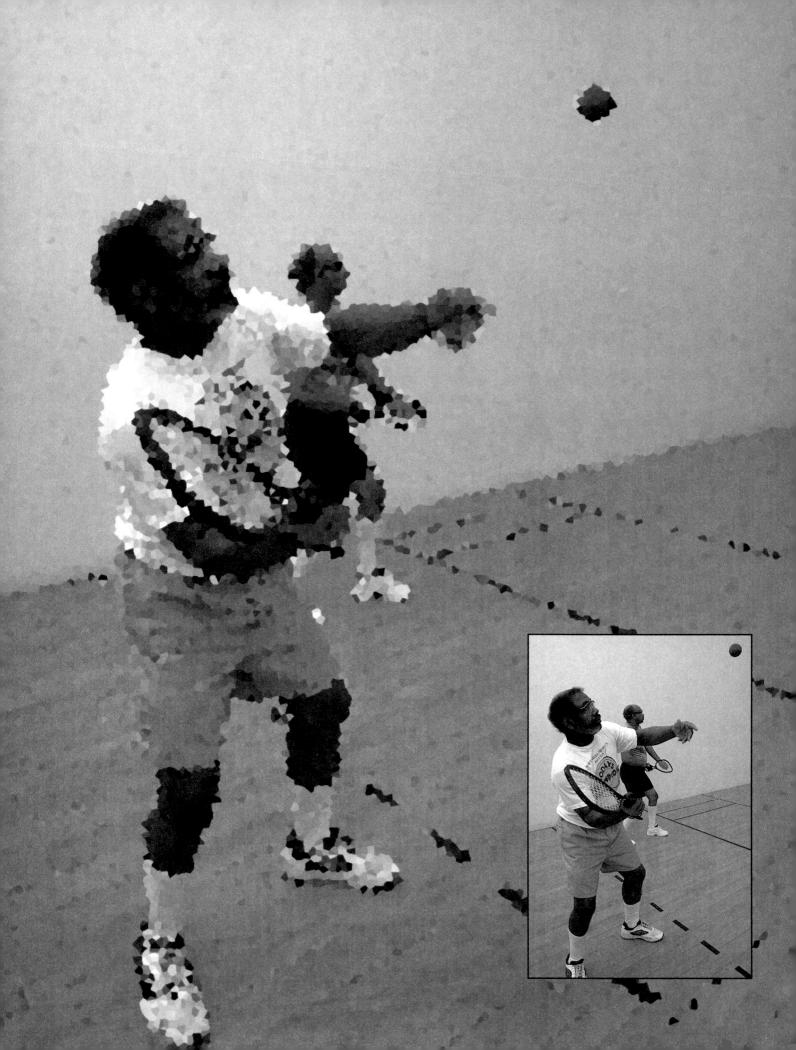

CHAPTER 15

Participating in Sports and Recreation

Participating in sports is an excellent way to be physically active. All sports activities count as exercise—planned activities for the single purpose of improving physical fitness. Although sports activities exercise the muscles, burn calories, and reduce stress, they are unique in providing opportunities for fun, friendly competition, and socialization.

You're probably thinking, "I can't play sports. Sports are for athletes. I'm too clumsy, and anyway, I don't like competition." But we emphasize participation and doing what you enjoy. Sports are opportunities for doing what you like and feel comfortable with. And sports are for everyone, not just athletes. Although some sports are best left to the young, you can participate in most sports throughout your lifetime. And, you're never too old to begin. In the senior Olympics each year, thousands of people in their 70s, 80s, and 90s participate at various levels in all kinds of sports from basketball to sprinting to racewalking.

This chapter provides you with guidelines for getting started in sports activities. There are three general categories of sports:

- *Individual sports* (walking, running, cycling, swimming) can be performed alone.

- *One-on-one sports* (tennis, and racquetball) are played with one or more persons.

- *Team sports* (basketball, volleyball, softball) always require more than two people.

Categories of Sports

Individual sports include:

- Walking
- Jogging/running
- Bicycling
- Swimming
- Dancing
- Skating
- Skiing
- T'ai-chi

One-on-one sports include:

- Tennis
- Racquetball
- Squash
- Golf

Team sports include:

- Volleyball
- Basketball
- Softball

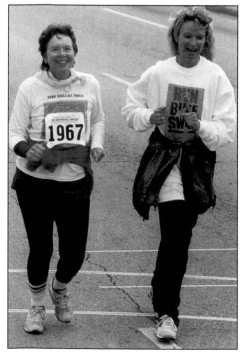

Finishing a road race brings satisfaction and a great sense of accomplishment.

The principal focus of this chapter is on individual sports, which people typically play for fun and enjoyment rather than for competition. Also, as you will see, we are more enthusiastic about sports that have low injury rates. Sports are good for your health only if you can participate safely, without harm or injury.

Choosing a Sports Activity

When you choose a sports activity, consider the following factors:

- *Competition.* Competition is the last reason to participate in sports. You don't have to compete. Or if you like, you can compete with yourself by setting goals as part of your overall fitness program.

- *Level of skill or difficulty.* People enjoy what they do well. Your enjoyment of a sport depends on your current level of skill.

- *Physical conditioning.* Your physical condition determines what sport suits you most. As your conditioning improves, you can branch out and participate spontaneously in many sports.

- *Experience and knowledge.* Your experience with and understanding of a sport will make you more comfortable about participating in it.

- *Benefits.* The sport you choose should meet your special needs for health and enjoyment.

- *Risks.* Your knowledge and perception of risk influence how you negotiate it, so that you participate in sports safely and without injury.

- *Environmental factors.* Consider the conditions and location in which the sport is best played.

Competition

The term *competition* is often misused, abused, and misunderstood. Most of us are competitive to some degree, either as a way to measure our abilities compared with others' or to test ourselves to see how far we can excel. We like to compete with ourselves because we can control our expectations of ourselves, whereas we can't control the expectations of others. Even if we fail to reach a goal, we know when we've done our best.

You don't have to be competitive to participate in a sport. Millions of people jog but don't participate in road races. And there are many reasons for entering road races that have nothing to do with competition. Many people run road races for the exercise and camaraderie rather than to beat the clock or other competitors. Their goal is only to finish the race and feel good about their accomplishment. Many road races have "fun runs" or walks in addition to the main events, just for people who aren't interested in carrying off the laurel crown. Some runners participate in road races as part of their weekly exercise programs to break up their routines. Others enter sponsored races to raise money for charity. Only a small portion of road race participants run competitively because they want to finish at the front of the pack, or at least high in their age groups.

Level of Skill

In addition to the four measures of physical fitness—cardiovascular endurance (aerobic fitness), muscle strength, joint flexibility, and balance—coordination and level of skill are also important components of performance in sports activities. Whether you're starting or resuming sports activities, consider your strengths and weaknesses in each of these areas and choose a sport that requires skills that match your abilities. For example, if you have poor balance, you may not want to start out skating or skiing, both sports that require very good balance. You may eventually be able to ski, but initially, at least, you should begin with exercises that improve your balance, such as t'ai-chi, and work up to participating on the ski slopes. If you want to ski next winter, you may want to enroll in a t'ai-chi class in the spring to build appropriate balancing skills.

Most important, if you are in good health, reasonably fit, and don't have specific physical limitations, you can probably begin to participate at low intensities in any of the sports discussed in this book. The chart on the following page weighs the skills various sports require and may help you to select the sport that suits you best. The chart is intended only as a guide, because as long as you enjoy a sport, your level of skill doesn't matter.

Physical Conditioning and Sport-Specific Conditioning

Physical conditioning refers to your general fitness level. You arrive at this level as a direct result of all the activities in which you participate. Some of these activities are probably *sport specific*. For example, if you started your exercise program years ago by walking, then progressed to jogging, then increased your speed and distance and finally competed in 10-km (6.2-mile) road races, you may be in good physical condition overall and in excellent *sport-specific* condition. That is, you are in excellent shape to run. Let's assume that because you are in excellent physical condition, you decide you want to participate in a mile-long swimming race. To your dismay, you find that when you begin training, you're exhausted after swimming only a few laps and have to quit. Part of the reason for your exhaustion is that swimming uses muscle groups in both the upper and lower body while running uses muscle groups only in the lower body. Although you are in excellent cardiovascular condition (required for both sports), the demands on your upper body in a swimming race are more than your current condition can meet. Similarly, if you were to step onto a racquetball court, you

Requirements for Starting Participation in Sports

Find the sport that interests you. Determine the extent to which each factor is required for participating in that sport. Evaluate your general abilities or resources in each area and decide which sport is right for you. If you enjoy the sport and have fun, being good at it isn't important, but you should be able to participate comfortably.

	Aerobic Fitness	Strength	Flexibility	Balance	Coordination	Knowledge/ Skills	Risk of Injury	Expense
Walk	●●	●	●	●	●	●	●	●
Jog/run	●●●	●	●	●	●	●	●●	●
Cycle	●●	●	●	●	●	●	●●●	●●
Swim	●●●	●●	●●	●	●●	●	●	●●
Dance	●	●	●	●●	●●	●	●	●●
T'ai-chi	●	●●	●●	●●	●●	●	●	●
Skate	●●	●●	●	●●●	●●●	●●●	●●●	●●
Cross-country skiing	●●	●●	●●	●●	●●	●●	●●	●●
Downhill skiing	●●●	●●	●●	●●●	●●●	●●●	●●●	●●●
Golf	●	●	●●	●●	●●●	●●●	●	●●
Tennis	●●	●	●●	●●	●●●	●●●	●	●●●
Racquetball/ squash	●●	●●	●●	●●	●●●	●●	●●	●●
Volleyball	●	●	●●	●	●●●	●●	●	●
Basketball	●●	●●	●●	●●	●●●	●●●	●●	●
Softball	●	●	●●	●	●●	●●	●	●

Key: ● = Low ●● = Moderate ●●● = High

would find that although you would be using the same lower body muscle groups that you use in running, you would be using different fibers in the same muscles, so you would tire much more quickly than you had anticipated.

Because each sport has specific conditioning requirements, it is important to start each one slowly and take the time to develop sport-specific conditioning. You need good cardiovascular conditioning for many sports, but you'll enjoy them more if you consider the specific physical requirements of each sport and train for it appropriately. Almost anyone can improve his or her golf swing, tennis backhand, or basketball shot with sport-specific training. The goal is to develop the muscle groups that are most instrumental to the sport you are playing. Eventually, if you train in many sports, you achieve all-around muscle fitness.

Developing all-around conditioning will give you more options and will allow you to participate spontaneously in sports and recreational activities. The better condition you are in, the more freely and confidently you will participate. If you cycle regularly and someone asks you to go on a bike tour through the wine country, you'll feel confident accepting the invitation. If you swim regularly and want to try snorkeling on vacation, you can do it without worrying. Conditioning gives you freedom and increases your options to enjoy life and friends. This is why cross-training is becoming so popular. *Cross-training* is participating and training in more than one sport with the object of using all your major muscle groups. If you swim, bike, and play racquetball, you use not only all your major muscle groups but also both types of muscle fibers: fast twitch and slow twitch.

Fast-Twitch and Slow-Twitch Muscles

What are fast- and slow-twitch muscles? All skeletal muscle groups are composed of slow-twitch and fast-twitch fibers. The endurance and power of a given muscle group depend on the type and distribution of muscle fibers and the way muscles use energy during exercise.

Slow-twitch fibers contract at a slower rate than fast-twitch fibers and function predominantly "aerobically," extracting oxygen directly from the blood to create energy. Slow-twitch muscles are slow to fatigue and are used for continuous activities such as walking, cycling, jogging, and swimming.

Fast-twitch fibers contract at a fast rate and release energy by a predominantly "anaerobic" process (without oxygen), processing glycogen to release energy. Fast-twitch muscles have great power but less endurance. These types of muscles equip you well for high-intensity work and sports that require speed and power, such as sprinting, racquetball, and squash.

As you age, you lose muscle fiber, but you lose more fast-twitch than slow-twitch fibers. As a result, activities that require

---

Anaerobic versus Aerobic Exercises

Anaerobic Exercise

- Exercise in which energy is released without the use of oxygen
- Short, intense
- Requires more power and coordination, less endurance
- *Examples:*
  Weight lifting
  Sports that require sprinting
  Calisthenics
  Squash
  Racquetball

Aerobic Exercise

- Exercise in which energy is released by using oxygen
- Continuous, rhythmic
- Requires more endurance, less power
- *Examples:*
  Brisk walking
  Jogging/running
  Swimming
  Cycling
  Inline skating

speed and power are more affected by aging than activities that require continuous exertion. However, you can improve the performance of both fast- and slow-twitch fibers with training.

Understanding the characteristics of muscle composition should help you select sports that match your abilities, identify target areas for improvement, and set realistic expectations regarding your level of performance.

Experience and Knowledge

Have you ever tried a new activity or resumed an old one after a long interval and noticed how quickly you became exhausted? While your level of conditioning has a great deal to do with how fast you tire, experience plays a large role as well. If you've had experience with a particular sport, such as swimming, you will remember proper technique and quickly regain efficiency and skill. As you use less energy per stroke, your general swimming conditioning, speed, and distance will all improve.

Similarly, if you rode a bike as a child and resume cycling in middle or late adulthood, you will use less energy than someone who has never ridden a bike. The value of experience applies to all sports and exercises. There's a strong case for again trying some sports and physical activities you participated in before, perhaps as a teenager or a young adult.

Be cautious, however, when you return to sports you played years before. Our knowledge of fitness and training and how the body reacts to exercise has increased greatly over the years, so don't practice the same training and conditioning techniques you did when you participated years ago. In the 1960s, for example, water was not freely given during training workouts, only at set times, and often it was heavily salted. Today, we do exactly the opposite. We now know that it is critical to drink water regularly during exercise and that heavily salted drinks, even sports drinks, are unnecessary. We've benefited from research and today play sports safely and confidently.

Benefits

Sports offer opportunities to participate in an activity of choice with others who enjoy the same activities and values. There are many reasons to recommend sports and recreational activities as part of a fitness program:

- Energy expended through sports improves cardiovascular endurance, strength, flexibility, balance, and motor skills and helps you to control your weight. Meanwhile, because you're also having fun, sports activities don't seem like exercise.

- Opportunities for social activities with family and friends can be planned around sports events. When you are traveling or on vacation, sports events give you access to new friends and local culture that otherwise you would not encounter.

Do You Have a Functional Limitation?

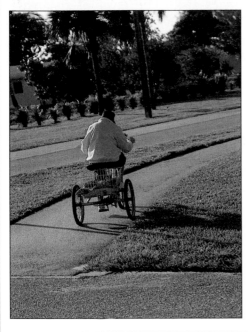

Does an injury to a bone or joint, or a functional limitation such as poor hearing or eyesight, limit your ability to participate in sports? It need not prevent you from joining in. It simply means that you must carefully consider what's involved and what's safe for you. For example, if you have a problem with your inner ear and balance, you may not want to bicycle. You could, however, ride a stationary or a three-wheel bike.

- You may become very skilled at a sport you can enjoy alone and from which you can derive great satisfaction.

- Sports activities are fun, so you are more likely to stay motivated and participate. The time flies, and you don't mind the effort. As you begin to focus on strategy and tactics, you learn to listen to your body and understand what it can and can't do.

- Sports are a healthy outlet for competition if you want to compete.

- Participation in sports activities increases self-esteem and helps with stress management. There are few greater feelings of self-satisfaction than finishing an event you never contemplated entering just a short time before. Only those who have had the satisfaction understand the exhilaration of finishing their first road races or triathlons.

- Some organizations maintain clubhouses where participants can store equipment, share information, and plan outings or trips that extend beyond the sports activities.

Risk

As we grow older, we tend to be reluctant to participate in sports because we think the risk is too high. *Risk* is a relative term. We face some risk everyday when we get in our cars, walk across a mall parking lot, or venture out to shop for groceries on an icy winter day. The risks we take daily are known to us, and because

Don't Be a Weekend Warrior

Weekend warriors jump right in with maximum effort. We're all guilty of overdoing it. What comes over us? There's nothing we can tell you about this phenomenon because we have been as guilty as you. The one thing we all must realize is that the older we are, the more severe are the consequences of "overdoing it."

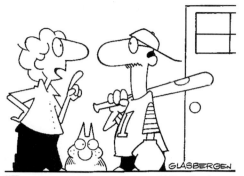

"Try to act your age, dear. What's the sense of behaving like a 15-year-old on the weekend if it makes you feel like a 150-year-old all week?"

we have negotiated them successfully for years, we regard them as relatively harmless.

Each sport, to be sure, carries risk. The level of risk varies from very low (walking or golf) to very high (inline skating or downhill skiing). The risk of injury, in general, increases with the speed of movement, risk of falling, and amount of body contact.

All risk is relative, however, and depends on the sport and on your level of skill, conditioning, and experience. Whether you choose to cycle or ski, think about what is required and use good judgment to negotiate risk and enjoy your chosen sport without harm or injury. For example, if you participate in a brisk walking program on a track at the neighborhood school, your risk of injury is low. But if you go hiking in a remote mountainous area with difficult access, your risk is much higher. Even if you are an experienced hiker who is conditioned to high altitude, has the right kind of gear, and knows the environment, you're at greater risk in the rough terrain than on the high-school track, but at lower risk than someone who is inexperienced.

Find the sport that interests you. Determine the extent to which each factor is required for participating in that sport. Evaluate your skills, resources, and experiences in each area and decide which sport is right for you.

Safety and Environmental Factors

Exercising safely is knowing and acknowledging the effects of your actions and the risks involved in the sport you choose. Concern for safety limits your participation in a sport only when you determine that the risk is greater than the benefit. For example, if you are thinking about walking through the park as you normally do, but the temperature is 5° F and the paths are icy, you may decide not to go because the risk is greater than the potential health benefits. If you live in an urban area that has a high incidence of crime, you may decide that the risk of taking a 2-mile walk is probably greater than the health benefits. Find a place that is safe to walk, like a mall, or, if you have transportation, a park in a safer neighborhood.

Here are some guidelines for participating safely in sports:

- *Weather.* Be careful if you are contemplating outdoor activities in very cold (below freezing) and windy or very hot (above 90s) and humid weather. Check the weather forecast if you're planning to be outdoors for an extended time. Dress appropriately for weather conditions. Avoid mid-day heat and use sunscreen.

- *Time of year.* The seasons vary greatly from region to region. If you are in a northern climate, you may venture outdoors to exercise in late April as the weather warms and flowers bloom. You may continue to enjoy outside exercise through the change of leaves in October. Look for indoor activities from November to March, except on warm days. If you are in a very hot cli-

Lessen the Risk: Think Ahead

- What fitness level do you need to participate?
- What motor skills do you need to participate?
- What experience and knowledge do you have?
- Is the activity high speed?
- Is there body contact or risk of falling?
- What environmental factors should you consider?

  Weather

  Terrain/altitude

- Do you have the right equipment and clothing?

mate, you may avoid outdoor activities in the summer months except early in the morning or late in the evening.

- *Time of day.* When you are venturing outside for sports activities, consider air quality—pollution from cars, pollen (if you have allergies), and ozone warnings. Early morning is often the best time of day for outdoor training. Don't walk, jog, or cycle outdoors after dark, unless you are in an off-road, lighted area. Even if you wear reflective clothing and equipment, being out on the road at night is very dangerous, and we don't recommend it for after-dark activity. Also, because night vision diminishes with age, you may be less able to see cracks and potholes in the road surface or other obstacles on the pathway.

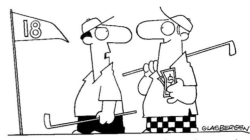

"How can you say that golf is a low-risk sport? My wallet gets injured every time I play!"

- *High altitude.* How people adjust to increases in altitude varies greatly, even among well-conditioned athletes. If you have poor health, particularly cardiac and pulmonary diseases, altitudes over 5,000 feet can contribute to acute or chronic problems. Initial symptoms of altitude sickness include shortness of breath, headaches, dizziness, and nausea. If you experience severe shortness of breath, descend immediately to lower altitudes, and if symptoms persist, seek medical attention. Usually, minor symptoms of breathlessness disappear within a day or two. To prevent altitude sickness while you adjust to higher elevations, reduce the intensity of your activity, ensure adequate rest, and avoid alcohol. Most important, if you haven't exercised before, don't start when you move to a high altitude but wait until you return to an altitude to which you're accustomed. Don't decide during the first week of summer vacation in the mountains at 8,000 feet that you're going to start jogging because you're inspired by the surroundings. Such an imprudent choice could cause severe health problems.

- *Location.* If you're not familiar with an area, ask about locations or facilities where you can participate in sports activities. Call a parks and recreation department, health/fitness club, or YMCA to learn about recreational facilities in the area. Hotel concierges or health club managers can advise you as well. If you decide to go off road, pick a terrain that fits your experience and conditioning level. In wooded areas or state parks, take a trail map and compass unless the trails are clearly marked. Be aware of traffic, road hazards, and unleashed dogs. Always carry identification with you. Do not wear jewelry or carry valuables. Take 25¢ or 50¢ with you so that you can make a phone call if you need help or if the weather changes and you need a ride home.

- *Protective gear.* Learn a lesson from the pros. They wear the best protective gear available. Choose appropriate protective gear for your sport. Wear a helmet if you are biking or skating and knee, elbow, and hand pads if you are skating outside. Goggles or protective eyewear are important if you are biking, swimming, or playing racquetball.

Hydration

Seventy percent of your body weight is water. Meeting the body's need for water is critical. The body requires approximately 2 to 3 quarts of water each day to function properly. You get some of the daily requirement for water from the foods you eat, but more than half the requirement comes from beverages. Milk, juices, sodas, coffee, tea, and alcoholic and other beverages all provide water. Beverages that contain caffeine and colas, coffee, tea, and alcohol act as diuretics and remove water from the body by increasing urination. If you don't replace lost fluid, you become dehydrated.

You lose water all the time through breathing, urination, and sweating from ordinary daily activity. If you are physically active, you lose more water through sweating, and your need for fluids increases. The best source of fluid is plain water. Numerous sports drinks are available that replace minerals lost through sweating, but you should use them only for long endurance events such as 20-mile bike rides, 6.2-mile runs, and marathons. For most people, these drinks don't offer any benefit over plain water. They contain additional calories (which you may not want or need), and they cost more than water.

How much and how often should you drink? Drink water before, during, and after engaging in physical activity, especially

---

Factors That Predispose to Dehydration

- *High-intensity activity.* The more intense the activity, the more water you need.

- *Warm and hot air temperature.* The higher the temperature, the more water you need.

- *Humidity.* You need more water at any temperature in conditions of very low or very high humidity.

- *Altitude.* The higher the altitude, the lower the humidity. Therefore, the higher you go, the more frequently you need water.

- *Alcohol and caffeine consumption.* Alcohol and caffeine pull water out of cells and dehydrate the body. If you drink alcohol after a workout, drink two large containers of water first.

- *Drugs.* Some prescription drugs, such as diuretics, antihistamines, and antidepressants, have dehydrating side effects. If you are taking diuretics, consult your physician before exercising heavily.

sports activities that last longer than 1 hour. Drink 1 cup of water every 10 to 20 minutes if you're participating in vigorous activity and sweating heavily. You may need to drink more in extremely hot and humid conditions or at high altitudes.

Choosing the Exercise That's Right for You

With such a wide range of sports and recreational activities, how does one choose which ones to pursue? The first rule in choosing a sport or an activity is to do something you like. Whatever you do, you should enjoy it. If you don't know what type of exercise you like, you may have to try several to find out. If you've never exercised or played sports, we recommend trying several. You may be surprised how many of them you enjoy. Don't be caught in the trap of thinking the harder the exercise, the better. Running is not always better than walking. Be sure to try one type of sport long enough to be sure you like it, especially if it involves investing in special shoes, clothing, or equipment. Don't make the mistake of deciding that an exercise is for you based on 5 minutes on a tread-mill, step machine, or rowing machine. Try an activity for at least 20 to 30 minutes to see if it's comfortable. Remember, you're committing yourself to exercising at least three times a week for the rest of your life, so you want to choose an activity that won't bore you. Thousands of exercise machines are gathering dust in people's basements because the individuals who bought them discovered too late that the machines didn't interest them. We don't discourage you from buying equipment; we want to be sure you enjoy yourself, because staying active is a lifetime commitment that's easier to keep when you're enjoying yourself.

If you buy an exercise machine, there are ways to counter the monotony and boredom of repetitious exercises. If you exercise alone, listen to music or sports on the radio. Position the machine in front of the television and watch the news or your favorite show. Some people read while they're using stationary bicycles or step machines, but we realize that the knack of reading and exercising at the same time is unusual.

Individual exercises are often more enjoyable when people have companions. You can make a pact with a friend or your spouse to walk or bicycle together every day. The daily walk is a good way to spend time together and provide mutual support for new health endeavors. Team sports likewise enjoy a large following because they provide similar opportunities for society and mutual support.

Vary your activities to help break the monotony of repetitive exercise and enhance your enjoyment of exercise. You might walk with one friend on Monday, bike with another on Wednesday, and swim with a third friend on Friday. Or you can walk twice during the work week and bicycle through your neighborhood on weekends, or rent a canoe at a local lake and paddle around for an hour or more. Every kind of exercise counts toward an active life-style.

Walking

Walking is the most popular exercise, the simplest to do, and the least expensive. If you haven't been very active, walking is a good way to start your exercise program. A model walking program is described on pp. 22–24. Walking can form the core component of your program, and as you improve your fitness level, it can evolve into a recreational sport.

Walking Events

You may enjoy walking so much that after a while, you may enter walking events. Walking has become a popular recreational sport. There are walking clubs, competitive walking races, "fun walks," and fund-raising walks for charities. Race walking, orienteering, volksmarches, and hiking are all variations of walking.

Race Walking. Elite race walkers can move nearly as fast as runners (6 to 8 mph). If you are interested in race walking, you must learn the proper technique. Race walking is not difficult to learn, but you would probably benefit by taking a class or working with a coach. It takes effort and concentration to synchronize the vigorous arm movements and accentuated hip movements required to increase your speed and lengthen your stride for race walking. We've all seen pictures of the "race walker's wiggle." Correct walking technique decreases the risk of injury due to the accentuated hip movement and the greater stress placed on the legs.

Orienteering. This sport combines the physical skills of walking or running with the intellectual skills of reading a compass and map. Point-to-point or cross-country orienteering is the official competition of the International Orienteering Federation. Courses are graded so that beginners and accomplished practitioners alike

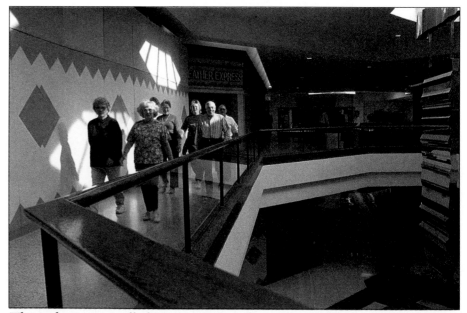

The indoor, controlled environment of a mall provides an ideal setting for walking.

can participate with equal challenge. Distances range from 2 to 12 km.

Volksmarches. "People walking" originated in Germany. Volksmarches are noncompetitive events for walkers. These outings are open to people of all ages and physical abilities. The American Volksport Association has more 550 chapters nationwide that promote walking for fun and fitness.

Rugged Trail Walking. Hiking is another variation of walking. Depending on the condition of the trail, incline, and altitude, hiking may require a high level of fitness. Additionally, you must be prepared to deal with changing environmental conditions (rain, snow, falling temperatures), especially if you are planning an extended hiking trip.

Running

Running is an excellent form of exercise. It is one of the most efficient forms of aerobic training and burns a high number of calories per hour. When performed properly, running is extremely safe. A recent research study showed that middle-aged or older people who run have fewer joint and tendon problems and less disability than nonrunners. Running requires a moderate level of aerobic fitness, so if you have been very inactive, you may want to start with the walking program described on pp. 22–24 and then progress to running after you've improved your level of fitness.

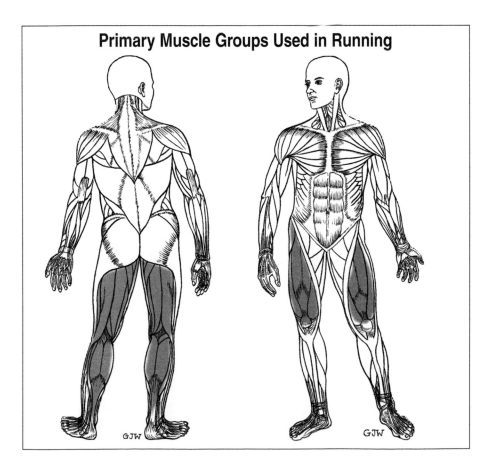

Primary Muscle Groups Used in Running

Calorie Expenditure for Strolling, Walking, Jogging, and Running

	Pace (mph)	Time for 1 Mile (min)	Calories Burned (kcal/hr)*
Strolling	2	30	196
Walking	3.5	17	330
Jogging	5.5	10	690
Running	7	8.5	894

*This example assumes a body weight of 175 pounds. If you weigh less, you'll burn fewer calories at the same pace; if you weigh more, you'll burn more.

A Running Program

- *Equipment and clothing.* Because running is a high-impact activity, it's imperative to have a good pair of running shoes right from the start. The right shoes reduce the chances of injury to the bones, tendons, and muscles of the feet, lower legs, lower back, and hips.

- *Place.* Most people run outdoors, but you can also run on an indoor track or treadmill. Running on a machine is monotonous, and boredom can become a deterrent. When you run outdoors, a track is a good place to start because if you get too tired, you're not too far from your starting place. If you run on the road, avoid heavy traffic and be sure that there is always a place where you can get off the road quickly if a car comes too close.

- *Technique.* Warm up and cool down for at least 5 minutes before and after you run to avoid soreness and injury. Start with a 3- to 5-minute walk at a brisk pace to warm up. Always stretch after you run.

  After 5 minutes of brisk walking, start your run at a pace that is just a little faster than your brisk walk. Increase your pace as your conditioning improves. You should be working at the 15 to 17 level (hard) on the Borg Scale of Perceived Exertion (see p. 14), and you will breathe somewhat heavily. Expect to break out in a sweat.

  Stop after 15 minutes, even if you feel you could go farther. Walk for 5 minutes and then stretch the muscles in your lower extremities. Stretching after running is essential to avoid shortening the muscles and pain and injury.

- *Schedule.* Begin your running program with a goal of running for 15 minutes three times a week. Increase this time by 5 minutes per day every 2 weeks. Your final goal should be to run 30 minutes or more three times a week. Once you reach this level, run 4 days a week for 6 weeks, at which point you should be ready to increase your schedule to running for 30 minutes, 5 days per week.

- You may find you can advance more quickly than we have suggested. However, don't hurry to increase either your pace or your distance. If you advance your training too quickly, you're more likely to injure yourself.

Running Events

Hundreds of special running events are advertised in the back of running magazines and in the sports pages of local newspapers. These unique races are fun because there is usually a carnival atmosphere around the event that lasts from a day or two before the race to the day after. The following events draw participants from all over their regions and beyond:

- *Pikes Peak Run (Colorado).* Participants run up Pikes Peak (elevation, 14,110 feet) or they run both up and down.

- *Bay to Breakers (San Francisco).* This 7-plus mile course follows the hills of the peninsula through the streets of San

---

Common Distances for Walking and Running Events

- 1-mile "fun run" or walk
- 5 km (equals 3.2 miles)
- 10 km (equals 6.2 miles)
- 15 km (equals 9.4 miles)
- A half marathon is 13.1 miles
- A marathon is 26.2 miles
- A century race is 100 miles

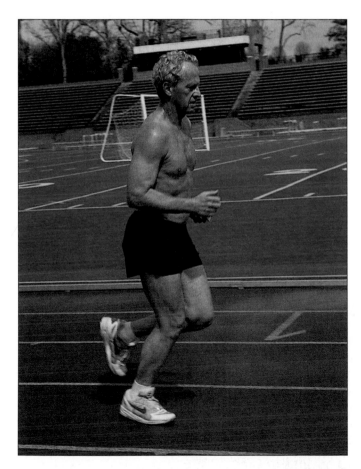
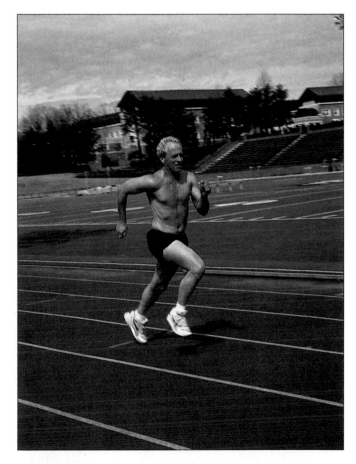

Running Posture and Pace

For paces up to 5.5 miles per hour (10-minute mile), run with your body erect, your arms bent at 90° angles, and your hands cupped loosely. Swing your arms slightly with each stride.

As you increase your pace to 7 miles per hour (8-minute mile), lean your body into the run, close your fists loosely, bend your arms, and swing them with each stride.

Demands of Athletic Activities

Activity	Level of Impact	Repeated Motion	Lateral Motion	Risk of Sprain
Walking	Low	Moderate/high	Low	Low
Running	Moderate/high	Moderate/high	Low/moderate	Low
Tennis	Moderate/high	Moderate/high	High	Moderate
Basketball	High	High	High	High
Aerobics/dance	Low/moderate	High	Low/moderate	Low/moderate

Francisco and Golden Gate Park to the ocean. Groups of walkers and joggers dress in costumes and form centipedes.

- *River to River Run (Southern Illinois).* Relay teams of eight people run 80 miles from the Mississippi River to the Ohio River.

- *Peach Tree Road Race.* Held on the Fourth of July in Atlanta, Georgia, this race draws one of the largest group of participants in the world.

- *New York Marathon.* Held every fall, this 26.2-mile race is run through all three boroughs of New York City.

- *Boston Marathon.* One of the oldest and most prestigious road races, this marathon is held on Patriot's Day every spring and is a social and sports event like no other.

- *Ironman Triathlon.* Held on the Big Island of Hawaii every year in October, this race includes an ocean swim of 2.4 miles, a bike race of 112 miles, and a full marathon of 26.2 miles. Many consider the Ironman to be the ultimate test of courage and conditioning. The entire week in which it is held is filled with festivities and fun for participants and their families. Many people over 50 and some in their 70s participate.

Selecting Shoes for Sports Activities

Different activities put different demands on the foot. It is important to select shoes that can meet the demands of the specific activity you are performing. Athletic shoes are designed with features that withstand the stresses of different movements required by different sports:

- *Impact.* The amount of force under the foot when it hits the ground

- *Repeated motion.* The amount of repeated movement of the foot

- *Lateral motion.* The amount of side-to-side movement

- *Risk of ankle sprain.* The risk of twisting the ankle during an activity

Characteristics of Athletic Shoes

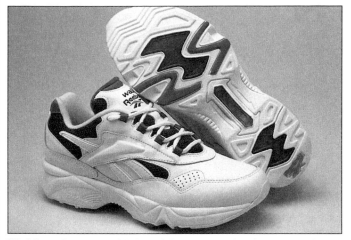

Walking shoes need lightweight construction for repeated motion, a roomy toe box, and a beveled heel to accommodate the heel strike. Extra flexibility in the forefoot makes for an easier pushoff.

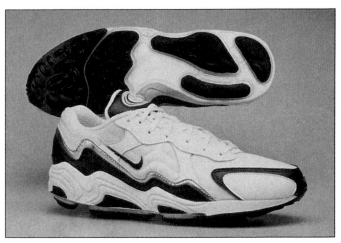

Running shoes need extra cushioning in the heel and forefoot. Some runners need a shoe with a stiffer material on the inside of the heel to help control pronation (the foot leans inward).

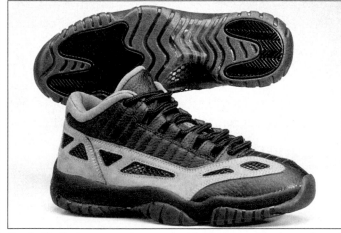

Basketball shoes need a good midsole for cushioning, a broad base of support in the outsole for stability, and additional support, from a stiff upper. Basketball shoes need added ankle support.

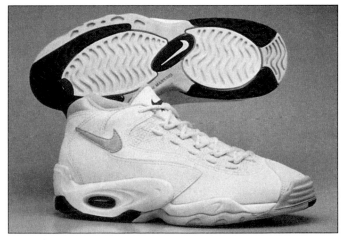

Tennis shoes need adequate cushioning in the midsole to absorb the shock in both the heel and forefoot. A durable outsole is needed to resist the wear from starting and stopping. A special toe cap can limit abrasion from the toe drag that occurs during the serve. Tennis shoes also need a broad base of support for side-to-side movements and extra ankle support.

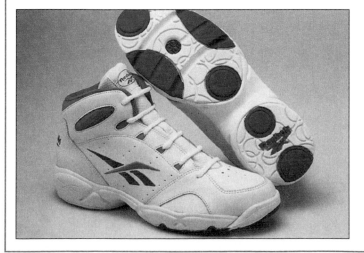

Aerobic workout shoes need plenty of cushioning in the midsole, especially in the forefoot where the impact is concentrated. Good forefoot flexibility and a broad base of support are also important.

You Need New Shoes When:

- Tread pattern is worn
- Heel support wears on either side
- Toe box is thin or worn
- Your feet feel tired after activity, especially in the arches
- You feel pain in the shins, knees, and hips after activity

Buying Athletic Shoes

- Shop for shoes at the end of the day when your feet are likely to be larger.

- Take along the type of socks that you'll be wearing with the shoes.

- Select a shoe with a removable insole if you'll be wearing orthotic devices.

- Spread and wiggle your toes to be sure there is ample room in the toe box. Your longest toe should be about a thumbnail's width from the end of the shoe.

- Lace your shoes and check the space between the lace holes across the tongue of the shoe. There should be about 1 inch of space for appropriate fit. Less space means you don't have room for adjustments like tightening, and more than an inch may mean the shoes are too narrow or tight.

- Stand on your tiptoes to be sure the heels don't slip.

- Check the arch of the shoe. It should support the arch of your foot.

- Walk or jog around the store to test for comfort and cushioning, preferably on a hard surface instead of carpet.

- If you find a shoe that works well for you, stay with that model. Buy an extra pair for future use or to alternate with another pair. If your feet perspire heavily, alternate pairs each time you run to allow one pair to air and dry thoroughly. Two

Do You Have Special Footwear Requirements?

Pay attention to how your shoes wear to determine if you have special footwear requirements. Place your shoes side by side on a flat surface.

- If your forefoot and heel are perfectly aligned with the ground and lower leg when in motion, your shoes will wear evenly and sit relatively straight. You don't need specific footwear stability or motion-control features.

- Do you overpronate? If your foot leans excessively inward, your shoes will tilt to the inside. The outer side of your foot hits the ground first and rolls inward with each stride. You will need shoes that provide extra stability and motion-control features.

- Do you underpronate? If your foot leans excessively outward, your shoes tilt to the outside. The outer side of your foot hits the ground first and continues to roll outward to push off. You don't need any additional stability or motion-control features, but durable cushioning is essential because the impact forces are concentrated on the side of the foot.

pairs of shoes worn on alternate days will last more than twice as long as one pair of shoes worn every day.

Gearing Up and Dressing Up for Outdoor Activity

Gear

If you're hiking or biking in the woods or going on a long excursion, be prepared for unexpected weather or other emergencies. Think about the planned location and terrain and, if appropriate, pack a waterproof tote containing all or some of the following items:

- First-aid kit (clean, dry bandages; elastic bandages; antibiotic ointment)
- Medical emergency information
- Matches (in waterproof container)
- Compass
- Map or trail guide
- Rain gear
- Pocket knife
- Flashlight
- Water container
- Sunscreen/lip protection
- Insect repellent
- Whistle
- Snacks
- Wristwatch
- Personal identification/phone numbers
- Twine/small rope
- Blanket

Clothes

- If the air is warm, dress in loose-fitting, light-colored, quick-drying fabrics. Don't forget your sunglasses and a sun-shedding hat that won't blow away.
- If the air is cold, dress in lightweight layers. Insulated air trapped beneath several thin layers of clothing keeps you warmer than a single thick layer. You can add or subtract layers as needed.
- If you are likely to get wet, take special precautions, especially if the weather is cold.

The 4 Ls for Outdoor Wear

- Light colored
- Loose fitting
- Light weight
- Layered

---

1 + 2 + 3 Layers for Comfort Outdoors

- *Layer 1.* Avoid wearing cotton or wool, which absorb perspiration and keep it next to your skin so that you feel clammy or cold. Polypropylene fabric wicks perspiration away from the skin or toward an outer layer of clothing.

- *Layer 2.* Add a layer of wool or synthetic fabric for warmth. Keep it loose for freedom of movement.

- *Layer 3.* An outer shell can keep wind and water out and inner layers dry. Rainwear should have latex-rubber gaskets at neck, wrists, and ankles to prevent cold water from penetrating to skin and clothing. Front zippers can be a source of leaks, so consider a pullover jacket with a hood.

Calories Expended During Outdoor Bicycling*

Speed (mph)	Calories (per min)	(per hr)
5.5	5.3	318
9.5	8.3	498
13.1	13.0	780

*Estimates are for someone who weighs 175 pounds.

Bicycling

Bicycling is an excellent and safe way to be physically active. Bicycling burns calories more efficiently than walking. Biking about 3 miles on flat terrain with no wind expends the same number of calories as walking 1 mile.

There are numerous advantages to both indoor and outdoor bicycling. Either type of exercise is an excellent choice if you have bone or joint problems that weight-bearing activity such as walking or jogging could aggravate. Outdoor bicycling can be an inexpensive and fun method of transportation, and it allows you to enjoy the environment and participate in special events and competitions.

Bicycles

Modern bicycles are lightweight and have a range of gears, which allows you to pedal comfortably with relatively constant effort over varying terrains and conditions. A high-quality bicycle costs between $300 and $600. It's worth buying a bicycle at a bicycle specialty shop because the bike can be fitted properly to your body. An informed salesperson can answer your questions and help you select a bike to meet your specific needs. Because a bicycle is an investment, always lock your bike when you leave it outdoors. There are several types of bicycles on the market.

Bicycle Maintenance

How well you take care of your bike will determine how long it will last and how much enjoyment you'll get out of it.

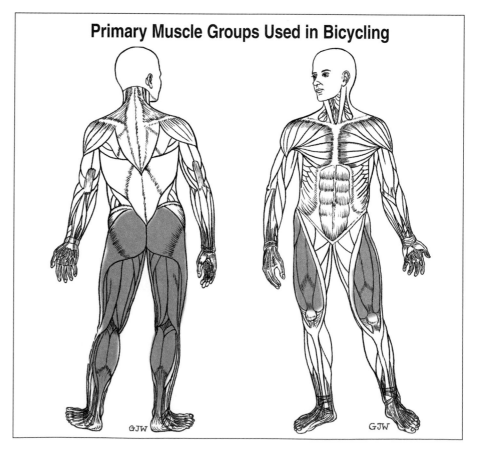

Primary Muscle Groups Used in Bicycling

Some Contemporary Bicycles

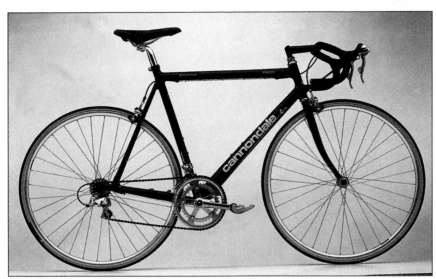

Racing bikes have lightweight, thin frames and wheels, no fenders, and dropped handlebars. They are designed for use only on paved surfaces. They usually have 10, 12, 15, 18, or 21 speeds.

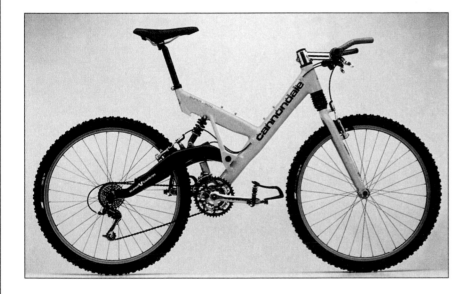

All-terrain bikes (mountain bikes) have sturdier frames and considerably wider tires to absorb the shock of riding on rough surfaces. These bikes can have as many as 15 to 21 speeds. Whereas the racing bike is designed for high speeds, the mountain bike is designed for hill climbing and for riding over obstacles. Mountain bikes also can be ridden on paved surfaces and bike paths.

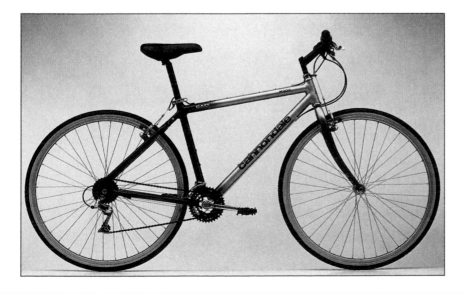

Hybrid bikes look a little like mountain bikes but have old-fashioned upright handlebars. This handlebar configuration provides comfortable riding in an upright position. The hybrid bike has a frame that is a cross between the mountain bike and the racing bike. Its tubing is intermediate in strength and weight, and its tires are intermediate in size. The hybrid bike has become popular for people who wish to ride off road, on paths, and on roadways.

Adjusting Your Bicycle for Proper Fit

Just as your shoes must fit properly, your bike must also fit your body so that you can exercise comfortably and safely.

Handlebar tilt. The bottom portion of the handlebars should be parallel to the ground or sloping slightly from parallel.

Handlebar height. This is a matter of personal preference.

Saddle height. With the ball of your foot on the pedal, your knee should be slightly bent at the bottom of each pedal stroke. If you are rocking your hips from side to side to reach the bottom of the pedal stroke, the saddle is too high.

If you ride with a saddle that's too high, you won't be able to spin the pedals easily. This position may feel good at first because it allows you to use the same muscles you use for walking, but, with time, you'll experience pain.

If you ride with a saddle that's too low, you won't get the maximum benefit from your leg muscles. You'll be unable to spin the pedals at a fast cadence, and the stress placed on your knees may result in injury.

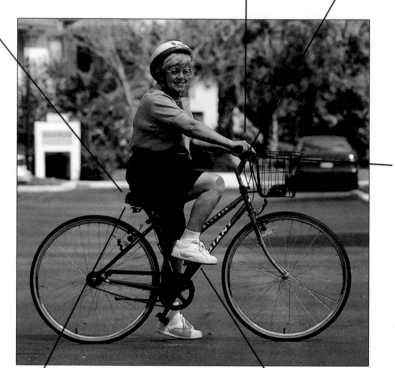

Handlebar reach. Your distance from the handlebars is critical for control. Brake levers should be placed where you can feel comfortable grabbing them from above. Looking down toward the front wheel while you are seated, the handlebar should conceal the front wheel axle.

Foot position. Place the ball of your foot directly atop the pedal spindle. This position allows the two calf muscles in each leg to help you point your toes downward and move the pedal through its range of motion.

Saddle tilt. Most cyclists prefer the saddle to be perfectly parallel to the ground. Riding with the nose of the saddle angled up is uncomfortable. A saddle with the nose angled down forces you to lean too far forward into the handlebars. If you feel you want your saddle pointing downward, the saddle is probably too high. Lower it until you feel comfortable with it parallel to the ground.

Toe clips. Toe clips are appropriate for long-distance touring or racing bikes but not for mountain bikes or all-terrain bikes. Toe clips come in small, medium, and large sizes. Look for toe clips that snugly hold your foot in the proper position without sliding forward on the pedals.

Chain. Keep the chin clean. A dirty chain causes premature wear and makes pedaling more difficult. Have the chain checked at a bike shop if it stretches and begins to skip when you change gears or climb hills.

Tire pressure. Check your tires before each ride and inflate them to the desired air pressure. This is usually printed on the tire. Adequately inflated tires reduce the risk of flats.

Brakes. Check the brakes before each ride. Brakes should be firm. Replace brake pads when they wear.

Other Bicycling Gear

Here are some things you need in addition to a bike to make bicycling safe, comfortable, and enjoyable:

Shoes. If you're not racing or using toe clips, select a soft-upper, comfortable shoe. The sole should be firm enough for efficient transfer of power to the peddle but flexible enough for you to walk on it. You can purchase racing shoes that clip directly onto the pedals or use toe clamps. Clips and toe clamps, however, are not mandatory and can increase the risk of falling when you come to a stop.

Biking shorts. Lycra biking shorts are tight yet stretch with your movements. A pad in the crotch provides cushioning, absorbs perspiration, and reduces chafing. If you are riding for leisure rather than long distances, wear any shorts that are comfortable. Some touring shorts that look like regular shorts with pockets are specially constructed for biking.

Shirt. Racing suits of Lycra or a synthetic fabric fit snugly to minimize wind resistance and allow your body to breathe. There is usually a pocket on the back of the shirt for carrying food and water bottles.

Helmet. Mandatory! Head injuries from falls account for the most serious biking injuries.

Gloves. Although not required, padded cycling gloves provide cushioning and reduce pressure on the heel of the palm. Pressure can cause numbness and nerve injury. Gloves also protect your hands in a fall.

Water bottle. You lose a great deal of water during biking, so you should buy at least one water bottle to mount on the frame or handlebars. People who compete usually mount two water bottles and carry a third in the back pocket of a racing shirt.

Eyewear. Bicycling eyewear has clear plastic lenses that wrap around the eyes to protect them from flying rocks, dirt, and insects.

Car rack. If you want to transport your bike out of the city for a ride in the country, go to a cycling event, or take it with you on vacation, you'll want a car rack. Car racks are easy to install and use.

Selecting and Fitting Helmets

- *Size.* Buy the smallest size that fits comfortably. The helmet should touch your head at the crown, sides, front, and back.

- *Straps.* Independently adjustable straps and quick-release buckles are recommended. Straps should meet just below the hinge of the jaw, in front of the ear. The chin strap should feel tight when you open your mouth.

- *Ventilation.* Select a helmet that allows air to flow through vents under the rim to dispel heat.

- *Standards.* Look for the American National Standards Institute (ANSI) and Snell Foundation stickers for voluntary compliance with industry standards.

Bicycling Skills

Beginning bicycling requires a minimum fitness and skill level.

- *Pedaling and spinning.* Pedal in a circular, spinning motion, pulling up on one pedal as you push down on the other. Try not to think of pedaling as a push-pull motion. Concentrate on the "roundness" of your pedaling. In the beginning, a cadence (or rhythm) of 60 to 70 revolutions per minute will probably work best for you. You can find this cadence by shifting gears. Over time, try to develop your legs so they can spin comfortably at a brisk cadence of around 80 to 90 revolutions per minute. Shift to a lower gear if it helps you to spin. Don't pedal too slowly because your legs will tire more quickly. If you pedal too fast, you'll spend too much energy just fanning the pedals. Keep your cadence smooth and steady by choosing the right gear for the terrain.

- *Shifting gears.* Practice shifting the gears under light pedal pressure. Go to a parking lot where you're free of distractions to practice until shifting feels natural to you. Learn which shifter controls the front or rear derailleur. Look down and see the chain move (derail) from one chainwheel or cog to the others. Practice squeezing the brake gently. Note which brake controls which wheel and apply the rear wheel brake first. If you apply the front wheel brake first, you may fly over the handlebars. Use middle gears at first. Don't try to increase your distance or time too rapidly.

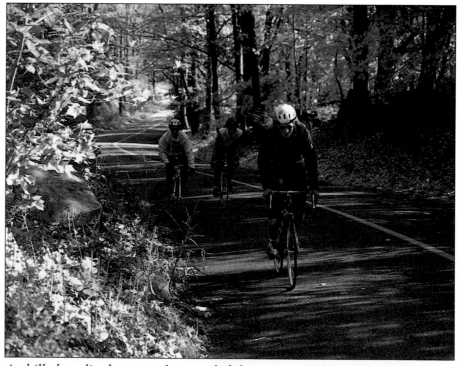

A skilled cyclist knows when to shift by paying attention to slight variations in cadence and looking ahead at the terrain.

- *Pace.* Start slowly on a flat course. Warm up by turning the pedals easily for 5 to 10 minutes to increase blood flow and prevent straining your muscles. Cool down the same way to prevent muscle cramps. Ride 15 to 30 minutes three times per week, and increase this time by 5 minutes every 2 weeks. Your goal is to ride 30 or more minutes four or five times each week. After 6 to 8 weeks you may begin to include modest hill riding in your schedule. However, the hills should never be so steep as to require your lowest gear or your maximum exertion. Remember, the less wind resistance, the easier it is to peddle.

- *Cycling form.* Develop your cycling form, handling skills, and balance. Concentrate on your position and cadence. Practice a brisk cadence and, for now, stay out of high gears (the gears that make peddling harder).

Precautions

Bicycling is one of the safest sports, but you should be aware of the risks:

- Because of the air circulating around you when cycling outdoors, you may not be aware that you are sweating and becoming dehydrated. Carry a water bottle, and drink water frequently—about every 30 minutes. Dehydration is the most common but preventable reason for cycling fatigue.

- Keep your bike in good repair. Learn proper maintenance and make adjustments or repairs immediately on returning from your ride so you won't need to delay your next excursion.

- If you ride at sundown or dawn, install an appropriate lighting system and wear reflective clothing. There are advantages to riding at these times—clean, cool, calm air and minimal traffic. However, the light at these times of day is often deceiving, and riding on the roads is more dangerous.

- Wear a helmet and eyewear for protection from the sun, flying objects, and irritants.

- Use mirrors to allow you to observe overtaking vehicles without having to turn your head.

- If you are riding for an hour or more, take some bananas or high-calorie bars to replenish your energy stores. Don't take candy or foods that are high in sugar or sucrose. Sugar is the least sustaining form of carbohydrate or energy food.

Hiking and Biking Etiquette

Hiking

- Travel in groups of four or fewer.
- Hike in single file down the center of the trail.

- Don't contribute to erosion by hiking off the trail.

- Take rest stops only in areas where your presence won't damage vegetation.

- Carry out all that you carry in.

- Pick up litter when you find it.

- Use established latrines when available.

Off-Road Biking

- Ride only on open, designated trails.

- Respect and abide by all trail closures, private property notices and fences, and all requirements for use permits and authorization.

- Don't skid tires or ride on ground that is rain soaked and easily scarred.

- Yield the right of way to other nonmotorized recreationalists.

- Use caution when overtaking another person (especially equestrians), and make your presence known well in advance.

- Don't disturb wildlife and livestock.

- Don't litter.

Bicycling Events

Bike races around the country vary considerably. "Citizen races" are for the casual racer. To race in competitive events, you must be a member of the United States Cycling Federation. You can get a membership application at any bike shop. Most cyclists who compete join a team for strategic advantages. Strategy during a bike race is one of the most enjoyable aspects of the competition.

Swimming

Swimming is an excellent sport for overall conditioning and for keeping a variety of muscles strong. As a survival skill, swimming also allows you to participate confidently in numerous other recreational activities such as sailing, water skiing, canoeing, and scuba diving. Proficient swimmers may participate in water aerobics or water games.

If you didn't learn to swim as a child, it's not too late to learn. Many people in their 50s and 60s take swimming lessons for the first time in their lives. The principal disadvantage of swimming is that you need a pool within a convenient distance. Schools, universities, hotels, recreation centers, YMCAs, YWCAs, and JCCAs are likely to have public facilities. If you travel frequently for business, swimming is an excellent sport because most hotels have pools.

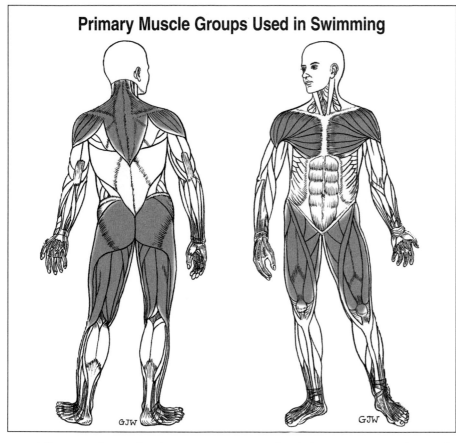

Primary Muscle Groups Used in Swimming

The number of calories you expend while swimming depends on what stroke you use, how fast you swim, your swimming skills, and your body composition. A poor swimmer is less efficient and burns more calories than a skilled swimmer. Women burn fewer calories than men because they have more body fat (which contributes to buoyancy in the water). Water buoyancy reduces your apparent body weight by 10 percent of your actual body weight.

Swimming Gear

In addition to a swimsuit, you might consider the following equipment:

- *Swim cap*. To keep your hair relatively dry and out of your face
- *Goggles*. To protect your eyes from chlorine in pool water and from debris in open water and to allow you to see under water
- *Waterproof stopwatch*. To time your workouts
- *Kickboard*. To support your upper body while kicking
- *Hand paddles*. To increase arm and shoulder strength
- *Swim fins*. To increase ankle and leg strength
- *Pull-buoy*. To support your feet while using only your arms

Tips for Swimming

- Feeling anxious or afraid of the water is the greatest problem most beginning swimmers must overcome. It's important to

Advantages of Swimming

- Uses most major muscle groups
- Provides greater upper body exercise than walking, jogging, or cycling
- Reduces the risk of stress fractures (swimming is a nonimpact and nonweight-bearing exercise)
- Burns a moderate amount of calories and aids in weight control
- Improves cardiovascular conditioning
- Allows participation at various levels of skill

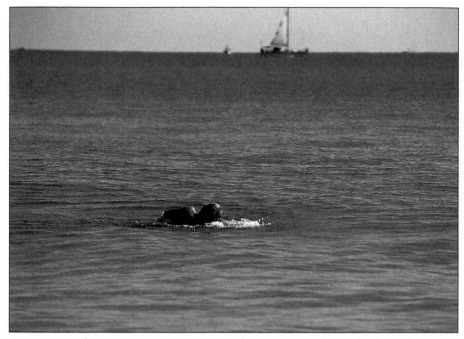

A warm, calm ocean invites practiced swimmers. Stay close to shore to avoid currents and sudden changes in water temperature.

learn to relax in the water, immersing yourself in it and moving through it. Trying to stay on top of the water tires you and makes you feel tense.

- Take lessons to learn to swim correctly. Group and private lessons are usually available through the YMCA, the YWCA, a city recreational center, or a school.

- Swim in a pool that has a comfortable water temperature. Cool water can contribute to stiffness, especially if you have arthritis. Get wet gradually to help your body adjust to the cooler water temperature.

- Learn to float face down and practice floating on your back so you know you can rest any time you need to.

- Learn to feel comfortable with your face in the water. Submerge with your eyes open. Wear goggles if the chlorine bothers your eyes.

- Practice bobbing to learn to control your breathing.

- Take time to do a few easy stretches before and after your swim. Flexibility is necessary for making full strokes and for relaxation.

- Be courteous to other swimmers if you are sharing lanes in a lap pool.

- If you have an allergy to chlorine in pool water or you develop one, use goggles, a nose clip, or a mask to protect your eyes and nose. Alternatively, find a pool that uses less harsh chemicals.

Precautions

- Be aware of the depth of the water and any potential hazards before going in. Know where the pool ladder or steps are. Swimming in open water has its own set of risks, including rocks, pollution, currents, and sudden changes in water temperature.

- Never swim alone, regardless of your skill level.

- The injury rate for recreational swimming is very low. Occasionally, pain occurs from the abnormal stresses of strokes and kicking. Vary your strokes to avoid pain from overusing joints in the foot, knee, or shoulder.

- Pool chemicals can irritate and dry the skin. Shower immediately after swimming with soap and water and apply a moisturizing lotion to your skin to prevent excessive drying.

- Wear goggles to prevent irritating the lining of your eyes. Goggles should fit properly and be comfortable.

- Infection of the ear canal—swimmer's ear (otitis externa)—is caused by excessive pool water in the ear canal, which provides a hospitable alkaline environment for bacterial growth. In most cases, over-the-counter drops containing acetic acid will cure the infection. If pain persists, ask your physician for prescription medication.

- Although you are surrounded by water, you still need to replace lost fluid during long swims. Because your perspiration is being washed away and your skin is being cooled by the water, you aren't aware of being dehydrated. Take your water bottle to the pool with you if there is no water fountain close by, and drink as with any other workout.

Swimming Events

If you want to participate in swimming events, numerous programs are available through the YMCA, the YWCA, or JCCAs. Most cities have a masters swimming program that organizes competitions by ability levels and age groups.

Dance and Other Movement Sports

Dancing for fitness has become more popular in the past 10 years. Popular forms of fitness dancing include jazz, aerobic dancing, and step aerobic dancing. Ballroom dancing, square dancing, and line dancing are also excellent and fun forms of aerobic exercise. The fitness and skill level required to participate varies from minimal

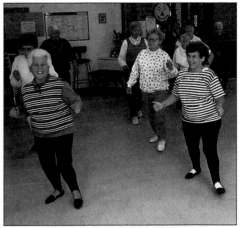

Line dancing requires coordination, rhythm, and a sense of fun.

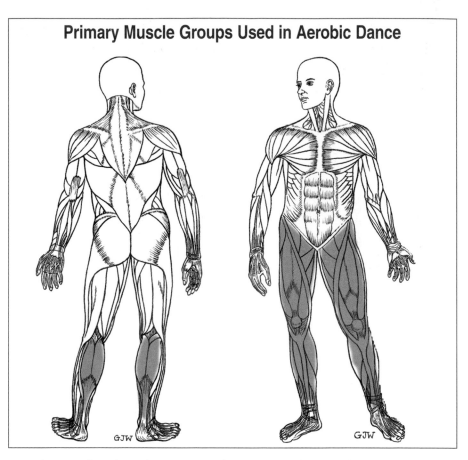

Primary Muscle Groups Used in Aerobic Dance

to advanced. Several programs have been designed specifically for older people and those with chronic diseases.

For many people, aerobics dance classes provide opportunities for exercising with a group of people. You're less likely to miss a session if you enjoy the fellowship of the group. A trained fitness instructor usually leads the group in a series of dance steps set to music. Dance classes are usually offered at health/fitness centers, YMCAs, and recreation centers, and there is a fee to

Benefits of Dance Exercise

- Uses large muscle groups of legs and burns calories
- Improves aerobic fitness
- Strengthens leg muscles and bones
- Increases flexibility
- Improves coordination and balance
- Provides social support and motivation (group classes)

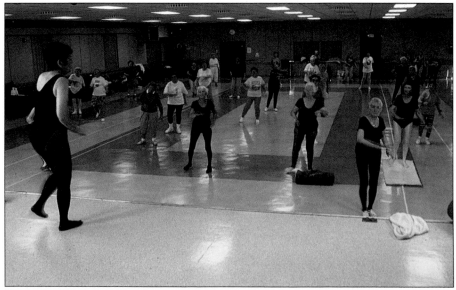

Low-impact step aerobics are safe for almost everyone.

Do You Want to Improve Your Balance?

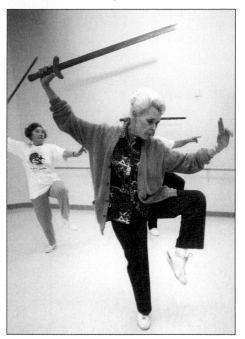

T'ai-chi quan (pronounced tie chee qwan), an individual movement sport, is rapidly gaining in popularity. This centuries-old martial art form enhances balance and body awareness. T'ai-chi involves repetitive movements and, if practiced regularly, can increase respiratory fitness and balance. It has been shown to reduce the frequency of falls in older people. T'ai-chi must be taught by a certified instructor, but once you learn the movements, you can practice anywhere—in your backyard or living room, at the beach, or in the woods. People who perform these types of routines say they also reduce stress and promote relaxation.

cover the expense of the instructor and use of the facility. If you don't want to spend the money for dance classes, you can tune in to a dance class on television or purchase a videotape for use at your convenience. Most videos are inexpensive ($9 to $15). A disadvantage of videos is that you may become bored with the same routine. Alternating between an organized class and a home video is a good plan.

Dancing Gear

The only equipment you need for aerobic dance is proper footwear. Aerobic dance shoes have a strong heel support and a smooth sole to help prevent falls. If you want to participate in step aerobics, you may want to purchase a small plastic platform costing less than $40.

Benefits of Skating

- Uses large muscle groups of the legs and buttocks
- Burns significant number of calories
- Improves cardiovascular fitness
- Build strength in leg and hip muscles and bones

Precautions

- The impact associated with dance movements varies. Most moves in dance aerobics result in an impact force of one to three times your body weight. The impact force of step aerobics is approximately two times your body weight. Avoid step aerobics if you have any problems with your knee or ankle joints or if your coordination or balance is poor. High-impact routines are not recommended. If you desire a higher-intensity workout, add arm movements and handheld weights.

- Performing dance movements on a special floor that provides resilience may help prevent overuse injuries, especially stress fractures.

Skating

There are three types of skating: roller skating, ice skating, and inline skating. All are excellent ways to burn calories without stressing joints and bones. All, however, require a significant level of skill to skate safely. If you skated as a child, you'll find it easier to take up skating again as an adult.

Skating Gear

- A good pair of inline skates cost between $100 and $200, or more. Ice skates cost between $80 and $120. You'll also need

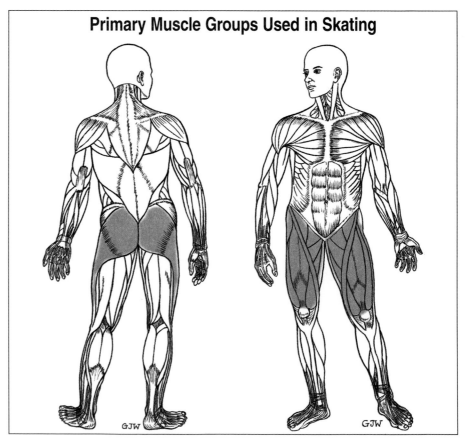

Primary Muscle Groups Used in Skating

a helmet and padding to protect your wrists, elbows, and knees. You can use the same helmet for bicycling.

- Dress appropriately. Consider the weather, environmental conditions, and other guidelines for dressing for physical activities.

Tips for Skating

- *Relax*. Skating is a graceful, rhythmic sport. The basic motion sequence is step—glide—push. As you step forward with one foot, push away with the other. Always move your body weight over the foot you are stepping with. As you bring the other leg forward to step again, allow yourself to glide. Work on making this a smooth and rhythmic motion. Watch other skaters to observe the rhythm of their movements.

Inline Skating

This contemporary form of roller skating has gained enormous popularity in the United States over the past 5 years. A distinguishing feature of inline skating is the design of the boot, which aligns all wheels in one straight line rather than two by two and parallel as on the roller skating boot. Like other forms of skating, inline skating can be done indoors in a rink, but the usual practice is to skate outdoors on paths, sidewalks, parking lots, and roads.

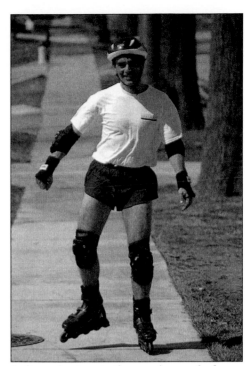

Inline skating is favored mostly by the young, but older enthusiasts are not exempt from participating.

Precautions

- Inline skating requires modest fitness and skill to get started and a high degree of skill to skate safely. Because of the high speeds achieved (sometimes as much as 20 mph or 40 mph in competition) and the inherent difficulty in stopping, there are significant risks to inline skating. Injuries are common and often severe. Fractures of the arms and wrists are the most frequent serious injuries because of falls on outstretched hands. Leg fractures, road burns, and head injuries are also common.

- If you want to take up inline skating, seek formal instruction on proper technique, especially how to stop. Stopping usually requires dragging a brake pad on the skate or dragging the entire skate. Newer brake systems are being developed, including handheld brakes, but these are still quite difficult to use.

- Don't skate on traffic roadways; choose low-traffic paths with large expanses of grass on both sides. Some communities encourage skating on bike paths.

Ice Skating

Ice skating is a good way to deal with the doldrums of winter. Participation is relatively inexpensive because skates can usually be rented for a nominal fee at public ice skating rinks.

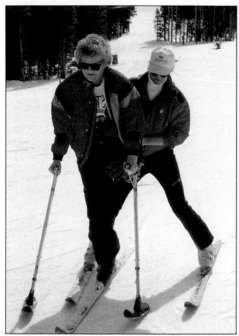

Skiing improves all-around fitness and is therefore ideal exercise for people with special needs.

Ice skating requires a modest level of skill and fitness and is safer than inline skating. Injuries can occur, however, from falls on the hard surface. The most common injuries are sprains or fractures of the arms, bruises to the buttocks area, and injuries to the face. Ironically, some of the worst accidents occur when people are standing still and not paying attention to others on the ice. If you want to stop to talk or rest, move to the side of the rink or off the ice.

Skating Events

There are competitive events for inline skating (racing), ice skating (racing and figure skating), and roller skating (figure skating). Contact your local sporting goods store to locate local clubs and organizations that sponsor events.

Skiing

Downhill (Alpine) Skiing

Downhill skiing is a moderately strenuous sport that requires a modest level of physical fitness and muscle flexibility and tone. Skiing offers unique challenges. Many people with impaired function (blindness, loss of hearing or limbs) participate and even compete in this demanding sport.

Downhill Skiing Gear

• Skiing can be one of the most expensive sports in which to participate, requiring special warm clothes, boots and bindings,

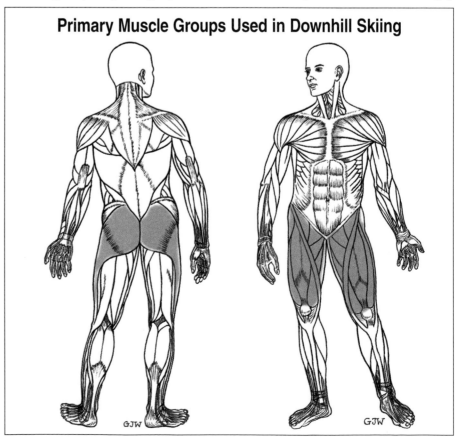

Primary Muscle Groups Used in Downhill Skiing

skis, poles, goggles, lift tickets, and transportation to and from a ski area. Ski equipment can cost over $500 but can be rented for approximately $20 per day. Ski passes at major resorts cost $30 to $50 per day. If you're more than 65, many ski resorts allow you to ski without charge or at a significantly reduced fee.

Tips for Downhill Skiing

- Skiing makes unique demands on your muscles. To participate successfully and comfortably, you'll need to develop muscle groups in the thighs and hips. Start to prepare 4 to 6 weeks before your ski trip by performing stretching and strength-building exercises (*see appendices 1 and 2 of this book*). Jumping rope and step aerobics are excellent exercises to prepare for skiing. Work up to 10-minute sessions of stretching or exercising primary muscle groups.

- Some exercise machines simulate the motion of skiing. You can simulate the same motion by jumping from side to side while keeping your feet together. This conditions the same muscle groups you use in skiing.

- A specially textured plastic mat that comes with sock boots is also available and allows you to slide from side to side to simulate the motions used in skating. This exercise also conditions the muscles used for skiing.

Precautions

- If you have never skied or if you are beginning again after a period of inactivity, take lessons to learn techniques, especially for turning and stopping.

- Injuries for downhill skiing are high. A study at a Vermont ski resort showed that there were 3 to 7 injuries per day per 1,000 alpine skiers. Many of these injuries were serious, including broken bones and torn ligaments, especially of the knees.

- Don't ski when you're overly tired. The later in the day, the greater your risk for fatigue and accidents.

- Stay on the slopes that are appropriate to your level of expertise and where you are always under control. Use the color-coded signs that indicate the level of difficulty of the trail. Green squares mark the trails for beginners. Trails marked with blue squares are for people who are able to stay upright, turn, and stop at will. Black diamonds mark the trails for experienced skiers; trails marked with double black diamonds are for highly skilled skiers. Stay away from these trails unless you have an appetite for cold fear.

- It is very important to plan your route from beginning to end before you start each run. Many trails can lead without warning to

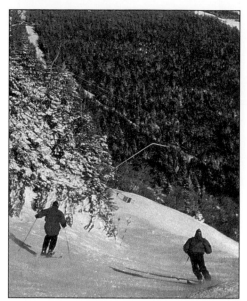

Like many high-speed sports, skiing safely requires skill, experience, and good judgment.

other trails of significantly greater difficulty. If you don't plan your route and don't know where you are going, a wrong turn can transform an easy, relaxed run into a terrifying experience in a matter of seconds. Therefore, make sure you get a detailed trail map from the ski lodge, ticket counter, or lift area, and always plan your route so that you know where you are going.

- Give yourself time to adjust to the higher altitude if you're not used to it. If you're skiing in the lower altitudes of Vermont, you may be able to ski from the top of the trail to the bottom without stopping. If you're skiing in Vail, Colorado, you may find that you need to rest every 100 yards until you get used to the higher altitude.

Skiing Events

There are ski competitions for amateurs, seniors, children, and people with special needs. Obtain more information about organized events in the ski area you plan to visit.

The three types of competitive events in alpine skiing are slalom, giant slalom, and downhill. All skiing races are against the clock, not another competitor. The fastest time wins.

The slalom is a short race on a course with flags. The skier must follow a specific path (the same for everyone) through gates (flags) to the bottom of the course. The downhill race involves getting to the bottom of the course as quickly as possible. There may be some markers, but generally the skier uses the whole trail. The giant slalom is a combination of the slalom and downhill races.

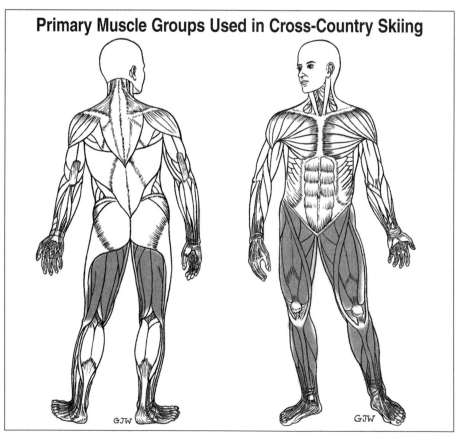

Primary Muscle Groups Used in Cross-Country Skiing

Benefits of Cross-Country Skiing

- Uses muscle groups of the lower body
- Provides excellent cardiovascular conditioning
- Strengthens muscles and bones (weight-bearing activity)
- Has low impact on joints
- Burns significant calories
- Provides full-body conditioning

The gates are farther apart so the speeds are faster than for the slalom course, but not as fast as for the downhill race.

Nordic (Cross-Country) Skiing

Cross-country skiing originated in northern Europe over 5,000 years ago and is an excellent aerobic exercise. It is a low-impact, weight-bearing sport that provides excellent aerobic conditioning and high calorie expenditure. Beginning Nordic skiers must have minimum skill levels and modest levels of fitness to participate successfully.

Nordic Skiing Gear

Cross-country skiing is less costly than downhill skiing because the equipment costs less (you can also rent it) and you don't pay fees for lift tickets. There may be a nominal fee to enter a Nordic ski area.

Tips for Nordic Skiing

- If you're a beginner, take a few lessons from a qualified instructor to master the techniques of cross-country skiing. The basic mechanics are step—forward—glide. Allow the heel of your trailing foot to raise off the ski, then smoothly step forward with that foot—pushing it into the lead and leaning your body weight over that leg. The key is to move rhythmically and smoothly at a comfortable pace.

Precautions

- Because the steep incline and potential for speed is not as great with cross-country skiing as with downhill skiing, it has a ten times lower injury rate than downhill skiing. However, injuries to the ankle or knee can occur during twisting falls.

- The same precautions apply to cross-country skiing as to other cold-weather activities. Dressing in layers is especially important, because cross-country skiing burns so many calories. You're likely to warm quickly and perspire heavily once you are moving. Perspiration on the skin can be very uncomfortable and even dangerous when the temperature is near freezing. Carry water, and drink frequently.

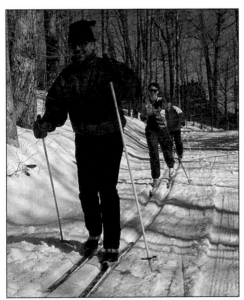

Cross-country skiing can be enjoyed in many local parks and recreation areas that are easily accessed and close to home.

- Because cross-country skiing might take you into fairly remote areas, keep in mind the tips you would follow in planning for a hiking trip. Take a map and compass so you don't get lost. The trails you take may not be heavily traveled.

- Ski areas are often in remote or rugged parts of the country where getting lost or being confronted by wild animals is not unheard of. Check with the ski patrol to learn about possible hazards.

Nordic Skiing Events

There are many types of cross-country events. All major ski areas have Nordic centers that sponsor events throughout the winter. Races are run at various distances and against the clock. The starts are staggered (each person starts 2 minutes after the one ahead), and racers all use the same track (trail) through the snow. The person with the best time wins.

Sports with Partners

Tennis

Tennis is a popular sport that can be played as singles (one-on-one) or doubles (two-on-two). When played as a leisure sport, tennis, especially doubles tennis, requires modest to advanced skills and only minimal levels of fitness. The higher your skill, and the higher your opponent's level of skill, the more strenuous your workout.

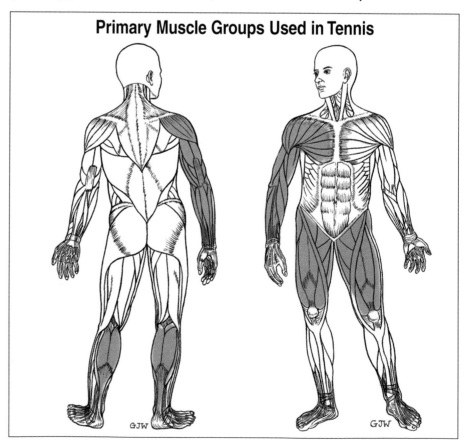

Primary Muscle Groups Used in Tennis

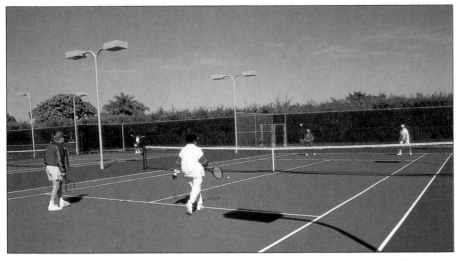

Doubles tennis is a leisurely sport which requires minimal skill and exertion.

Singles and doubles tennis are considerably different games. Singles tennis requires strenuous activity, burns calories, and contributes to aerobic fitness, balance, and coordination. Doubles tennis is less vigorous and usually has less effect on fitness. Don't let this discourage you from playing, however. Doubles tennis is an excellent opportunity for exercising, reducing stress, and enjoying the company of friends. Take lessons to learn the basics of the game if you haven't played before.

Gear

- *Shoes.* A good pair of tennis shoes may be your most important investment in tennis equipment. Singles tennis is a game with lots of full running strides. With each stride, the foot strikes the ground with a force three to five times your body weight. To avoid foot and other leg injuries, wear a good shoe with adequate cushioning in the midsole to absorb the shock in both the heel and forefoot *(see page 215)*. All racquet sports also require a high amount of side-to-side foot movement. A strong heel support is important to prevent strain. The front of the tennis shoe is built up to allow dragging of the toe during the serve.

- *Racquets.* The cost of tennis racquets ranges upward from $50.

- *Tennis court fees.* Many communities have public courts that require no fees. Clubs offer both indoor and outdoor tennis facilities.

Precautions

- Tennis is a safe sport. Occasional injuries include overuse stresses of the rotator cuff (shoulder muscles) or tennis elbow. Tennis elbow is caused by a stress of the wrist muscle that attaches along the outside of the elbow. Older people are at greater risk for developing tennis elbow. You can reduce this risk by using a racquet with an appropriate grip size. Using a metal racquet with strings that are too tight may contribute to tennis elbow.

- Lower back strain and pain are common complaints among tennis players and are due to overarching of the back and twisting motions used in hitting the ball on the run. Minimize this risk by stretching your lower back and thighs and warming up before you begin to play.

- Tennis played outdoors in the summer heat increases your exposure to the sun. Dress appropriately and wear sunscreen and a hat.

- Because tennis courts are made of material that absorbs heat, the temperature on the court can get much higher than in the surrounding area. It is not uncommon for the temperature on the court to be over 100° F when the temperature everywhere else is in the high 80s or 90s. As you sweat heavily, you will lose minerals and salts, which may result in leg cramps. You may want to consider a sports drink in addition to water, especially if you are playing for an hour or more.

Tennis Events

Most schools, recreation centers, and YMCAs, YWCAs, or JCCAs have tennis programs and competitions for different age groups and ability levels.

Racquetball and Squash

Racquetball and squash are played in a four-wall indoor court. People who have a wide range of skill levels can participate. It is important to find a partner with the same skill level as you. Your workout will be better, and you'll enjoy the game more. The racquet sports are excellent ways to burn calories, improve cardiovascular fitness, and develop coordination and agility. A beginner requires only a modest fitness level to play.

Beyond these commonalities, racquetball and squash are very different games. Generally, squash requires more strategy, skill, and endurance and is more strenuous at any level. Squash courts are more prevalent in the Northeast and Middle Atlantic states and in larger cities of the Midwest and West, while racquetball is relatively common throughout the country.

Gear

- Invest in a good pair of shoes. Shoes for racquetball and squash should have similar features as shoes for tennis (*see p. 215*).

- You will need a racquet, which costs between $50 to $100, and balls, which cost about $5 and can be found at most sporting goods stores.

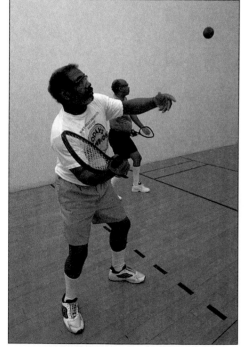

Racquetball is enjoyed most when it is played by partners with similar levels of skill.

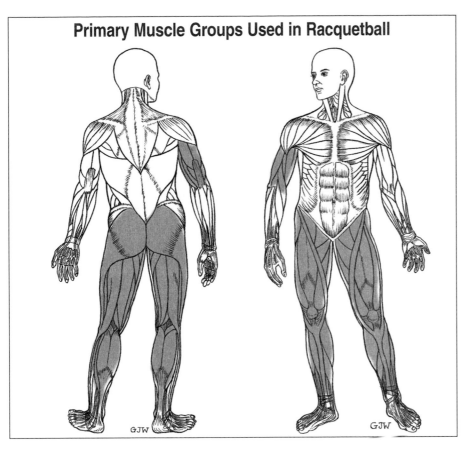

Primary Muscle Groups Used in Racquetball

- Squash and racquetball courts are found in YMCAs, JCCAs, community centers, and schools. In fitness clubs and health centers, membership fees are the major expense for participating in the game.

- Protective eyewear for racquetball and squash is mandatory in most sports clubs.

Precautions

- A principal hazard of playing indoor racquet sports is eye injuries from being hit with the ball. In an intense game, the ball travels more than 100 mph. All racquetball players should wear protective eyewear. The eyewear should wrap around the head and have lenses that are fixed to the surrounding frame. Open eyewear is not acceptable because the ball can squeeze through the holes in the frames and injure the eye.

- Low back strains and ankle sprains are other common injuries.

Golf

Golf is a popular, low-intensity sport that requires a moderate to high level of skill. The value of golf as physical activity increases if you walk the course and carry your own clubs rather than ride in a cart. Although you can play golf by yourself, people usually play in groups of two or four.

Gear

- Golfing expenses include a set of clubs and club fees, which can range from $15 to $50 per round.

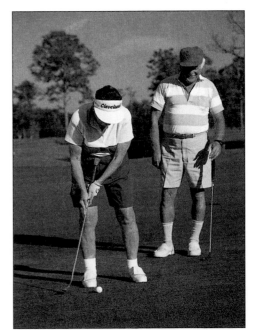

Sinking the ball for a birdie requires coordination, concentration, and often, plain luck.

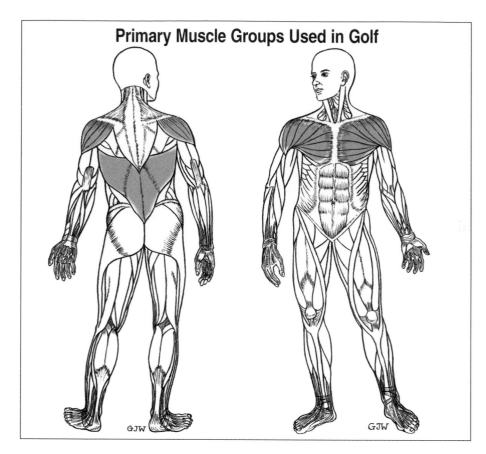

Primary Muscle Groups Used in Golf

Tips for Golfing

- As with other sports that require specific skills, taking lessons is the best way to begin. Even golfers who have played for years will take lessons from golf pros occasionally to adjust the mechanics of their games. Practice on a driving range until most of your shots go into the air and fairly straight. When you feel comfortable hitting the ball, try the golf course. (The golf course is not the place to learn the game!)

- Keep in mind that golf is a game of rhythm and timing, not speed and strength. Finding a smooth tempo to your swing results from a full turn and follow-through. Watch golfers on television. Their swings are one smooth, unbroken action. To find the right tempo for your swing, complete the swing as you count from 1 to 3 at a normal speed. At the count of 1, bring the club back; at the count of 2, at the top of the backswing, start to bring the club forward; at 3, swing through the ball, not at it.

- Learning to play golf is worth the effort and frustration. It's an ideal sport for retirement, when you have the time to spend on the course. Also, playing golf on vacation can take you into a variety of beautiful settings—mountains, lakes, beaches, and deserts.

Precautions

Golfing injuries are rare. The most common injury is low back strain due to extension and rotation of the back. Wrist, elbow, and shoulder strains also are common complaints. Flexibility exercises can help prevent stiffness and improve your swing. A less-appreciated hazard of golf is skin cancer caused by unprotected sun exposure. During one round of golf, you can be exposed to the sun for several hours. Be sure to use sunscreen and protective clothing to prevent skin cancer.

Team Sports

Team sports have both social and fitness benefits. You can organize teams to play spontaneously, for example at picnics, family gatherings, or group outings. Or you can join a team that is part of a league and play regularly scheduled games for a complete season. If you commit to joining a team for league play, you must make the activity a priority. Your team members will count on you to show up for the game. There's nothing more disappointing than forfeiting a game because there aren't enough players.

All the environmental and safety precautions that apply to individual sports apply to team sports as well.

Team sports seem to bring out the weekend warriors in people. If you are at a picnic or filling in at a regular local game, and if your level of fitness is fair but not good, resist the temptation to play "all out." As you grow older, sports that require sudden starts and stops—as team sports often do—take a greater toll on your body. Risk of injury is greater in team sports, partly for this reason and partly because there is more body contact. If you're playing baseball at a picnic, remember it's a picnic, not the World Series. You can pull a muscle or hamstring in a second, but the injury can take weeks or months to heal.

Volleyball

Volleyball is a team sport in which a ball is batted back and forth across a net approximately 8 feet above the ground. It is inexpensive, requiring only a ball and a net and a large area to play. Volley-

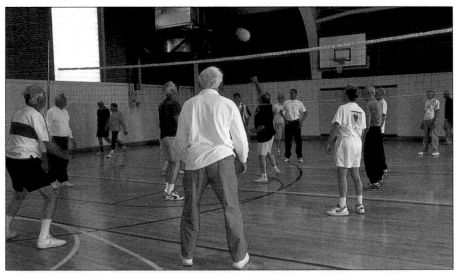

Volleyball is a team sport that has few requirements but many rewards.

ball can be played indoors on the gym floor or outdoors on grass or sand. A variation of the game is played in the swimming pool.

Minimal skills are required, and players of varying abilities and conditioning can play on the same team. Volleyball requires low to moderate fitness, depending on the intensity with which the game is played.

The game has a low injury rate, and the relatively few injuries that do occur are usually related to stresses and strains on the wrists and arms, which are used for hitting the ball. Twisted or sprained ankles from landing wrong after jumping to hit the ball over the 8-foot net are also common.

Basketball

Basketball is a popular U.S. sport that is becoming more popular worldwide. Low-level skills need not prevent you from participating and enjoying the game. Participation can range from shooting baskets, to playing one-on-one with someone of equal ability, to playing a rigorous, full-court running game with full teams.

The injury rate for basketball is relatively low. Sprained ankles are the most common injury. Wear protective eyewear if you're playing in a group. In the excitement of play, it's also easy to get poked in the eye.

Softball

Softball is similar to baseball but is played with a larger and softer ball and a larger bat. There are slow- and fast-pitch versions, but

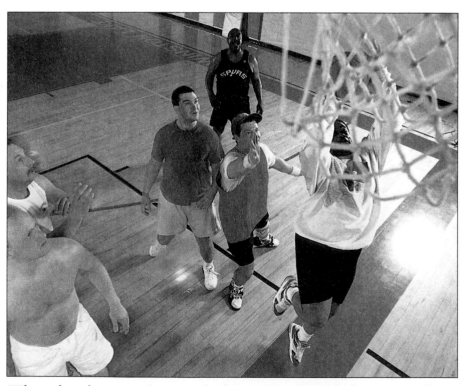

When played at a moderate or high intensity, basketball is an excellent way to burn calories and improve aerobic conditioning.

slow-pitch is the more popular game. You need only minimal skill to begin playing softball. Although not particularly rigorous, the game demands hand-eye coordination and some running. The principal value of softball is as an outlet for competition and social interaction. Injuries are rare if sliding into the bases is prohibited and if you do some stretches to warm up before you play.

Add Sports and Recreation to Your Fitness Program

All physical activity is good for your health. Some sports contribute more to physical fitness than others, but even those that don't build fitness promote movement, flexibility, and coordination. Above all, no matter how competent or skilled you become at a sport, you should enjoy it. Play to have fun.

Adding sports and recreational activities to your fitness program broadens your options for participating in different kinds of physical and social activity. Social interaction is as important to general well-being as physical fitness, and recreational sports provide an excellent opportunity to spend time with friends. The social benefits of sports are significant at any age. Sports help you to stay active and fit as you grow older.

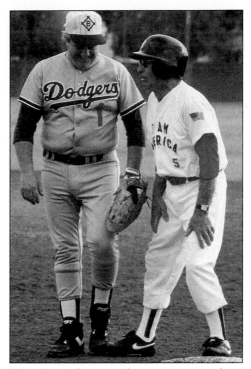

You don't have to be young or athletic to participate in a softball league. Just keep your eye on the ball and swing that bat.

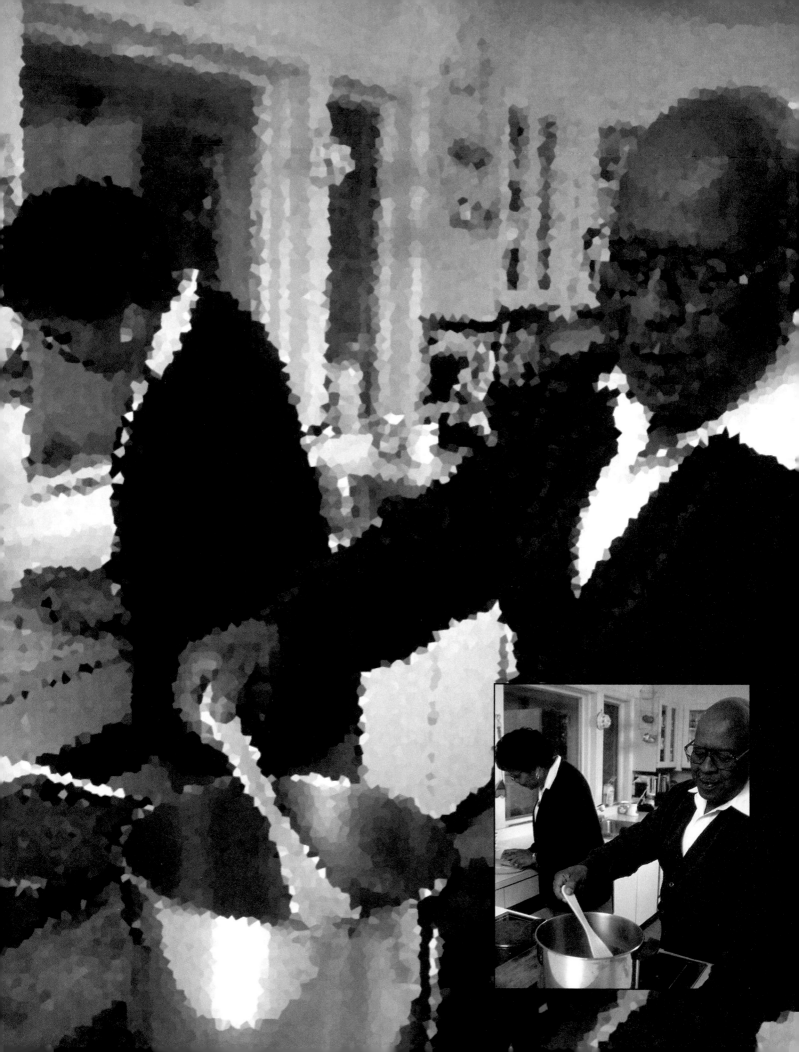

CHAPTER 16

Eating, Nutrition, and Weight Control

Diet and nutrition are important to our health at every age and stage of life, but good nutrition is especially important as we age. Eating a balanced diet and controlling our weight can offset the effects of age-related alterations in metabolism and declining physiological function. And, good nutrition, like exercise, can help protect us from many common problems that occur with aging. Exercise, a balanced diet, and weight control are protective measures that help to ensure our continued health and independence.

Essential Nutrients

What are the essential nutrients and how do we get them? Five major food groups supply the body with essential nutrients: carbohydrates, fats, proteins, vitamins, and minerals. In addition to these essential nutrients, we need adequate fiber and water to function efficiently.

Carbohydrates

Carbohydrates, the body's chief source of energy, are metabolized to provide glucose, the primary fuel the body uses to do its work. Food sources of carbohydrates are almost exclusively from plants: fruits, vegetables, and whole–grain breads and cereals. Carbohydrates are categorized as simple or complex. Simple carbohydrates are sugars we get mostly from fruits and sucrose

What Are Essential Nutrients?

Our bodies can make certain nutrients on demand but require adequate amounts of food to obtain "essential" nutrients. These essential nutrients must be derived from our diet.

The Energy Nutrients

The nutrients that provide us with calories for energy include carbohydrates, fat, and protein.

- **Carbohydrates—4 calories per gram**
- **Fat—9 calories per gram**
- **Proteins—4 calories per gram**

Food Sources of Complex Carbohydrates

- Cereals, rice, pasta
- Breads
- Beans (kidney, white, split peas, black-eyed peas, lentils)
- Corn, peas, potatoes, winter squash, sweet potatoes, yams

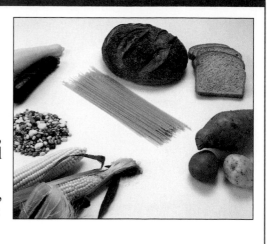

(honey, molasses, syrup, and cane sugar). Although sucrose is a source of energy, it is otherwise low in nutrient value. Complex carbohydrates are starches and fiber and are found mostly in vegetables and grains. Because complex carbohydrates also provide the body with fiber, and because carbohydrate foods give us calories with very little fat, they are the preferred source of energy. When carbohydrate stores are low, the body uses fat stores or, if these fail, proteins as a source of energy. A low-carbohydrate diet can lead to breakdown of muscle protein, loss of sodium, and dehydration. Reduced reserves of muscle protein can lead to a compromised immune response and greater vulnerability to disease.

The National Academy of Sciences recommends a high-carbohydrate diet because eating generous amounts of complex carbohydrates, in addition to protecting protein stores, increases dietary levels of important vitamins, minerals, and fiber and decreases the amount of dietary fat. For these reasons, it is recommended that Americans obtain more than 55 percent of their calories from carbohydrates.

FAT!

What is it?
Why do we need it?
What does it do?

Fats

As a nation, we have learned to love fat: high fat, flavorsome red meat; hamburger; sour cream; whipped cream; butter; cookies; cakes; chips; french fries—anything fried. But fat is undoubtedly bad for us. It adds unwanted calories, raises our cholesterol, clogs our arteries, and contributes to the diseases that lead to premature death—heart disease, diabetes, and cancer—which also result in billions of dollars in health care expenditures. If there's a health habit we should change along with inactivity, it's eating too much fat.

We should not plan to give up fat completely. We need a certain amount of it for critical body functions. Fat insulates our bodies against heat loss, cushions and protects our internal organs from damage or trauma, and, most important, provides a compact source of quickly mobilized energy. Stored fat contains more than twice as many calories per gram as carbohydrate or protein does. But excess body fat is bad for our health.

Saturated and Unsaturated Fats

Fat is a generic term referring to a number of compounds that contain fatty acids, each having a different chemical structure. Depending on their chemical structure, fatty acids comprise either saturated or unsaturated fat. Saturated fats are generally animal fats and are solid at room temperature. Butter is an example of a saturated fat. Unsaturated fats are generally derived from plants and are liquid at room temperature. Corn oil and olive oil are examples of unsaturated fats. Exceptions are coconut oil and palm oil, which are saturated fats even though they are liquid at room temperature.

Knowing the difference between saturated and unsaturated fats is important because saturated fat is associated with elevated blood cholesterol levels. Cholesterol, a white, waxy substance, is manufactured naturally by our bodies. It belongs to a group of chemical substances called sterols and is essential for the formation

It's the saturated fat in food—more than the cholesterol—that has the greatest impact on cholesterol levels.

Lipoproteins and Cholesterol

Blood cholesterol and triglyceride (*triglyceride* is the medical term for fat in the blood) are carried by protein particles that can be separated in the laboratory by density and sorted into three categories: low-density lipoprotein (LDL), high-density lipoprotein (HDL), and very low-density lipoprotein (VLDL).

LDL—the so-called "bad" cholesterol—tends to be deposited in the blood vessel walls. High levels (above 159 mg/dl) indicate an increased risk for high blood pressure and heart attack.

HDL—the so-called "good" cholesterol—serves a "clean-up" role by sweeping deposits from the blood vessel walls. High levels protect against heart disease, and low levels (less than 35 mg/dl) increase your risk for heart disease.

VLDL—carries most of the triglyceride in the blood. High levels of VLDL or triglyceride are not a risk factor for heart-disease.

Total Cholesterol—is your combined VLDL, LDL, and HDL values. If your total cholesterol is high, your LDL will be too. The accompanying table lists desirable and undesirable levels of HDL, LDL, and total blood cholesterol.

Risk	Total Cholesterol (mg/dl)	LDL (mg/dl)	HDL (mg/dl)
High	above 239	above 159	less than 35
Borderline	200–239	130–159	n/a
Desirable	below 200	below 130	above 60

of cell membranes and certain hormones. Cholesterol is not an essential nutrient because our bodies constantly manufacture it, mostly in the liver and kidneys, but we also ingest it from foods of animal origin. Too much cholesterol clogs our arteries. Cholesterol travels in the bloodstream with triglyceride bound to protein particles, called lipoproteins. When lipoprotein levels become too high, cholesterol accumulates in the blood vessel walls, much like lime deposits accumulate on the inside of a water pipe. This process—called atherosclerosis or hardening of the arteries—causes narrowing of the blood vessels, which impedes blood flow and may lead to high blood pressure, heart attack, or stroke.

Reducing Dietary Fat

Because the fat in your diet more than dietary cholesterol leads to high blood cholesterol levels, reducing blood cholesterol levels means reducing your intake of fat, especially saturated fat. Most Americans get 40 percent of their calories from fat. The Dietary Guidelines for Older Americans recommend that we get no more than 30 percent of our total daily calories from fat and less than 8 percent of our calories from saturated fat, or no more than 18 grams per day of saturated fat. *(See Action Box 1 on p. 250 to track your daily fat grams.)* Reducing the fat in your diet will help you lower your blood cholesterol levels, reduce your risk for coronary heart disease, and may reduce your risk for certain types of cancer. It will also reduce your caloric intake and help you control your weight. Remember, fat contains the most calories per gram of all three major energy nutrients. In addition to limiting fat in your diet, the Food and Nutrition Board recommends that you limit your intake of dietary cholesterol to less than 300 mg/day.

One of the easiest ways to reduce the amount of saturated fat you eat is to limit your intake of animal products, especially high-fat meats. The major sources of saturated fats are found in beef, lamb, pork, veal, and whole milk or dairy products including butter and cheese. Fortunately, there are now low–fat or fat–free versions of many dairy products.

Tips for Reducing Saturated Fat

- Choose leans cuts of meat, poultry, and fish.

- Trim all visible fat from meat.

- Remove the skin from poultry.

- Keep your portion size of cooked meat to a 3-oz serving—about the size of a deck of cards.

- Eat fewer servings of red meat; replace red meats with skinless poultry and fish.

- Eat more meatless meals.

- Choose low-fat or fat-free dairy products.

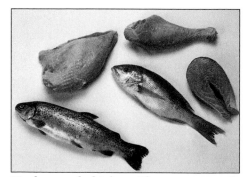

Turkey and chicken (if you remove the skin before serving) and fish (if you don't cook it in fat) contain the least amount of saturated and total fat.

Meats—Fat and Lean

Following is a sampling of meats from fattiest to leanest. Unless otherwise noted, all serving sizes are 4 oz of meat from cooked, skinless poultry or from cooked, carefully trimmed beef, pork, veal, or lamb. Remember, most people over 50 should eat no more than 18 g of saturated fat per day.

	Saturated Fat (g)	Total Fat (g)	Calories
Fattiest (more than 10 g saturated fat)			
Pork spareribs, untrimmed	13	34	449
Duck with skin	11	32	381
Very Fatty (5 to 10 g of saturated fat)			
Ground beef (27 percent fat)	9	23	327
Ground beef (20 percent fat)	8	21	307
Beef top sirloin (choice), untrimmed	8	19	304
Ground beef (17 percent fat)	7	19	289
Beef tenderloin (choice)	6	16	276
Ham, leg, rump, half, untrimmed	6	16	285
Pork center loin, untrimmed	5	15	271
Perdue ground chicken	5	16	240
Lean (1 to 4 g saturated fat)			
Lamb loin	4	11	244
Chicken thigh	3	12	236
Ham, leg, rump half	3	9	233
Ground turkey	3	11	226
Beef top round (choice)	3	8	244
Veal sirloin	3	7	190
Chicken breast with skin	3	9	223
Pork tenderloin	3	7	211
Turkey breast with skin	2	8	214
Chicken drumstick	2	6	194
Beef eye round (select)	2	5	182
Chicken breast	1	4	186
Very Lean (less than 1 g saturated fat)			
Extra-lean ground turkey breast	0	1	146
Turkey breast	0	1	153
For Comparison			
Flounder	0	2	132
Pink salmon	1	5	168

ACTION BOX 1

Track Your Daily Fat Grams

Keep a record of the foods you eat. Track your intake of fat, saturated fats, and dietary cholesterol. You can find the grams of fat contained in foods on the "Nutrition Facts" labels. Determine the number of recommended grams of fat and saturated fat you should eat each day based on your total calorie intake. The recommended daily energy allowance (total calories per day) for people over 50 is 2,300 for men and 1,900 for women.

Recommended Fat Intake

Total Calories/Day	Total Fat (g)	Saturated Fat (g)
1200	40	11–13
1400	47	12–15
1600	53	14–18
1800	60	16–20
2000	67	18–22
2200	73	20–24
2400	80	21–26
2600	87	23–29
2800	93	25–31

Food	Amount	Total Fat (g)	Saturated Fat (g)	Dietary Cholesterol (mg)
Your Goal:		_____ g	_____ g	300 mg

- Limit fried foods (french fries, fried meats and vegetables, doughnuts).

- Choose low-fat or fat-free salad dressings, margarines, and sauces.

- Avoid baked goods and desserts that contain shortening, palm oil, and coconut oil.

Proteins

Dietary protein supplies the body with amino acids, the building blocks from which the body manufactures its own protein stores. Proteins are essential for a number of vital bodily functions. They repair or support the growth of new body tissue including bones, muscles, blood vessels, skin, hair, and nails; they manufacture bodily secretions and fluids needed for most bodily functions; and, in their role as enzymes and hormones, they maintain cellular and organ function throughout the body.

The body manufactures amino acids to build protein. Of the 22 known amino acids needed to build proteins, 9 must be supplied through diet because our bodies cannot manufacture them independently. Proteins supplied by diet are categorized as complete and incomplete proteins. Complete proteins supply the body with all nine essential amino acids in the right amounts and proportions required for protein synthesis. Sources of complete

Food Sources of Complete and Incomplete Protein

Complete	Incomplete
Meat	Grains (rice, breads, pasta, couscous)
Poultry	Beans (kidney, baked, black-eyed peas, lentils, chickpeas)
Fish	Seeds/nuts (sesame, sunflower)
Dairy	Vegetables and fruits (broccoli, corn)
Eggs	

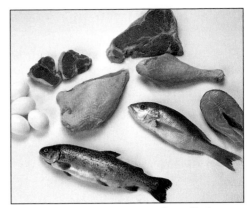

Complete protein provides all the essential amino acids.

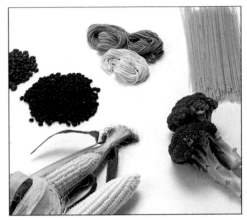

Incomplete protein lacks one or more essential amino acids.

proteins include animal products: meat, poultry, fish, eggs, and dairy products. Incomplete proteins lack one or two essential amino acids and, when eaten alone, cannot provide the body with the building blocks it needs to manufacture proteins. Sources of incomplete proteins are beans, grains, nuts, seeds, and vegetables. Because these foods contain different types and amounts of amino acids, they can be combined to provide complete proteins. For example, beans and rice in the right amounts combine to provide sufficient quantities and proportions of essential amino acids for protein synthesis. Animal sources of protein are often considered "best" because of their complete amino acid composition. Often, however, when we eat complementary proteins in the same meal, we make a higher-quality protein than that derived solely from meat or eggs. Moreover, protein derived from grains and vegetables is likely to contain less fat.

The recommended daily allowance (RDA) of protein for adults over age 50 is 63 g for men and 50 g for women. Most adults over 50 meet their protein needs when protein supplies about 15 percent of their total daily calories.

Vitamins

Vitamins are organic substances that we require in very small amounts for two purposes: to perform specific metabolic functions and to help manufacture components of body tissue (bone, hair, skin, nerves, brain). Vitamins are necessary for life and health. They are essential nutrients because we derive them exclusively from our diet. The body cannot manufacture them. Because we need only very small amounts, they are usually measured in milligrams (mg), which are 1/1,000 of a gram, or micrograms (μg), which are 1/1,000 of a milligram.

Vitamins can be categorized according to their solubility. Fat-soluble vitamins are absorbed in fat and include vitamins A, D, E, and K. Water-soluble vitamins are absorbed in water and include vitamins C, B_1 (thiamin), B_2 (riboflavin), B_3 (niacin), B_5 (pantothenic acid), B_6 (pyridoxine), B_9 (folate, folacin, folic acid), and B_{12} (cobalamin or cyanocobalamin).

Vitamin Requirements for Older Adults

Vitamin	Recommended Daily Allowance	Function	Common Sources
Fat-Soluble Vitamins			
Vitamin A (retinol, carotene)	*Men:* 1000 µg *Women:* 800 µg	Maintains structure of all cell membranes Essential for good vision, especially night vision Helps in normal formation of bones and teeth	*Food sources:* Dark green and yellow vegetables (sweet potatoes, winter squash, carrots, broccoli, fruits [like peaches, apricots, cantaloupe]); the liver oils of cod and other fish; liver; fortified milk and dairy products [cheese, butter, egg yolk])
Vitamin D (calciferol, cholecalciferol)	*Men and women:* 5 µg or 200 IU	Essential for normal formation of bones and teeth Helps our bodies absorb calcium and phosphorus from food and maintain normal calcium levels in tissues	Our bodies manufacture a certain amount of vitamin D through exposure to sunlight. The ultraviolet (UV) rays activate 7-dehydrocholesterol, a form of cholesterol in our skin, converting it to vitamin D, which our bodies then absorb *Food sources:* Saltwater fish such as herring, salmon, and sardines; organ meats; fish-liver oils; egg yolks; fortified dairy products
Vitamin E (tocopherol)	*Men:* 10 mg *Women:* 8 mg	Functions as a potent antioxidant, a chemical that prevents oxidation (breakdown) of fatty acids, a principal component of cells and tissues. Some researchers believe that these substances can help slow the aging process. Helps maintain the chemical stability of fat-like substances in the body, including vitamin D and several hormones.	*Food sources:* Wheat germ; plant fats (soybean, cottonseed, peanut, and corn oils); margarine made from vegetable oils; whole raw seeds and nuts; soybeans; eggs; butter; liver; sweet potatoes; green leafy vegetables

µg = microgram(s); mg = milligram(s); IU = International Units

Signs of Deficiency	Signs of Excess/Toxicity	Comments
Night blindness, excessive dryness of the conjunctiva and cornea of the eye	Fatigue, headache, joint pain, hair loss, weight loss	As we age, our bodies dispose of vitamin A less efficiently, and it is more likely to remain stored in our body tissue. For this reason, some doctors believe that the RDA of 800 to 1,000 µg is too high for older adults. Although some older adults believe that taking vitamin A supplements will improve their night vision (that is, their ability to adapt to decreasing light and changes in light and dark), this is not the case. Beta carotene, a derivative of vitamin A, may protect against the development of heart disease and some cancers.
Osteomalacia (a condition in which bones lose calcium and become softer) can contribute to osteoporosis and a greater risk of bone fractures	Although older adults as a group tend to consume too little calcium, excess consumption of vitamin D can lead to excess stores of this vitamin and excess blood calcium. Abnormally high levels of calcium can result in excessive calcification of bones, kidney stones, and possible damage to the heart and kidneys.	As we age, our skin becomes less efficient at manufacturing vitamin D. Compounding this problem is the fact that many older people spend less time outside. With less exposure to sunlight, people who are unable to leave their homes, or hospitalized patients and others who spend little time outside, are at risk for vitamin D deficiency. People who are unable to leave their homes should boost their intake of vitamin D to at least 10 µg (400 IU) per day. Another option is to spend more time outside, although there is little agreement about how much time must be spent in the sun to manufacture adequate stores of vitamin D. Estimates range from a minimum of 10 minutes twice a week to a maximum of 30 minutes every day.
Deficiency is rare	Relatively nontoxic; at extremely high doses (more than 900 mg/day) can cause depression, fatigue, diarrhea, blurred vision, headaches, and dizziness	The amount of vitamin E in the body appears to remain constant as we age. Some studies suggest that high doses of vitamin E may protect against heart disease and some cancers.

Continues on the following page

Vitamin Requirements for Older Adults *(continued)*

Vitamin	Recommended Daily Allowance	Function	Common Sources
Fat Soluble Vitamins continued			
Vitamin K (phylloquinone)	*Men:* 80 µg *Women:* 65 µg	Essential for formation of substances involved in blood clotting	Bacteria in our intestines can manufacture this vitamin in the form of substances called menaquinones *Food sources:* Green leafy vegetables and members of the cabbage family; pork; liver; yogurt; egg yolks; kelp; alfalfa; fish-liver oils; blackstrap molasses
Water Soluble Vitamins			
Vitamin C (ascorbic acid)	*Men and women:* 60 mg	Essential for formation of collagen and fibrous tissue in teeth, bone, cartilage, connective tissue, and skin Helps maintain structure of capillary walls	*Food sources:* Citrus fruits; tomatoes; green peppers; berries; potatoes; fresh, green leafy vegetables such as broccoli, brussel sprouts, collards, turnip greens, parsley, and cabbage
Vitamin B$_1$ (thiamin)	*Men:* 1.2 mg *Women:* 1 mg	Involved in the breakdown of carbohydrates, fats, and protein Essential for normal cardiovascular and nervous system function	*Food sources:* Pork; organ meats; green leafy vegetables; legumes; sweet corn; egg yolks; corn meal; brown rice; yeast; the germ and husks of grains; berries; nuts
Vitamin B$_2$ (riboflavin)	*Men:* 1.4 mg *Women:* 1.2 mg	Essential in the breakdown of carbohydrates, fats, and proteins Helps the body use vitamins B$_6$ and B$_9$ Can help prevent some eye conditions, such as cataracts	Widely distributed in foods, but only in small amounts *Food sources:* Organ meats; milk; cheese; eggs; green leafy vegetables; meat; whole-grain and fortified cereals and breads; legumes

µg = microgram(s); mg = milligram(s); IU = International Units

Signs of Deficiency	Signs of Excess/Toxicity	Comments
Bleeding, slowed clotting; deficiency is rare in healthy older adults but fairly common in people with severe liver disease	Excessive doses are usually non-toxic; however, vitamin K in food supplements may be a problem for those who take the blood-thinning drug warfarin (brand name: Coumadin)	Research indicates that intestinal manufacture of this vitamin is not sufficient to meet vitamin K requirements in older adults whose dietary intake is restricted; intake may be inadequate in those who eat few green leafy vegetables because of cost, chewing problems, or food preferences.
Bleeding gums, easy bruising, swollen or painful joints, nosebleeds, anemia, lowered resistance to infections, and slow healing of wounds and fractures Severe deficiency can result in scurvy (characterized by weakness, anemia, and spongy gums; often teeth will loosen); particularly at risk are alcoholics, smokers, and people who do not eat enough fruits and vegetables	When levels of vitamin C are too high, kidney stones may form. The body may also absorb vitamin B_{12} less efficiently	Although popularly touted as preventing colds and even cancer, there is no consistent evidence that large doses of vitamin C have health benefits. Blood levels of vitamin C tend to decrease with age. Large doses of vitamin C can interfere with blood sugar measurements; therefore, people with diabetes should not take more than 1 g of vitamin C per day.
Severe deficiency results in beriberi (characterized by irritability, loss of appetite, nausea, increased pulse rate, confusion, insomnia, memory disturbances, irregular heart rate, and muscular weakness); although deficiency is rare in healthy older adults in the United States, alcoholics and people who do not eat enough vegetables and grains may not get enough vitamin B_1	No known toxic effects	Little is known about age-related changes in requirements and metabolism of thiamin.
Local inflammation, oral lesions, cracks in skin at corners of the mouth and fissuring of the lips, opaque corneas, sluggishness, and dizziness; deficiency is rare in healthy older adults whose calorie intake is adequate	No known toxic effects	Absorption appears to remain constant as we age

Continues on the following page

Vitamin Requirements for Older Adults *(continued)*

Vitamin	Recommended Daily Allowance	Function	Common Sources
***Water Soluble Vitamins* continued**			
Vitamin B$_3$ (niacin)	*Men:* 15 mg *Women:* 13 mg	Helps the body break down and use all major nutrients Required for healthy skin, normal gastrointestinal tract function, maintenance of the nervous system, and production of sex hormones	*Food sources:* Lean meats, poultry, fish, liver, kidney, eggs, peanut butter, and brewer's yeast are excellent sources; enriched and whole-grain breads and cereals, wheat germ, dried peas and beans, and nuts contain lesser amounts
Vitamin B$_5$ (pantothenic acid)	*Men and women:* 4 to 7 mg (estimated guideline)	Helps break down carbohydrates, fats, and protein Essential to most living things	*Food sources:* Widely distributed in plant and animal products; the richest sources are meats, whole-grain cereals, and legumes
Vitamin B$_6$ (pyridoxine)	*Men:* 2.0 mg *Women:* 1.6 mg	Essential roles include: formation and breakdown of amino acids; formation of neurotransmitters and hormones important to brain function; regulation of body fluids; and functioning of nervous and musculoskeletal systems	*Food sources:* Meats, especially organ meats; eggs; whole-grain cereals; soybeans; peanuts; walnuts; wheat germ; unmilled rice; brewer's yeast
Vitamin B$_9$ (folate, folacin, folic acid)	*Men:* 200 μg *Women:* 180 μg	Promotes formation of RNA and DNA and amino acid metabolism	*Food sources:* Green leafy vegetables, asparagus, broccoli, liver, milk, eggs, yeast, wheat germ, kidney beans; also found in lesser amounts in potatoes, dried peas and beans, whole-grain cereals, nuts, bananas, cantaloupe, lemons, and strawberries
Vitamin B$_{12}$ (cobalamin or cyanocobalamin)	*Men and women:* 2 μg	Essential for normal function of all cells Plays a role in manufacture of RNA and DNA Helps the body break down protein, fats, and carbohydrates Required for blood formation and neural function	*Food sources:* Liver; kidney; meats; fish; shrimp; oysters; dairy products, particularly eggs

μg = microgram(s); mg = milligram(s); IU = International Units

Signs of Deficiency	Signs of Excess/Toxicity	Comments
Muscular weakness, general fatigue, indigestion, loss of appetite, and skin lesions Severe deficiency results in pellagra, a condition characterized by dermatitis, diarrhea, dementia, and—if untreated—death Deficiency is rare in healthy older adults in the United States; however, alcoholics may be at risk	Gastrointestinal distress (nausea, vomiting, diarrhea), itching, flushing, fainting, and liver damage	Large doses of vitamin B_3 have been used, along with other measures, to manage high cholesterol levels in those who do not respond adequately to dietary management.
Deficiency is unlikely in healthy older adults who consume varied diets	No known toxic effects, although excess may cause diarrhea	Pantothenic acid supplements have been used to treat the "burning foot" syndrome, a neurological disorder.
Anemia; skin inflammation around nose, eyes, and mouth and behind ears; nervousness; and depression; although this is a rare deficiency, alcoholics and people who eat diets low in other B vitamins may be at risk	Neurological problems, including difficulty walking and numbness of feet and hands, have developed in people who take high supplemental doses for months or years; however, toxicity is uncommon	Pyridoxine-deficient individuals have shown improvements in memory when this vitamin is replaced. Research indicates that the requirement for older women may be closer to that for older men (1.9 mg/day).
Anemia; although folate deficiency is widespread in many parts of the world, it is rare in the United States in healthy older adults who eat varied diets; most at risk are alcoholics	No known toxic effects; excess folate may mask vitamin B_{12} deficiency	Many older adults take less than the RDA; however, most seem to have adequate levels of folate.
Pernicious anemia (low hemoglobin count in the blood), nerve inflammation, poor muscular coordination, depressive symptoms, and cognitive impairment; early treatment is necessary to prevent irreversible nervous system damage	Appears to be nontoxic	Although deficiency is rare, except in pure vegetarians who eat no animal products and do not supplement their diets, its prevalence increases with age. It can take 6 to 12 years for the deficiency to develop because the liver stores large amounts of the vitamin. Cobalamin deficiency may be more common than was formerly thought. The vitamin is best replaced by intramuscular injections, because people who are cobalamin deficient often have trouble absorbing it from foods.

Mineral Requirements for Older Adults

Mineral	Recommended Daily Allowance	Function	Common Sources
Calcium	*Men:* 800 mg *Premenopausal women:* 1000 mg *Postmenopausal women:* 1500 mg (Although the RDA for adults aged 51 and older is 800 mg, most doctors recommend that women take 1000 mg daily before menopause and 1500 daily after menopause to slow the loss of bone mass)	Essential roles include: Maintenance of skeletal muscle rigidity (99 percent of the calcium in the body is found in bone); nerve impulse transmission; muscle contraction and relaxation; blood clotting; heart function	*Food sources:* Dairy products (richest source); calcium-fortified citrus juices; canned fish (with bones); green leafy vegetables *Supplements:* Although there are academic arguments about the best form of calcium, common antacids containing calcium carbonate (such as TUMS) are one of the least expensive options
Iron	*Men and postmenopausal women:* 10 mg	Essential for formation of hemoglobin, the substance in the blood that carries oxygen to the cells	*Food sources:* Liver; lean meats; dried beans; fortified cereals; raisins; figs
Zinc	*Men:* 15 mg *Women:* 12 mg	Essential for a variety of metabolic processes, including tissue growth, development, and healing; the breakdown of protein, fats, and carbohydrates; the senses of smell and taste; and immune reactions	*Food sources:* Foods high in protein, such as meats, milk, egg yolks, oysters, liver, seafood; legumes, nuts, peanut butter, and whole-grain cereals are good sources but are less well absorbed

RDAs for Other Essential Minerals

Phosphorus	800 mg
Magnesium	*Men:* 350 mg *Women:* 280 mg
Iodine	150 µg
Selenium	*Men:* 70 µg *Women:* 55 µg

µg = microgram(s); mg = milligram(s); IU = International Units

Signs of Deficiency	Signs of Excess/Toxicity	Comments
Reduced bone mass and weak bones; particularly at risk are post-menopausal white women, who have a greater chance of developing osteoporosis and bone fractures as a result of this disease	Can cause kidney stones; high intake without sufficient water can lead to constipation	Our bones serve as a reservoir of calcium for the body, continually taking and releasing calcium to keep blood levels within an acceptable range. When dietary intake is inadequate, bone losses occur. We absorb only about one third of the calcium we consume, and vitamin D plays an important role in this process. Calcium absorption decreases with age, perhaps because our body levels of vitamin D decline. For this reason, we recommend calcium supplementation for older adults, particularly women. However, older adults with a history of kidney stones or high calcium levels should avoid taking calcium supplements.
Anemia, pallor, fatigue, spooning of nails; although deficiency is rare in healthy older adults, people who limit their intake of red meat or use antacids excessively (impairing iron absorption) may be at risk	Uncommon except in people who are receiving multiple blood transfusions, those with a genetic defect of iron metabolism, or those who are alcoholics Signs of acute toxicity are intestinal cramping, vomiting, nausea	Iron deficiency due to poor diet is rare. Iron deficiency is almost always due to blood loss and can be a sign of serious disease, such as cancer.
Fatigue, decreased alertness, poor appetite, prolonged healing of wounds, flaking dermatitis, and susceptibility to infections and injury	Lack of muscle coordination, gastrointestinal irritation, vomiting, diarrhea, dizziness, lethargy, kidney failure, and anemia; uncommon except in people who take large supplemental doses of zinc	The average intake of zinc tends to fall well below the RDA of 15 mg/day. The best way to ensure adequate zinc intake is to ensure adequate dietary intake.

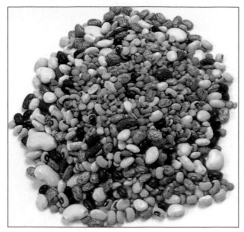

Legumes (peas or beans) are an excellent source of minerals including calcium, phosphorus, potassium, magnesium, iron, and zinc.

Minerals

Unlike the energy nutrients and vitamins, minerals are inorganic elements widely distributed in the natural world. Of the 92 known elements in the periodic table of elements, 25 are found in the human body. As such, minerals are not metabolized by the body but have a variety of vital functions, forming part of the body's structure and regulating body processes. The principal minerals necessary for good health are calcium, iron, zinc, phosphorus, magnesium, iodine, and selenium.

Recommended Dietary Allowances for Adults Over 50 Years of Age

How much of these nutrients to do we need? There is little agreement about the amount of essential nutrients that the body needs after age 50. The influence of the aging metabolism on the requirements for nutrients isn't well understood. The Food and Nutrition Board has determined RDAs for adults aged 51 and older, but these amounts differ very little from the recommended amounts for the general population. A number of vitamin and mineral deficiencies are a source of concern in adults aged 50 and older. Studies have suggested that there is an increased need for vitamins D, B_6, and B_{12} and for calcium, iron, and zinc, but a decreased need for vitamin A. Other nutrients of concern in older adults are fat (too much of it can accelerate heart disease), calories (carbohydrates are the pre-

Calcium-Rich Foods

	Serving Size	Calcium (mg)	Fat Calories (% Total Daily Calories)
Dairy Products			
Yogurt, plain, low-fat	1 cup	415	25
Milk, skim	1 cup	316	0
Milk, whole	1 cup	313	48
Mozzarella, part skim	1 oz	207	56
Cheddar	1 oz	204	74
Vegetables			
Spinach, cooked	1 cup	244	0
Broccoli, cooked	1 cup	178	0
Canned Fish			
Sardines, in water with bones	3 1/2 oz	240	72
Salmon, with bones	3 1/2 oz	237	38

ferred source of calories and energy), and protein (too little of it can increase vulnerability to disease).

RDAs are the standards for determining the essential nutrients Americans need to be healthy. These standards take into account variations among most normal healthy people. They are based on the best available scientific knowledge and are reviewed from time to time in light of new findings.

The RDAs are not established for all the nutrients that you need, and you don't have to consume 100 percent of the RDA for every nutrient each day. If you meet the RDAs for the essential nutrients through a balanced diet, you will get the other nutrients you need. You are at risk for a nutrient deficiency only when you consume less than 67 percent of any RDA for an extended period of time.

Nutritional Supplements

Nutritional supplements are big business in the United States. People spend billions of dollars every year on over-the-counter nutritional supplements to enhance their health or prevent disease. Nutritional supplements are useful for people who must bring their weight up to normal or who have specific nutrient deficiencies. However, on the whole, if you are healthy and eat a nutritionally balanced diet, you are unlikely to need nutritional supplements.

There are three forms of nutritional supplements: caloric or energy supplements, vitamins and minerals, and ergogenic aids.

Caloric or Energy Supplements

The most common caloric supplements are the liquids sold premixed in cans. Some of the better-known brands include Ensure, Sustecal, and Osmolite. Energy bars—candy bars with some protein and vitamins added—are another form of caloric supplement. These supplements were originally developed to provide essential nutrients for people who are unable to eat normal diets because of illness or surgery and who must bring their body weight back to normal. However, companies that make caloric supplements recently have been marketing them aggressively as nutritional supplements for healthy people. In addition to calories, these supplements often have high fat contents and little fiber. They are also very expensive. You don't need caloric supplements unless you have a specific medical need. Most people eat too many calories and too much fat. If you need an energy boost, eat an apple, banana, bagel, or serving of low-fat yogurt. They cost less and taste a lot better.

Vitamin and Mineral Supplements

Large doses of antioxidants such as vitamin E, vitamin C, and beta carotene have been advocated to prevent the onset of conditions such as heart disease and cancer. However, there is no conclusive evidence that antioxidants reduce the risk of these diseases. Antioxidant vitamins may eventually prove to be good preventive medicine; in the meantime, they are inexpensive and safe, but their effectiveness is unknown.

If you want to be sure you are getting the necessary amount of all vitamins and minerals, use a multivitamin supplement containing 100 percent of the RDA of vitamins and minerals for adults. There is no advantage to buying "natural" vitamins, brand-name vitamins, or those composed especially for middle-aged or older people. Use multivitamins to complement a healthy balanced diet. Vitamin supplements are not substitutes for poor eating habits.

Ergogenic Aids

Ergogenic is a term that has been applied to a variety of nutritional products that claim to be "life enhancing." Examples included lecithin, ginseng, and chromium. There is no reliable scientific evidence that these substances confer any health benefit. To the contrary, as well as being expensive, some may be dangerous in large doses.

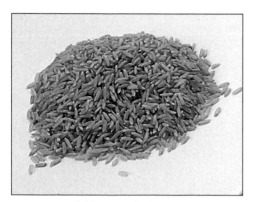

Sources of fiber include grains, such as rice...

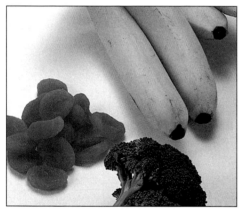

fruits and vegetables...

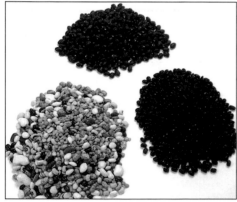

and legumes.

Fiber

In addition to the essential nutrients, we also need fiber and water to function efficiently. Fiber is found only in plant foods. Humans, unlike cows or horses, can't digest fiber. Because it resists digestive enzymes, fiber passes through our stomach and small intestines and enters the large intestines basically unchanged. Because it is not digested or absorbed, fiber does not contribute any nutrients to the body, but it is important, nonetheless. Fiber performs valuable functions precisely because it is not digested. Fiber, along with adequate fluid intake, is the safest and most effective way to prevent and treat constipation. A high-fiber diet also protects against heart disease, lowers "bad" blood cholesterol, helps control blood sugar in people who have diabetes, and reduces the risk of some forms of cancer.

There are two basic types of fiber—soluble and insoluble—and many different forms.

Two Types of Fiber

Insoluble Fiber

- Absorbs many times its weight in water, swelling within the intestines

- Prevents constipation; increases stool bulk and promotes more efficient elimination

- May alleviate some digestive disorders (diverticulitis and irritable bowel syndrome)

- May prevent colon cancer and breast cancer

- Controls appetite

Soluble Fiber

- Appears to lower LDL ("bad") blood cholesterol levels

- Prevents constipation; helps produce a softer stool but does less to help the passage of food

- Retards the entry of glucose into the bloodstream and helps improve glucose tolerance (important for diabetics)

- Controls appetite

Although the U.S. nutritional guidelines have not established exactly how much fiber we need, the National Cancer Institute and the American Dietetic Association both recommend 20 to 35 g of fiber per day. That means you should try to eat a minimum of five servings of fruit or vegetables and six servings of whole grain products daily. Increase your fiber intake slowly to prevent cramping and bloating. Remember to drink plenty of fluids.

Sources of Dietary Fiber

Food	Serving Size	Dietary Fiber (g)
Grains		
Oat bran, dry	1/3 cup	4.0
Oatmeal, dry	1/3 cup	2.7
Rice, brown, cooked	1/2 cup	2.4
Bread, whole wheat	1 slice	1.5
Fruits		
Pear, with skin	1 large	5.8
Apricots, with skin	4 pieces	3.5
Apple, with skin	1 small	2.8
Banana	1 small	2.2
Grapefruit	1/2 fruit	1.6
Vegetable		
Peas, green, frozen, cooked	1/2 cup	4.3
Broccoli, cooked	1/2 cup	2.4
Carrots, cooked	1/2 cup	2.0
Potato, with skin	1/2 cup	1.5
Legumes		
Kidney beans, cooked	1/2 cup	6.9
Pinto beans, cooked	1/2 cup	5.9
Lentils, cooked	1/2 cup	5.2
Peas, black-eyed peas, canned	1/2 cup	4.7

Tips for Increasing Your Fiber Intake

- Eat a variety of foods, especially whole-grain cereals and fruits and vegetables. In addition to fiber, they contain important vitamins and minerals and are low in fat and calories.

- Choose foods that are unprocessed or unrefined. Processing and refining removes fiber.

- Eat the skins of fruits and vegetables whenever possible.

- Increase the amount of fiber you eat gradually to reduce the chances of intestinal gas due to fermentation in the colon.

- Be sure to drink plenty of liquids to move fiber through the intestines.

- Eat high-fiber foods at every meal. Fiber fills you without adding calories and can help you control your weight.

Water

Water is an essential nutrient. It is more essential to life than food because it cannot be made by or stored in the body and must be replaced as it is excreted. Yet water comprises about 60 percent of adult body weight. We can survive approximately 70 days without food but only 10 days without water. Water is involved in almost every body function, helping digestion and absorption of nutrients, carrying nutrients in the bloodstream and carrying waste products of metabolism from tissue and cells, providing a medium for chemical reactions, and regulating the body's temperature. An adequate water (fluid) intake is especially important because our thirst sensation diminishes as we age. Diuretic medications, caffeine, alcohol, infections, diarrhea, and living in a hot or dry climate also contribute to fluid loss and increase the need for water. At least 8

ACTION BOX 2

Test Your Knowledge of Nutrition

A. Provide two examples of food sources for each of the following nutrients:

1. Complex carbohydrate_____

2. Complete protein _____

3. Incomplete protein _____

4. Saturated fat _____

5. Calcium _____

6. Vitamin C _____

7. Iron _____

8. Fiber_____

B. Match each of the following terms with its definition: LDL; HDL; calorie; amino acids; saturated fat; complete protein; vitamins and minerals; essential nutrients; fiber; carbohydrate.

1. Unit of measurement that tells the amount of energy in a food. _____

2. Nutrients that are the preferred source of energy._____

3. Aids in the passage of food through the intestines._____

4. The building blocks of proteins. _____

5. Substance that increases blood cholesterol levels (found in meats, dairy products, coconut and palm oil). _____

   _____

6. "Good" blood cholesterol._____

7. "Bad" blood cholesterol. _____

8. Nutrients that we need in very small amounts. _____

9. Generic term for nutrients the body can't make. _____

10. Beans and rice make up one of these. _____

Answers: 1: calorie; 2: carbohydrates; 3: fiber; 4: amino acids; 5: saturated fat; 6: HDL; 7: LDL; 8: vitamins and minerals; 9: essential nutrients; 10: complete protein.

cups a day are recommended unless contraindicated by medical problems such as edema, congestive heart failure, or renal failure. Water, fruit juices, lemonade or other fruit beverages, crushed ice, and ice pops all meet the need for water. Drink at regular intervals throughout the day and during mealtimes to maintain adequate hydration.

The signs of dehydration are cramps and loss of coordination, nausea, constipation, elevated body temperature, hypotension (low blood pressure), and mental confusion. If you are exposed to extreme heat, be especially careful to increase your fluid intake. Two thirds of heat stroke victims are aged 60 or older. Heat stroke can be fatal.

Eating a Balanced Diet

The body needs more than 40 different nutrients for good health. No single food group can supply all these nutrients, so you must consume a variety of foods to meet your daily nutrient requirements. The United States Department of Agriculture's (USDA) Food Guide Pyramid will help you obtain a balanced diet from a variety of foods. The pyramid graphic *(see p. 266)* illustrates how much food from each food group we should eat each day. Note that carbohydrates are recommended as the foundation of the diet, and fats and sugars, shown at the tip of the pyramid, are recommended "sparingly." This planning and tracking tool shows the serving sizes of different foods from each of the five food groups.

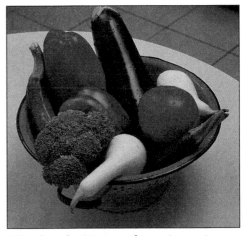

Think color! Eat at least 1 serving of a colorful food (red, orange, yellow, green, purple) at every meal.

Putting the Food Guide Into Practice

The recommendations in the Food Guide Pyramid are based on the following established dietary guidelines:

- Each day choose foods from all five major food groups shown in the pyramid. Begin with plentiful grains, vegetables, and fruits, which provide carbohydrates, vitamins, minerals, and dietary fiber.

- Choose foods that are low in fat, saturated fat, and cholesterol to protect against heart disease, excess weight, and cancer.

- Use sugar in moderation. Sugar supplies calories but no nutrients.

- Moderate your use of salt and sodium. Table salt contains sodium and chloride, which are essential to good health. Most Americans, however, eat more salt than they need— between 2 to 5 teaspoons of salt every day—more than twice the recommended amount. About half the sodium you eat comes from the salt you add to food at the table or during preparation.

- Finally, if you drink alcoholic beverages, do so in moderation. Alcoholic beverages contain calories but few or no nutrients.

Calories in Alcohol

There are 7 calories per gram of alcohol, almost as many calories as in a gram of fat.

Food Guide Pyramid

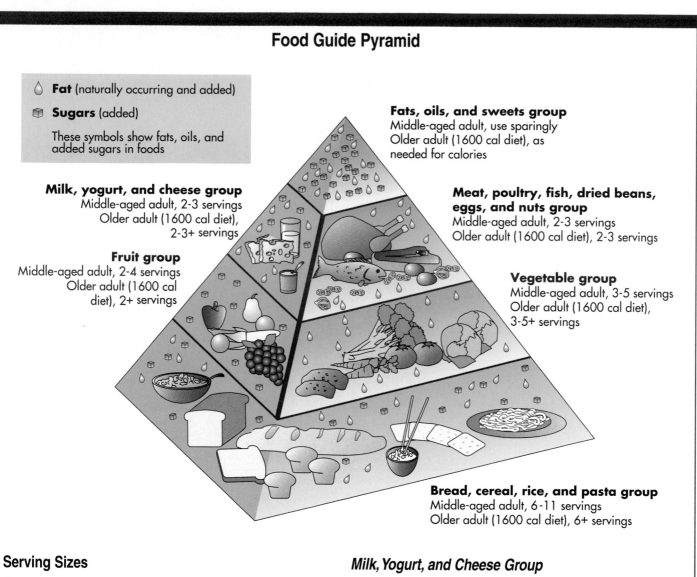

◊ Fat (naturally occurring and added)

▢ Sugars (added)

These symbols show fats, oils, and added sugars in foods

Milk, yogurt, and cheese group
Middle-aged adult, 2-3 servings
Older adult (1600 cal diet),
2-3+ servings

Fruit group
Middle-aged adult, 2-4 servings
Older adult (1600 cal diet), 2+ servings

Fats, oils, and sweets group
Middle-aged adult, use sparingly
Older adult (1600 cal diet), as needed for calories

Meat, poultry, fish, dried beans, eggs, and nuts group
Middle-aged adult, 2-3 servings
Older adult (1600 cal diet), 2-3 servings

Vegetable group
Middle-aged adult, 3-5 servings
Older adult (1600 cal diet), 3-5+ servings

Bread, cereal, rice, and pasta group
Middle-aged adult, 6-11 servings
Older adult (1600 cal diet), 6+ servings

Serving Sizes

Bread, Cereal, Rice, and Pasta Group

- 1 slice bread
- 1 oz ready-to-eat cereal
- 1/2 cup cooked cereal, rice, or pasta

Vegetable Group

- 1 cup raw leafy vegetables
- 1/2 cup other vegetables, cooked or chopped raw
- 3/4 cup vegetable juice

Fruit Group

- 1 medium piece fruit
- 1/2 cup chopped, cooked, or canned fruit
- 3/4 cup fruit juice

Milk, Yogurt, and Cheese Group

- 1 cup milk or yogurt
- 1 1/2 oz natural cheese
- 2 oz processed cheese

Lean Meat, Poultry, Fish, Dried Beans, Eggs, and Nuts

- 2 1/2 to 3 oz cooked lean meat, poultry, or fish
- 1/2 cup cooked dried beans
- 1 egg
- 2 tablespoons peanut butter

Visual guide

- 1 oz of meat is the size of a matchbox
- 3-oz portion is the size of a deck of cards
- 8-oz portion is the size of a medium-sized paperback book

Based on *Nutrition and Your Health: Dietary Guidelines for Americans*, 3rd ed., Home and Garden Bulletin No. 232, by the U.S. Department of Agriculture/U.S. Department of Health and Human Services, 1990, Washington, DC: U.S. Government Printing Office.

Tips to Reduce Sodium

- Remove the salt shaker from the table.

- Don't add salt to foods while cooking.

- Limit the use of baking soda, baking power, and monosodium glutamate (MSG) when you cook. These substances are high in sodium.

- Read food labels to know which foods are high in sodium.

- Avoid processed or packaged foods.

- If you salt your food, try using pepper, spice blends, or lemon juice on meats and vegetables as alternative ways to enhance food flavors.

- When eating out, request that your food be prepared without MSG, butter or margarine, or other heavy sauces.

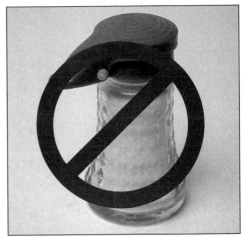

To reduce your salt intake, remove the salt shaker from the table.

Limit Your Alcohol Consumption

Too much alcohol can raise blood pressure, increase your weight, increase your risk for liver disease and some types of cancer, and cause falls and other accidents. Overuse of alcohol is also linked to social and emotional problems.

- Limit your alcohol to no more than 2 drinks per day. One drink is defined as 1 oz of 100-proof liquor, 12 oz of beer, or 4 oz of wine.

- If you are drinking at social functions, mix your own drink to control the amount of alcohol added.

- Add extra parts of fruit juice, soda, or tonic water to liquor.

- Make a wine cooler by adding soda and fruit juice to wine.

- Try nonalcoholic beers and wines.

- Alternate alcoholic drinks with nonalcoholic beverages.

- Don't drink on an empty stomach. The effects of alcohol will be more exaggerated.

- Drink extra water to avoid dehydration.

- Say "no" or drink club soda when you don't want to drink or have had enough.

- NEVER DRIVE AFTER YOU HAVE BEEN DRINKING ALCOHOL.

Evaluate Your Nutrition

Do you eat a variety of foods every day from each of the five food groups?

- Do you regularly eat 5 servings of high-fiber foods like whole-grain breads and cereals, fruits, beans, and greens and other vegetables?

Foods High in Sodium

- Frozen entrees or TV dinners
- Pizza and other fast food
- Cured meats or luncheon meats
- Sausages, frankfurters, hot dogs
- Canned fish or shellfish (in oil or brine)
- Canned soups
- Canned vegetables and juices
- Salted nuts
- Salted crackers, chips, pretzels, popcorn
- Commercially prepared baked goods, cookies, rolls
- Catsup
- Olives, pickles, relish
- Mayonnaise, commercial salad dressings
- Meat tenderizers, MSG

- Do you try to limit the amount of fat you eat to no more than 30 percent of your total daily calories?

- Is your daily dietary cholesterol intake less than 300 mg/day?

- Do you limit your intake of salt (sodium) to less than 1 teaspoon per day?

- Do you use sugar sparingly by adding little or none to the foods you eat and by limiting your consumption of candy, sugar-sweetened soft drinks, and rich desserts?

- Do you avoid alcohol or limit your consumption to no more than 2 drinks per day?

Planning Meals

The way you eat today is probably very different from the way you ate when you were a teenager or young adult. These changes in eating habits present some real challenges as you attempt to adopt and maintain a healthy life-style. If you are like most adults, you probably:

- Eat fewer meals at home

- Eat "mini-meals" while engaging in other activities throughout the day

- Eat alone or in shifts, rather than with the family gathered around the dining room table at home

- Use more convenience foods—take-out, ordered-in, and microwaveable foods

Everything is changing—how we shop and cook, what we eat, and when and where we eat. With new food technologies, vending machines can include refrigerated foods that require no heating. Supermarkets have expanded to offer fully cooked entrees that are ready to eat or only require reheating. In some parts of the country, home-delivered meals are available 7 days a week, making cooking and shopping almost unnecessary.

How do you eat healthfully in today's fast-paced world?

- Practice meal planning

- Have healthy foods readily available or carry them with you

- Choose healthy snacks

- Read labels carefully

- Know portion sizes

Plan meals to ensure a healthy diet. Learn to organize your time, money, equipment, and food to produce meals that are low-fat and nutritionally balanced. Successful meal planning doesn't mean that you must prepare all your meals from "scratch" or only eat at home. Purchasing prepared food products or eating out can provide a healthy balanced diet if you plan ahead.

Breakfast

If breakfast is so important, why do so many people skip it? The most common excuse given for skipping breakfast is lack of time. The benefits of a good breakfast far outweigh the benefits of sleeping an extra 15 minutes. Research has shown that people who skip breakfast are less likely to get an adequate supply of nutrients over the course of the day and are more likely to have reduced productivity late in the morning.

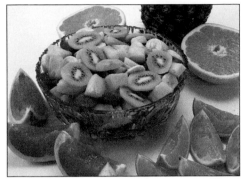

Breakfast fruits provide energy, fiber, and essential vitamins.

Tips for Planning Healthy Breakfasts

- Keep it simple but balanced. Choose foods from the grains (breads and cereals), the fruits, and the low-fat dairy groups. *(Complete Action Box 3 below.)* These foods will give you complex carbohydrates, fiber, calcium, and vitamin C. If you eat a hearty breakfast, include a low-fat meat.

- Try to consume 1/4 to 1/3 of your total daily calories at breakfast.

- Take breakfast with you if you're in a hurry. Leave the clean-up until later.

- Involve other family members. Everyone benefits from eating a good breakfast.

ACTION BOX 3

Plan a Healthy Breakfast

Think of the low-fat foods that you like for breakfast and list them in the appropriate food group below. Use this list to plan several days' breakfasts.

Breads/Cereals (whole-wheat bread, bagels, English muffin, bran flakes, hot or cold whole-grain cereal)	**Fruits** (juice [not "ade" or "cocktail"], orange, banana, peach, cantaloupe, nectarine, pear, grapefruit, berries)	**Low-Fat Dairy Foods or Meats** (nonfat milk, nonfat yogurt, part-skim mozzarella, nonfat cottage cheese) or low-fat meats (smoked chicken or fish)

	Breads/Cereals	Fruits	Low-Fat Dairy/Meats
Day 1			
Day 2			
Day 3			

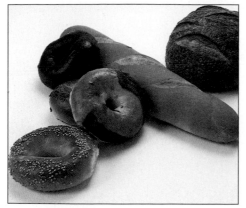

Try different breads to vary lunch menus.

Lunch

More than likely you'll frequently eat lunch away from home. If you do, taking your lunch, or "brown-bagging" it, will give you more control over the foods you eat and will probably cost less than purchasing food from a vending machine or restaurant. Lunch should include whole grains, meat, fish, or dairy products, and fruits or vegetables. *(Complete Action Box 4 below to plan a healthy lunch.)*

Tips for "Brown-Bagging"

- Prepare lunch the night before using leftovers from dinner that can be refrigerated and reheated. Thoroughly reheat foods to avoid contamination.

- Invest in the right utensils—containers that are freezer and microwave safe and insulated bags or coolers. Keep containers and utensils clean to prevent bacterial contamination of food.

- Vary your lunch menu. Try different breads and low-fat spreads and fillings for sandwiches, or try ready-to-eat cereal instead of a sandwich.

- Use healthy prepackaged foods.

ACTION BOX 4

Plan a Healthy Lunch

Think of the low-fat foods that you like for lunch and list them in the appropriate food group below. Use this list to plan several days' lunches.

Breads/Cereals/Rice/Pasta (whole-wheat bread, whole-wheat pita, tortilla, tabouli)	Fruits/Vegetables (apple, orange, banana, grapes, peach, nectarine, plum, pear, carrot sticks, broccoli or cauliflower flowerets, sliced bell peppers, radishes, cucumber rounds, vegetable juice [V-8])	Meats, Legumes, and Dairy (chicken, turkey, water-packed tuna, low-fat cheese, hard-boiled egg, three-bean salad, lentil soup, split-pea soup, cream of broccoli or cauliflower soup)

	Breads/Cereals	Fruits/Vegetables	Low-Fat Meats/Legumes/Dairy
Day 1			
Day 2			
Day 3			

Dinner

Today, many people consume 50 percent or more of their daily calories in the evening meal and in snacks before bedtime. Studies indicate that it is healthier to eat larger meals at breakfast and lunch and a lighter meal for dinner. *(Complete Action Box 5 below to plan a healthy dinner.)*

Tips for Planning Healthy Dinners

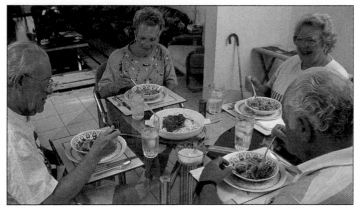

A dinner of pasta and vegetables is a low-fat, high-fiber, inexpensive alternative to red meat or poultry.

- Reduce your dietary fat, especially saturated fat and cholesterol, by preparing more meatless meals. If your family is not used to meatless meals, plan one meatless dinner per week and add more at intervals until you are consuming three meatless meals per week. The increased fiber content of meatless meals can help reduce blood cholesterol levels and reduce your risk for heart disease.

- Avoid the temptation to eat less red meat by increasing your consumption of high-fat dairy products. Choose low-fat cheeses or use meatless dishes that use plant sources of protein.

- Learn how to combine incomplete proteins from plant sources to make complete proteins.

ACTION BOX 5

Plan a Healthy Dinner

Think of the low-fat foods that you like for dinner and list them in the appropriate food group below. Use this list to plan several days' dinners.

Breads/Cereals/Rice/Pasta (rice, bulgur, cracked wheat, pasta, couscous, barley, baked potato)	**Fruits/Vegetables** (broccoli, cabbage, cauliflower, carrots, peas, string beans, squash, tomato, salad-type vegetables, cucumber, lettuce, sprouts)	**Meats, Legumes, and Dairy** (chicken, turkey, fish, chile with beans, lean cuts of red meat, low-fat cheese, egg, milk, yogurt)

	Breads/Cereals	Fruits/Vegetables	Low-Fat Meats/Legumes/Dairy
Day 1			
Day 2			
Day 3			

Complementing Proteins

Animal products provide complete proteins. They contain all the essential amino acids or building blocks of protein in the amounts we require. Plant foods contain some but not all the amino acids. You can combine plant foods to provide complete proteins. Some complementary protein sources include:

- Wheat bread or oatmeal + milk
- Broccoli + cheese
- Pinto beans + corn tortillas
- Red beans + rice

Snacks

You don't have to give up between-meal snacks. In fact, eating healthy snacks can contribute to a balanced diet if you choose nutrient-dense rather than empty-calorie foods. Eating healthy snacks can also help you control your urge to overeat at mealtimes. People who eat fewer than three meals a day are much more likely to overeat.

Tips for Healthy Snacking

- Keep only healthy snacks. Don't buy snack foods that are high in fat, sugar, or salt. If they're not available, you can't eat them!
- Choose high-nutrient, low-calorie snacks over high-calorie, low-nutrient snacks.

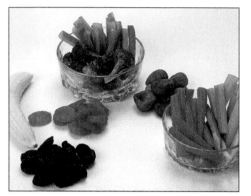

Plan healthy snacks.

High-Calorie versus High-Nutrient Snacks

High-Calorie (Low-Nutrient)	Provide few nutrients relative to the number of calories	Examples include candy and candy bars, chocolate, nondiet sodas, chips, pastries, cookies, cakes, doughnuts
High-Nutrient (Low-Calorie)	Contain a large amount of one or more nutrients for a relatively small number of calories	Examples include fruits (fresh, canned, dried, or juice); raw vegetables (fresh green beans, carrot and celery sticks, broccoli and cauliflower flowerets); vegetable juice; low-fat crackers (graham crackers, vanilla wafers); air-popped popcorn; whole-grain breads and ready-to-eat cereals; low-fat or fat-free dairy products (low-fat yogurt, low-fat cottage cheese, ice milk)

Tools, Products, and Resources for Healthy Eating

Tools and Equipment	*Uses*
Nonstick baking sheets, loaf pans, muffin cups, pots and pans	Allow you to bake and cook without adding fats and oils to prevent sticking.
Fat-separating measuring cups (spout is at the bottom of the cup)	You can pour off the liquid and discard the fat that floats on top. Useful in making soups, stews, and gravies.
Steam rack	Cooks vegetables with steam, retaining the color, taste, and vitamins.
Food processor or blender	For chopping and pureeing fruits and vegetables. You can use a food processor to make a delicious sour cream substitute with low-fat cottage cheese.
Wok (stovetop or electric version)	For stir-frying in small amounts of oil. Cooking on the sides of the wok allows excess fat to drain to the bottom.
Low-fat cookbooks (ones from the voluntary health organizations—American Heart Association, American Cancer Society, American Diabetes Association, American Dietetic Association—are excellent)	Provide recipes and healthful preparation methods for favorite foods. Many recipes feature foods that can be prepared quickly. Cooking healthy foods doesn't have to take extra time.
Microwave oven and microwave-safe containers	Many prepackaged foods can be prepared in the microwave. Read the label to be sure you know what you're eating. Use the microwave to reheat foods you have prepared (saves time and money).
Vegetable cooking spray	Reduces the amount of fat or oil in many recipes.

Shopping for Groceries

A shopping list like the one on the following page will help you minimize the purchase of high-fat, high-calorie foods. Keep an inventory of these foods to help you prepare quick, nutritious meals. Also as a reminder, keep a list of menus or favorite low-fat recipes that you can prepare at a moment's notice. *(Complete Action Box 6 on p. 275.)* Lack of time is one of the most common excuses people give for not eating healthfully.

Checklist for Smart Shopping

Dairy

- Skim milk
- Low-fat cheese
- Parmesan or Romano cheese
- Low-fat or fat-free cheese
- Low-fat yogurt
- Liquid margarine
- Egg substitute
- Ice milk or frozen, low-fat yogurt
- Nonfat evaporated milk

Meat/Seafood

- Sirloin or flank steak
- Tenderloin (beef or pork)
- Extra-lean ground beef
- Skinless chicken breast
- Ground turkey
- Fish fillets
- Lean luncheon meats
- Tuna or salmon packed in water

Fruits/Vegetables

- Fresh fruits and vegetables
- Frozen or canned fruit and fruit juices without added sugar
- Frozen or canned vegetables without added salt
- 100 percent juices with pulp

Breads/Bakery

- Whole-grain breads and muffins
- Bagels
- Tortillas
- Pita bread

Snacks/Crackers

- Animal crackers
- Graham crackers
- Vanilla wafers
- Pretzels
- Fig bars
- Popcorn (air-popped or low-fat microwaveable)

Cereals

- Pasta
- Brown rice, millet, bulgur, couscous, buckwheat
- Whole-grain, unsweetened, ready-to-eat cereals
- Oatmeal

Oils, Seasonings, Dressings

- Liquid vegetable oil or vegetable cooking spray
- Butter-flavored granules
- Reduced-calorie salad dressings
- Reduced-fat mayonnaise
- Low-salt chicken and beef bouillon
- Spices
- Mustard
- Vinegars

ACTION BOX 6

List Low-Fat Menu Items

Take this list with you when you go grocery shopping to give you healthy meal planning ideas.

Favorite Low-Fat Menu Items	*Menu Suggestions: Serve with...*

Meat Dishes

_____   _____

_____   _____

_____   _____

Meatless Dishes

_____   _____

_____   _____

_____   _____

Vegetables

_____   _____

_____   _____

_____   _____

Salads

_____   _____

_____   _____

_____   _____

Desserts

_____   _____

_____   _____

_____   _____

Breads

_____   _____

_____   _____

_____   _____

Soups

_____   _____

_____   _____

_____   _____

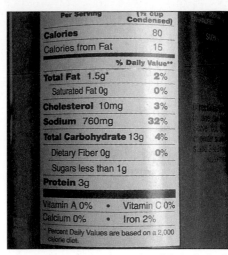

The information on food labels helps you make healthy food choices. Check the fat and saturated fat content, and compare total calories with calories from fat. Remember, you should obtain no more than 30 percent of your daily calories from fat.

"Cholesterol Free" Doesn't Mean "Fat Free"

Products made with vegetable fat may have no cholesterol, but they may still have a high-fat content. Check the label for total fat.

Deciphering Food Labels

Whether you plan meals in advance or fix meals at the last minute, what you buy at the supermarket largely determines what you eat. Shopping in today's supermarkets is a challenge. We are faced with claims that foods are "cholesterol free," "low fat," "high fiber," and "reduced sodium." What do these claims mean? The new food labeling eliminates much confusion in reading food labels.

Food labeling used to be voluntary, but today you'll find nutrition information on almost all the packaged foods you buy. The list of nutrients includes only those most important to today's consumers, most of whom must worry about getting too much of certain items, such as fat. The sample food label below shows you what a food label now looks like.

Sample Food Label

Nutrition Facts

Serving Size 1/2 cup (114 g)   Serving per container 4

Amount per Serving

Calories   260   Calories from Fat 120

	% Daily Value*
Total Fat 13 g	20%
Saturated Fat 5 g	25%
Cholesterol 30 mg	10%
Sodium 660 mg	28%
Total Carbohydrate 31 g	11%
Dietary Fiber 0 g	0%
Sugars 5 g	
Protein 5 g	

Vitamin A 4%	Vitamin C 2%
Calcium 15%	Iron 4%

---

*Percent Daily Values are based on a 2,000 calorie diet. Your daily values may be higher or lower depending on your calorie needs:

		2,000	2,500
Calories		2,000	2,500
Total Fat	Less than	65 g	80 g
Saturated Fat	Less than	20 g	25 g
Cholesterol	Less than	300 mg	300 mg
Sodium	Less than	2,400 mg	2,400 mg
Total Carbohydrate		300 g	375 g
Fiber		25 g	30 g

Calories per gram:

Fat 9   Carbohydrates 4   Protein 4

Standardized Serving Sizes

The serving sizes on food labels are now standardized and are based on food consumption surveys that have determined the amounts and portions of food that most people eat. You need to check the serving size, because your idea of an individual serving might be different from the average. If the serving size on the label is half what you eat in a single serving, you will get double the number of calories and nutrient amounts listed.

Saturated Fat

The labels list not only the grams of total fat, but also the grams of saturated fat. Remember, you should get no more than 18 g of saturated fat per day. A quick look at the grams of saturated fat will give you an idea of how much of your daily allowance you are getting from one food.

Percent Daily Values

In addition to grams, the label gives you the percent daily value of each nutrient you get from the food so you can estimate how different foods fit into your overall diet for the day. For example, if a product has a 25 percent daily value for fat, you are getting a full 25 percent of the fat you need in 1 day (if you consume 2,000 calories per day). This means that 2 servings of this food will meet half your fat needs for the whole day. You can also use these numbers to compare foods. For example, if a serving of Brand X's macaroni and cheese has a 27 percent daily value of fat compared to Brand Y's, which has 45 percent, you are better off buying Brand X, no matter how many calories per day you consume.

Tips for Choosing Food Products

The following tips may help you make healthy choices when you go food shopping:

Dairy

- *Milk.* Nonfat milk has 0 g of fat per cup. Low-fat (2 percent) milk has 5 g of fat per cup. Whole milk has 9 to 10 g of fat per cup.

- *Cheese.* It takes about 1 gallon of milk to make 1 pound of cheese. There are almost 2 pats of butter in every cup of whole milk (from which cheese is made). There are 16 cups in 1 gallon of milk; therefore, 1 pound of cheese has about 32 pats of butter. Cheddar, Monterey Jack, and Swiss are high in fat. Low-fat cheese should contain 3 g of fat per serving. Reduced-fat cheese should contain about 5 g of fat per serving.

- *Yogurt.* Look for nonfat milk at the top of the ingredient list. Adding your own fruit to plain yogurt will give you fewer calories and less sugar than fruit yogurts do.

- *Nondairy creamers.* These are useful if you are lactose intolerant but not if you want to lose weight. Mocha mix has 320 calories per cup and 9 teaspoons of sugar.

"Healthy" Doesn't Mean "Unappetizing"

Buy foods that are nutritious and that you enjoy eating. Foods are good for you only if you eat them!

- *Sour cream.* This is a high-fat product. Look for light sour creams, which have half the fat of regular sour cream, or, better still, look for fat-free sour creams.

- *Margarine.* Make sure that the first ingredient on the label is liquid oil, and that the ratio of polyunsaturated to saturated fats is 2:1. All margarines are 100 percent fat; the light versions have added water or air. There is less fat per serving because there is less margarine.

Meats

- *Fish and seafood.* These are lower in fat than almost all meat and poultry, unless you add fat during cooking.

- *Poultry.* Boneless, skinless chicken and turkey have the lowest fat content of all the meats. Dark meat is higher in fat. If you eat the skin, you eat double the fat calories.

- *Red meat.* The rule of thumb is to look for the words "loin," "round," "tip," or "flank." These are the leanest cuts. "Prime," and "choice" are the highest in fat. "Select" is usually the lowest grade, but also contains less fat.

- *Lunch meats.* Ham, corned beef, turkey breast, and chicken breast have less fat than regular cold cuts, but they are still high in sodium. So don't be fooled. Turkey salami and chicken bologna can have up to 18 g of fat per serving.

Produce

- *Go for the color*—dark orange and dark yellow fruits (papaya, apricots, cantaloupe, and mango); dark green, orange, or yellow vegetables (sweet potato and yams, spinach, broccoli, squash, peas).

- Don't forgo the humble potato which has vitamin C, iron, copper, and fiber.

Grains

- *Baked goods.* Breads that have the most fiber say "whole wheat." Light breads are light because the slice is half as thick as regular bread. There are fewer calories because there is less bread.

- *Cereals.* Hot cereals are generally lowest in fat and sugar.

- *Breads.* Avoid baked goods (croissants, biscuits, pastries, muffins), which have more fat and sugar than ordinary breads.

- *Frozen desserts.* Gourmet ice creams have as much as 10 teaspoons of fat per cup. Most fat-reduced frozen desserts have about 1/2 to 3 1/2 teaspoons of fat per cup—mostly because they are made with fat-free milk. Sorbets have the least fat but some are still heavy in calories because they have a high sugar content.

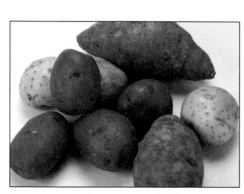

Potatoes and yams are high-energy foods and useful sources of vitamins and minerals.

Frozen Foods

- *Dinners.* Read the labels carefully. The light frozen dinners have about 300 calories, but if they have 10 g of fat, nearly 30 percent of the calories come from fat. Check the label for the content of fat as well as calories. You eat more healthfully if you eat 330 calories and 4 g of fat rather than 300 calories and 10 g of fat.

- *Frozen fruits and vegetables.* These are an excellent source of nutrients. Buy frozen produce with nothing added. Sauces, syrups, and flavorings add calories.

Eating Out

The practice of eating out is ingrained in our culture. It is predicted that by the year 2000, we will spend more than 60 percent of our food dollars of food prepared and obtained away from home. Yet, eating out or eating "on the run" may be hazardous to your efforts to eat a healthy diet and manage your weight. Make a quick assessment of how often you eat away from home. On a scale of 1 to 5, with *1* being least and *5* being most nutritionally balanced, how healthy are these meals?

Tips for Eating "On the Run"

- Don't eat in your car unless absolutely necessary. If you eat while you drive, bring food from home or stop at a supermarket rather than a fast-food restaurant for better choices.

- Order special meals on airlines (vegetarian, seafood, low-fat/low-calorie).

- Take a piece of fresh fruit or low-fat crackers to snack on between meals.

Watch Out for Hidden Sources of Fat
Most cookies, brownies, and other baked goods contain a lot of fat, as well as sugar.

Assessing Meals Eaten Away from Home

Reason/Occasion	How Often? (per month)	Dietary Rating
Lunches		
Snacks/ vending machines		
Fast-food meals		
Birthdays, anniversaries		
Business meals		
Vacations		
Social dining		

Eating in Restaurants

- If possible, choose a restaurant where you've eaten before. If you aren't familiar with the restaurant, call ahead to find out what's on the menu. Are a variety of foods available? Do they offer any heart-healthy choices? Ask how the food is prepared.

- Look for entrees that are broiled, grilled, steamed, or poached.

- Order either an appetizer (or alcoholic drink) before the meal or a dessert, but not both.

- Order smaller sizes of meats, soups (a cup rather than a bowl), or rich desserts.

- Order an appetizer as your entree.

- Eat only half your entree and take the rest home for lunch the next day.

- Share a dessert with a friend.

- Sip water throughout the meal, and stop eating when you're full.

- Look for healthy items in vending machines.

- Choose fruit or vegetable juice instead of a soft drink.

- If you are eating at a restaurant, plan ahead. Check out the menu and how the food is prepared.

Controlling Your Weight

Millions of people struggle to manage their weight to improve their appearance, feel better, and be healthier. Unfortunately, studies show that those who complete weight loss programs lose approximately 10 percent of their body weight, only to regain two thirds of it back within 1 year. Within 5 years, they are likely to have regained almost all the weight they lost, and perhaps more.

In the United States, obesity is a pervasive public health problem with health- and treatment-related costs exceeding $100 billion per year. Approximately 35 percent of women and 31 percent of men aged 20 and older are obese, and the middle and older age groups are more often affected.

What is a Healthy Weight?

The 1995 edition of the *Dietary Guidelines for Americans* provides a unisex version of the height and weight table with a wide range of weights considered desirable. *(See the box on the following page.)*

The most important difference between this table and its precursors is that the 1995 edition no longer allows for weight gain in middle age. Why is this? The original height and weight tables were put together by insurance companies to assess the risk of disease and premature death. The tables made allowances for age. They assumed you would naturally gain 10 or more pounds after age 35, and average weight gain was not considered a risk. Recently, however, large public health studies looking at the relation between age and weight gain show that even average weight gain can increase your risk of premature death from heart disease, diabetes, and some cancers. In other words, no matter what your age, health risk increases as your weight increases. Just a 15- to 20-pound weight gain over your weight at 18 years can increase your risk of premature death. Thus, the emphasis is on maintaining weight, not assessing how much you can "safely" gain.

Note that because the weights in the table are for both men and women, the range is wide. Weights at the lower end of the range are recommended for people who have a lower ratio of muscle and bone to fat. In other words, if you don't have a muscular physique—as most of us don't—your ideal weight will be closer to the lower range. Find your height in the table, then move across and find your desirable weight range. Your personal desirable weight will depend on a number of factors, including your weight at age 18, your physique, and your current health status.

1995 Weight Guidelines

Height (without shoes)	Weight (lbs)
4'10"	91–119
4'11"	94–124
5'0"	97–128
5'1"	101–132
5'2"	104–137
5'3"	107–141
5'4"	111–146
5'5"	114–150
5'6"	118–155
5'7"	121–160
5'8"	125–164
5'9"	129–169
5'10"	132–174
5'11"	136–179
6'0"	140–184

From the U.S. Department of Agriculture, U.S. Department of Health and Human Services.

Measuring Body Mass Index

A useful way to determine your desirable weight is to assess your weight in relation to your height. The Body Mass Index (BMI) provides a useful formula for this purpose. Research suggests that obesity-related problems begin to rise when BMI is greater than 25.

$$BMI = Weight\ (kilograms)/height\ (meters)^2$$

Measure your height and weight without shoes. Record height to the nearest 1/4 inch and weight to the nearest 1/2 pound.

1. Convert your weight in pounds to weight in kilograms (divide your weight in pounds by 2.2 [2.2 lbs = 1 kg]).

2. Convert your height in inches to centimeters and divide by 100 (1 inch = 2.54 cm) to get your height in meters.

3. Square your height in meters (multiply the number by itself).

4. Divide your body weight in kilograms by your height in meters squared.

Example:

1. Weight in pounds = 154/2.2 = 70 kg

2. Height in inches = 68 X 2.54/100 = 1.73 m

3. Height in meters squared = 1.73 X 1.73 = 2.99

4. BMI = 70/2.99 = 23.41

Tips for Weighing Yourself at Home

Weigh yourself no more than twice a week. Once is best. Weight does not change more than about 1 pound per day even during periods of rapid weight loss. More rapid weight gain or loss is due to change in body fluid.

- Weigh yourself at the same time of day.

- Wear the same clothing (minimal, with no shoes).

- Place the scale on a flat, hard, uncarpeted surface.

- Record your weight to the nearest 1/2 pound.

Measuring Body Fat

How much total body fat you have is important. Where fat is stored is also significant. People are either "apple shaped" or "pear shaped." The person who deposits excess weight in the abdomen has a body shape that resembles an apple, while the person who carries extra weight in the buttocks, hips, and thighs is shaped more like a pear. For health reasons, the "pear" is the preferred shape. Health risks increase when people store excess body fat in their abdomens or trunk regions. These people have an increased likelihood of developing high blood pressure, cardiovascular disease, and noninsulin-dependent diabetes.

Unfortunately, you can't change your body shape. That is part of your genetic makeup. But you can control your weight. If you tend to store excess pounds around the middle, it's especially important to keep your body weight within the healthy range.

Calculating Waist-to-Hip Ratio

You can determine if you have excess abdominal fat by measuring the circumferences of your waist and hips and computing a waist-to-hip ratio. You are within a healthy range for body fat if your waist-to-hip ratio is less than 1.0 for men or less than 0.8 for women.

It's easy to take these measurements yourself. You will need a flexible tape measure that does not stretch. It's best to take these measurements without clothing or in your underwear. Stand in front of a mirror while taking these measurements to help you determine that the tape is placed on your body correctly and that your measurements are accurate.

- Stand very straight with your feet together.

- Do not pull the tape too tightly. The tape should not compress your skin.

- Repeat the measurements to ensure accuracy.

- Record the measurements to the nearest 1/4 inch.

  Waist circumference. With your abdomen relaxed (after exhaling), place the tape around your body in a horizontal plane at the level of your natural waist. This level should be midway between the lower ribs and the top of your hip bone.

  Hip circumference. With your abdomen relaxed, place the tape around your hips in a horizontal plane at the level of the maximum width of the buttocks.

- Divide your waist measurement in inches by your hip measurement in inches to obtain a ratio.

  Example: Waist = 34 inches   Hip = 42 inches   Ratio = 0.81

What Is the Best Way to Lose Weight?

To determine if you need to lose weight, complete Action Box 7 below. Losing weight is a matter of energy balance. We gain weight when we take in more calories than we burn. We lose weight when we burn more calories than we take in—a process we call obtaining a negative energy balance. There are three ways to obtain a negative energy balance:

- *Eat less.* Take in fewer calories than you need for fueling body functions and activity.

- *Exercise more.* Burn more calories than you take in through physical activity.

- *Eat less and exercise more.* This is the preferred way to lose weight and keep it off.

To reduce your caloric intake:

- Follow the recommendations in the Food Guide Pyramid *(see p. 266)* for eating a variety of foods.

- Decrease alcohol intake.

- Eat fewer "empty calorie" foods (fats and simple sugars).

- Eat adequate protein.

    Don't let your caloric intake fall below 1,200 calories per day. Fewer than 1,200 calories will not provide you with all the nutrients you need to be healthy.

ACTION BOX 7

Do You Need to Lose Weight?

Answer the questions below to assess whether you should lose weight.	Yes	No
Is your weight above the range for your height shown in the 1995 Weight Guidelines on p. 281?		
Have you gained more than 10 pounds since reaching adult height?		
Is your waist-to-hip ratio more than 1.0 (for men) or 0.8 (for women)?		
Do you have any of the following health risk factors? High blood pressure (greater than 140/90 mm Hg)		
High blood cholesterol (above 240 mg/dl)		
Type II diabetes mellitus		
Osteoarthritis		
If you answered "yes" to two or more of these questions, weight loss may benefit your health.		

To increase your physical activity, follow the plan outlined in this book:

- Begin with low levels of activity and slowly progress to higher levels of activity.

- Gradually reshape patterns of activity rather than follow a strict, regimented exercise prescription.

- Consider a walking program.

- Develop a realistic goal and modify it over time.

- Progress up to 1 hour per day of moderate-intensity activity (brisk walking) accumulated each day.

- Develop an individualized program of activities that you enjoy.

- Engage in more vigorous activities (cycling, jogging, sports and recreation) as your capabilities improve.

- Evaluate different approaches until you develop a sustainable activity plan.

Evaluating Weight Loss Programs

In 1995, the Food and Nutrition Board of the Institute of Medicine published criteria for consumers to use in evaluating the effectiveness of various weight loss programs. The information provided in this section summarizes key points to help you make an informed decision.

Many different types of weight loss programs are available to consumers. They differ in intensity of treatment, cost, method of interventions, and staff credentials. All reputable weight loss programs, regardless of the type of intervention they offer, should voluntarily provide the following information and services:

Exercising More versus Eating Less—The Preferred Method of Weight Loss

Eating Less	Exercising More
People who lose weight through diet tend to regain all their weight and more.	People who lose weight through exercise and diet tend to keep their weight off.
The more restrictive the diet, the greater the risk of adverse effects. For example, rapid weight loss or very low-fat diets increase the risk of gallbladder disease.	Physical activity improves blood levels of cholesterol and sugar and protects against elevated blood pressure.
Women may be at greater risk for osteoporosis because of reduced calcium intake.	Weight-bearing exercise strengthens the bones and protects against osteoporosis.

Weight Loss Programs

Do-It-Yourself These comprise support groups such as Overeaters Anonymous or Take Off Pounds Sensibly (TOPS), in addition to numerous books, devices, and products that assist you to lose weight on your own.

Nonclinical These commercially franchised programs use materials prepared in consultation with health care professionals. However, the staff that deliver these programs are not health care providers.

Clinical These programs may or may not be part of a commercial franchise, and the staff may or may not have specialized training to treat overweight clients. Licensed professionals provide a variety of services including nutrition, medication, behavior therapy, exercise, psychological counseling, and even surgery.

• A truthful, unambiguous statement of the program's approach and goals, including known and hypothetical risks.

• A statement of the client population and who should and should not participate. For example, weight loss programs should discourage individuals who are underweight or anorexic from participating.

• A full disclosure of costs.

• A brief description of the credentials of the staff or the program's developers.

• A statement of procedures recommended for clients.

• Advice to individuals to know their health status and risk factors related to obesity and overweight.

• Advice to individuals with weight-related conditions (hypertension, diabetes, heart disease), risk factors for cardiovascular disease, or other health problems to contact their health care providers.

• Information about potential clients' state of health and weight loss goals.

• Medical supervision as a condition of entry for those with bulimia; significant cardiovascular, renal, or psychiatric disease; diabetes; or other significant medical problems. (Do-It-Yourself programs should advise consumers with these types of problems against attempting to lose weight without medical supervision.)

• Preassessment and continuing assessment including measurements of BMI and waist-to-hip ratio and interpretation of the results. (Do-It-Yourself programs should instruct clients how to measure height and weight and how to calculate BMI and waist-to-hip ratio.)

Weight-Related Health Risk Factors

The following conditions are aggravated by obesity and may improve with a weight loss program:

• High blood pressure
• Elevated blood cholesterol, triglycerides, or glucose
• Heart disease
• Diabetes mellitus
• Osteoarthritis in knees, hips, or feet
• Sleep apnea

- Simple checklists for clients to monitor their health status routinely, including easy-to-score psychological, dietary, and ongoing physical activity assessments.

Which Program Is Best for You?

It is not yet possible to match people with programs to improve significantly their chances of success. You must make your own evaluation. Here are some self-administered tasks you can use to determine whether you are right for a program and it is right for you:

- Obtain information about the program from the publisher or manufacturer to assess whether you are an appropriate candidate.

- Discuss the program or product with a knowledgeable health care provider to determine whether it is sound and appropriate.

- Determine whether the program focuses on long-term weight management. Is there a re-evaluation to assess your progress every 3 to 6 months?

- Determine whether the program provides guidance and skills training to help you change your behaviors.

- Assess evidence of the program's success.

- Last, but not least, make sure you understand what to expect from the program and that your expectations are realistic. Is the time right? Are you ready to devote the time and effort required?

Evaluating the Success of the Program

The primary purpose of weight management is to achieve and maintain good health. This goal includes weight loss but is not limited to it. Any good weight loss program should move the goal of treatment from weight loss alone to weight management, with the final goal of achieving the best weight possible in the context of overall health. Within the context of overall health, the success of any weight loss program is determined by the four following factors:

- *The weight you lose and are able to keep off.* Was the weight loss greater than or equal to 5 percent of body weight or a reduction in BMI of 1 or more units? Did you keep the weight off for more than 1 year?

- *Improvement in other obesity-related conditions/diseases.* Was there improvement in one or more of the following risk factors: high blood pressure, high blood cholesterol, high blood sugar/diabetes mellitus?

Predictors of Long-Term Success in Weight Management

Predictors of Sustained Weight Loss

- Regular habit of exercise
- Continued contact with the treatment program
- Eating a normal, balanced diet
- Continued self-monitoring of diet and exercise
- A positive, problem-solving attitude toward life's stressors

Predictors of Weight Rebound

- Family dysfunction
- Negative life events

- *Improvement in health practices.* Did you learn to practice and sustain good eating habits, learn to practice and sustain activity habits (engaging in 30 minutes or more of moderate-intensity activity four or more times a week and preferably daily), improve your outlook on life, increase your basic knowledge about weight gain and obesity?

- *Regular monitoring of weight and exercise patterns.* Did you monitor your weekly weight and activity?

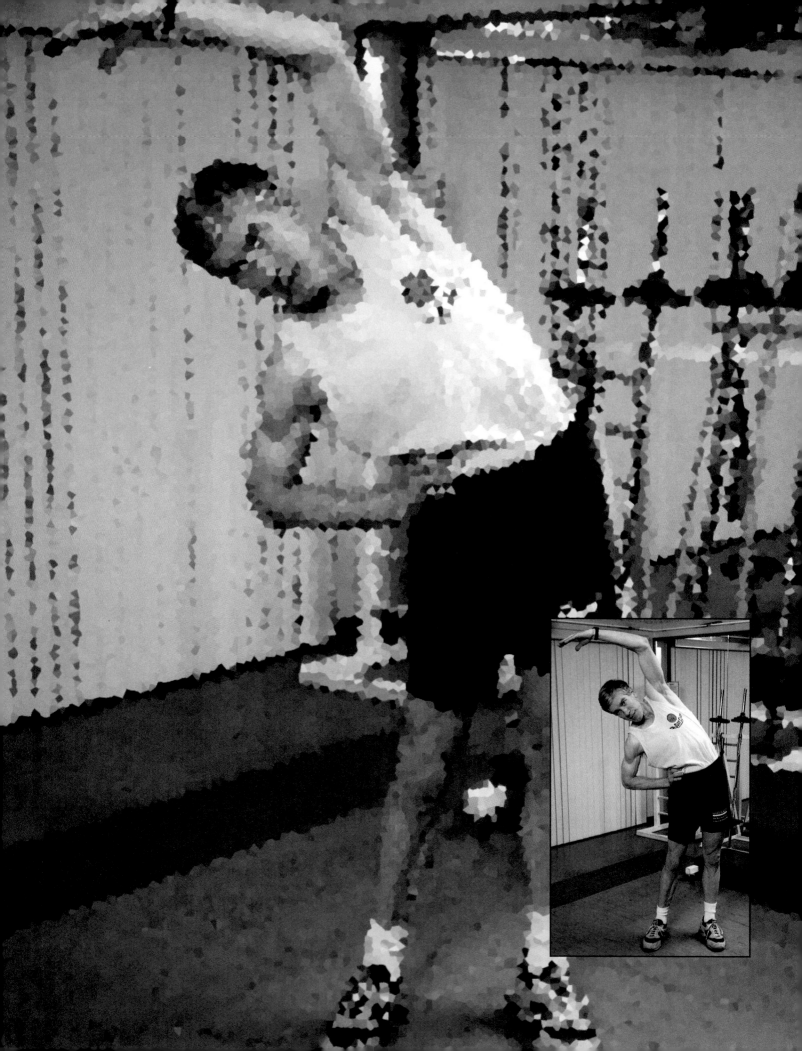

Stretching Exercises

General Instructions

- There are two phases to a stretch: active and static. The *active phase* is the moving phase of the stretch. As you move into the stretch, take it slowly and easily to a point of muscle tension. The *static phase* of the stretch begins at the point of tension.

- During the static phase of the stretch, maintain tension on the muscle, holding it for 10 to 20 seconds and then slowly release.

- Your goal is to perform each stretching exercise once. Stretch slowly and carefully, maintaining control from beginning to end.

- Never stretch to the point of pain.

- Don't bounce while the muscle is fully stretched. Bouncing can cause injury.

- Breathing correctly is important. Inhale before the stretch and exhale during the active phase of the stretch.

Stretches for Major Muscle Groups and Joints

Leg and Back Stretch

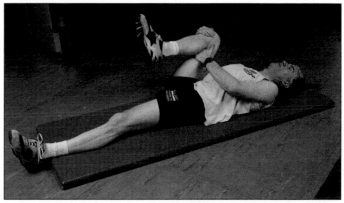

Lie on your back on the floor. With your knee bent, raise your right leg slowly and push it toward your chest with your knee pointing slightly out. Using both hands, grab your raised leg at the knee and pull so that you feel the stretch in the back of your leg and buttock area. Count to 20, then slowly return your leg to the extended position. Repeat with your left leg.

Hip Stretch

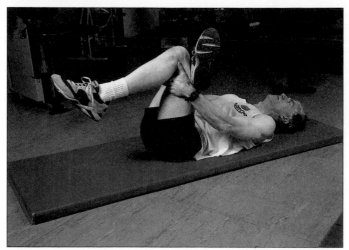

Lie on your back on the floor. Bend both legs at the hips and knees. Raising your right lower leg, place your right ankle in front of your left knee. Grab your left thigh and slowly pull on the thigh, feeling the stretch around the right hip area. Count to 20, then slowly release. Repeat with your left leg.

Hamstring Stretch

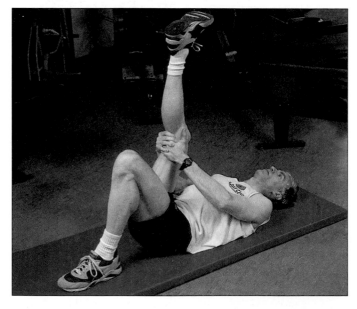

Lie on your back on the floor. Bend your left leg at the knee and place your left foot flat on the floor. Lift the right leg, bending it at the hip with the knee slightly bent. Grab the right leg behind the knee and pull, feeling the stretch from the hip to the knee area in the back of the leg. Count to 20 and repeat with the left leg.

Arched Back Stretch

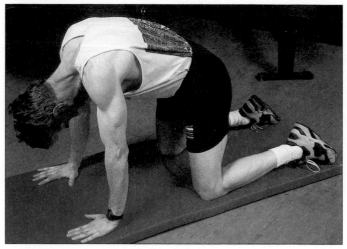

Kneel on your hands and knees and let your head hang down. Arch your back, feeling the pull from the shoulders to your lower back. Count to 20, then slowly return to your starting position.

Upper Back and Arm Stretch

Sit with your legs crossed and your back straight. Reach up with both arms, interlacing the fingers with your palms upward. Reach as high as you can, keeping your back and neck straight. Count to 20, then slowly return to your starting position.

Neck Stretch

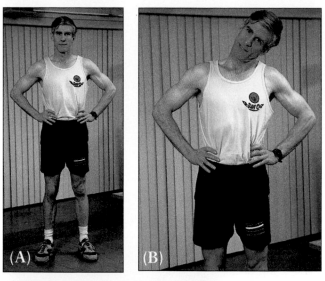

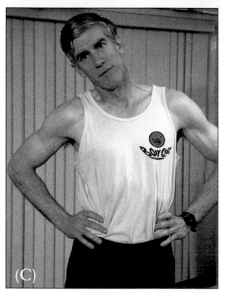

Stand with your hands on your hips and your feet apart to shoulder width (A). Slowly rotate your neck to the left, stretching it and holding it through a count of 5 (B). Then rotate your neck to the right (C). Rotate your neck four times to the left and four times to the right.

Trunk Stretch

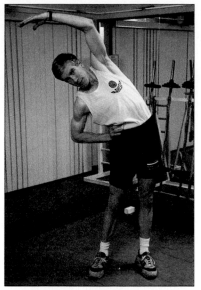

Stand with your feet apart to shoulder width and your back straight. Put your right hand on your right hip and extend your left arm in a circular, upward motion, raising it over your head with the elbow slightly bent. Bend your body to the right, arching your left arm over your head. Stretch the muscles in your left trunk for a count of 20. Repeat the exercise stretching the right trunk muscles.

Calf Stretch

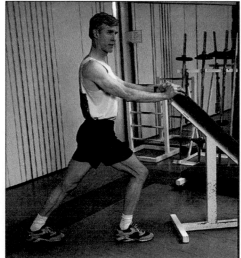

Stand facing a wall or a piece of equipment or furniture and support yourself with your hands almost at shoulder height. Extend your left leg directly behind you and slowly push down on the heel until the left foot is flat on the floor. Lean forward, slightly bending your right knee until you feel the stretch in the left leg. Count to 20, then repeat with the right leg.

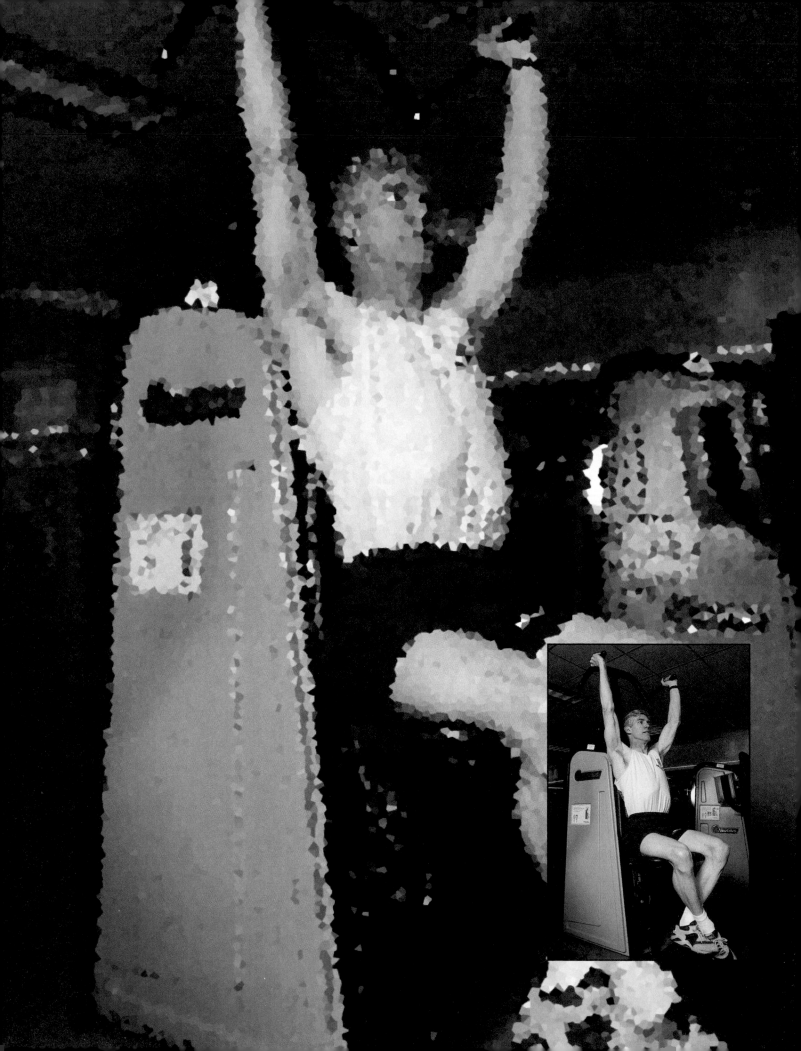

Strength-Building Exercises

General Instructions

- Wear comfortable shoes with rubber soles to provide secure footing.

- Wear light, loose-fitting clothing to give you freedom of movement and allow body heat to dissipate. Don't wear ties, scarves, jewelry, or anything that can get caught in weights or machines.

- Lift all weights from the floor using your legs rather than your lower back to avoid acute low back strain.

- Breathe properly. Don't hold your breath. Holding your breath can raise blood pressure and decreases blood supply to the brain, causing dizziness and fainting.

- Take your time. Do each repetition of an exercise through the full range of motion.

- Perform exercises in an appropriate sequence—from large to small muscles. If the small muscles become too tired, you'll be un-able to do the exercises that build the larger muscles.

- Your goal is to do a complete set of all the exercises. Complete 1 set before repeating any one exercise. This procedure will ensure that you work every muscle group at least once, and you can rest each muscle before you exercise it again.

- A *set* is 15 repetitions completed without paus-ing. Begin the exercise slowly with very low weights and at a resistance level that allows you to do 15 repetitions, or 1 set. When you are able to do 15 repetitions, increase the weight by a small increment (2 to 5 lbs) or to a level of resistance at which you can do 7 to 8 repetitions without pausing. Work up to 15 repetitions. When you can do a complete set at the new weight, increase the weight again.

- When you have worked up to a weight at which doing 2 complete sets is very difficult, stay at that weight for maintenance of muscle strength and endurance.

Calisthenics

Legs and Hips

This series improves strength, flexibility, and balance and assists in daily activities such as climbing stairs, walking, bending to lift or pick up objects, or rising from a chair. It also helps to prevent low back pain.

Squats: Strengthens the front of the thighs (*quadriceps*) and buttocks (*gluteus*).

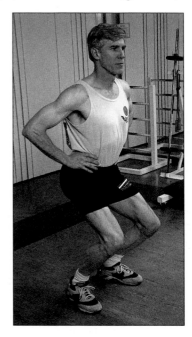

Stand with your feet apart to shoulder width. With your hands on your hips and keeping your back straight, bend your knees into a squatting position until your knees form 45° to 90° angles, depending on what feels comfortable, then slowly straighten. Repeat 15 times.

Chair Raises: If you have not been active, if you have knee problems, or if you are overweight, chair raises may be an easier alternative to squats. Chair raises use many of the same muscles as squats.

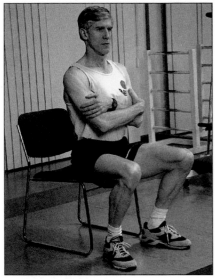

Choose a sturdy chair. Sit on the edge of it. With your arms folded across your chest, stand up straight, then slowly sit in one motion. Repeat 15 times.

Hip Raises: Strengthens the hip muscles and the buttocks (*gluteus*).

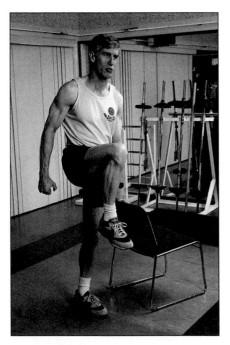

Stand, holding onto a chair for balance. Raise your right knee toward your chest as far as you can, then slowly lower the leg. Repeat 15 times. In a second set, repeat the exercise using the left leg.

Step-Up: Strengthens the calf muscles (*gastrocnemius*).

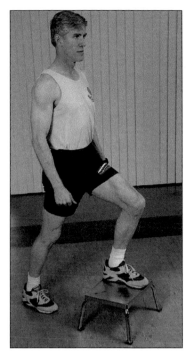

Find a set of steps or a sturdy bench or stool with an 8- to 12-inch step-up. Face the step, standing 10 to 12 inches from it. Planting the left foot firmly on the step, step up on the left leg, pause for 1 second, then step down on the right leg followed by the left. Repeat 15 times. In a second set, repeat the exercise using the right leg.

Abdomen and Trunk

This series assists in bending, lifting, carrying, and rising from a chair. It improves posture, helps you look trim and fit, stabilizes the lower back, and helps prevent low back pain, especially if you must spend a long time sitting.

Abdominal Crunch: Strengthens the abdominal muscles.

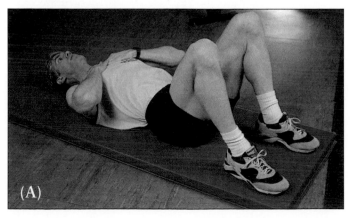

(A)

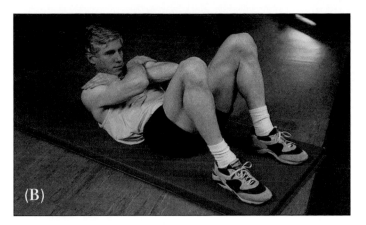

(B)

Lie on your back on the floor with your knees bent and your feet planted firmly on the floor. Rest both your hands on your upper chest (A). Lift your shoulders 3 to 4 inches from the floor by contracting your abdominal (stomach) muscles (B). Make sure the small of your back remains flat on the floor. Don't bend your neck, and don't sit all the way up. Return to your starting position. Repeat 15 times.

Pelvic Tilt: Strengthens the abdominal muscles.

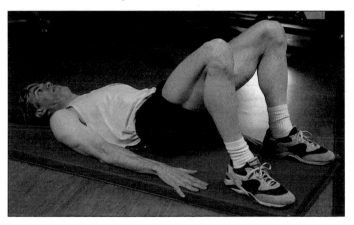

Lie on your back on the floor with your knees bent and your feet planted firmly on the floor. Your arms should be by your sides with the palms facing down. Tilt your pelvis backward by contracting your abdominal (stomach) muscles. Be sure the small of your back touches the floor. Your arms and legs should be relaxed and should not help with the exercise. Repeat 15 times.

Back, Shoulders, and Arms

This series assists in lifting objects above your head, carrying, and pushing and improves the ability to perform many daily activities.

Push-Ups: Strengthens the chest (*pectoralis*), shoulders (*deltoids*), and back of the arms (*triceps*).

Intermediate Push-Up

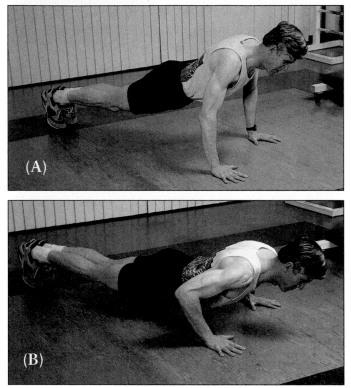

(A)

(B)

Lie face down on the floor with your legs and feet together and your toes curled under so that the soles of your feet are perpendicular (90°) to the floor. Place your hands flat on the floor, parallel to your shoulders, with your elbows bent slightly away from your body. Keeping your legs and trunk straight, slowly push up, keeping your body in alignment until your arms straighten (A). Keeping your trunk straight, bend your arms to slowly lower your body toward the floor (B). When you are close to the floor, raise your upper body by straightening your arms. Repeat 15 times.

There are several variations of the push-up. If you have limited strength in the upper body, try the beginner's push-up *(below)*, and when you have built up strength in your arms, graduate to the intermediate push-up *(see illustration above)*. Advanced push-ups are performed by supporting and lowering yourself on your fists or fingers or

on only one arm. Advanced push-ups require more strength than anyone needs for normal daily or recreational activities.

Beginners' Push-Up

Lie face down on the floor with your legs and feet together and your toes curled under so that the soles of your feet are perpendicular (90°) to the floor. Place your hands flat on the floor, parallel to your shoulders, with your elbows bent slightly away from your body. Keeping your knees on the floor, slowly push your upper body up until your arms straighten. Keeping your knees on the floor and your back straight, bend your arms at the elbows to slowly lower your body toward the floor. When you are close to the floor, raise your upper body by straightening your arms. Repeat 15 times.

Chair Dips: Strengthens the back of the arms (*triceps*) and the shoulders (*deltoids*).

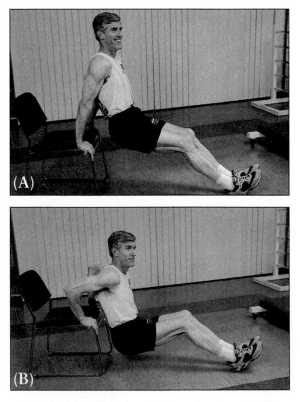

(A)

(B)

Extend your arms behind your body, placing your hands on the edge of a bench or sturdy chair. Your arms should be straight. Move your legs forward so that your knees are slightly bent (A). This is your starting position. Slowly lower your trunk by bending your arms at the elbows (B). Raise your body by straightening your arms to return to your starting position. Repeat 15 times.

Resistance Training with Handheld and Strap-On Weights

Equipment: Purchase three sets of dumbbells (2.2, 5.0, and 10 lbs) and two sets of strap-on weights (10 and 20 lbs). When you have gained strength, purchase a set of 15- and 20-lb dumbbells.

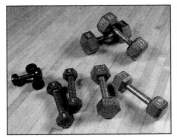
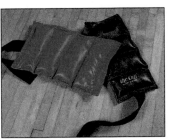

Dumbbells.   *Strap-on weights.*

Technique:

- Use slow, controlled movements.
- Don't jerk the weights or let your body sway.
- Count *1, 2* as you raise the weight(s) and *1, 2* as you lower it (them).
- Your goal is to do 2 sets of 15 repetitions for each exercise.
- Rest 30 to 60 seconds between each set.

Exercises for the Legs and Hips

This series improves balance and mobility and enhances ability to perform daily and recreational activities.

Leg Extensions: Strengthens the front of the thighs (*quadriceps*).

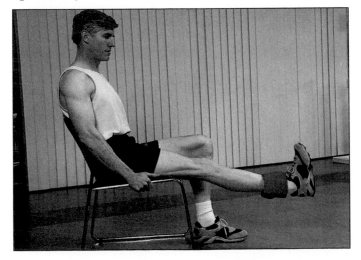

Strap a 10-lb weight securely around your ankle. Sit in a sturdy chair that supports your back. Raise your lower leg, straightening it at the knee, then slowly lower your leg to your starting position. Perform 15 repetitions for each leg.

Leg Curls: Strengthens the hamstring muscles.

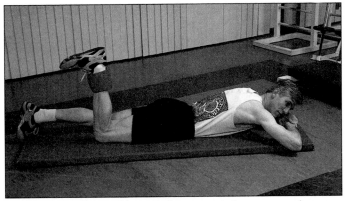

Strap a 5-lb cuff weight securely around your ankle. (Always lift half the weight you use for your leg extensions. For muscle balance, front thigh *[quadricep]* muscles should be maintained at twice the strength of the back thigh [hamstring] muscles.) Lie face down on the floor. Slowly raise your lower leg perpendicular (90°) to the floor. Lower your leg to your starting position. Perform 15 repetitions for each leg.

Heel Raises: Strengthens the calf (*gastrocnemius*) and the muscle below it (*soleus*).

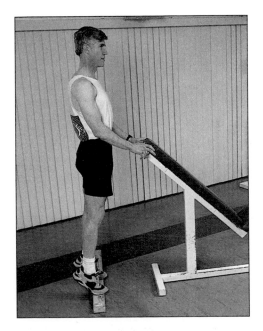

Standing erect and using a chair or wall for balance, rise on your toes as high as you can. Slowly lower yourself to your starting position. Place a 2-inch book or block of wood under your toes to create more resistance. Repeat 15 times.

Exercises for the Back, Shoulders, and Arms

This series improves strength, flexibility, mobility, and function. It also assists in many daily activities that require lifting objects above your head, carrying, pushing, and supporting yourself as you move or change positions.

Chest Fly: Strengthens the chest (*pectoralis*).

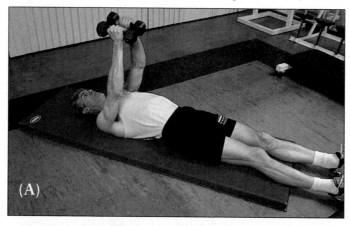

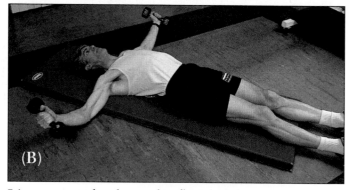

Lie on your back on the floor with your arms extended at right angles to your trunk. Grasping dumbbells in each hand, raise your arms above your chest with your palms facing in and your elbows slightly bent (A). This is your starting position. Using a semicircular motion, lower the weights to your sides until your elbows touch the floor (B). The weights should not touch the floor. Bring the weights back to your starting position. Repeat 15 times.

Military Press: Strengthens the shoulders (*deltoids*), upper shoulders below the neck (*trapezius*), and the back of the arms *(triceps)*.

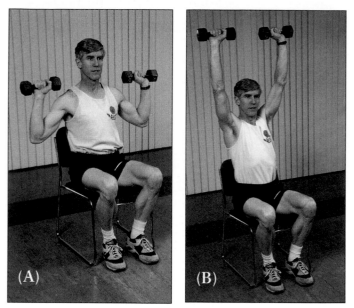

Sit in a stable chair that supports your back. Place your feet flat on the floor. Grasping a dumbbell in each hand, hold them by your sides. Raise the dumbbells to shoulder height by bending your arms at the elbows. Your palms should be facing forward and your thumbs facing in (A). This is your starting position. Raise the dumbbells above your head until your arms are fully extended (B). Lower the weights to your starting position. Repeat 15 times.

Upright Row: Strengthens the upper shoulders below the neck (*trapezius*), upper arms (*biceps*), and shoulders (*deltoids*).

Biceps Curl: Strengthens the upper arms (*biceps*).

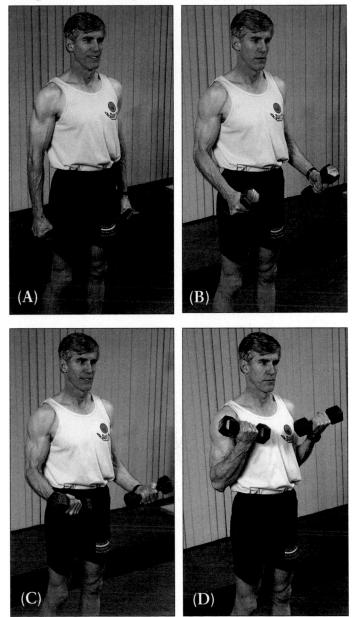

Stand with your feet apart to shoulder width. Grasping a dumbbell in each hand, hold them in front of your upper thighs, 8 to 10 inches apart, with your palms facing toward your body (A). This is your starting position. Pull the dumbbells up, bringing your elbows out to each side of your body until they are at the height of your ears (B). Pause, then lower the weights to your starting position. Repeat 15 times.

Stand with your feet apart to shoulder width. Grasping a dumbbell in each hand, hold them at your sides with the palms facing in (A). Raise the dumbbells by bending your arms at the elbows (B). When the weights are at about the height of your waist, turn your palms upward (C). This is your starting position. Raise the weights to shoulder height, keeping the elbows bent (D). Return to your starting position. Repeat 15 times.

Some people perform this exercise keeping the knees slightly bent. Locking the knees can place too much stress on the lower back.

Exercises Using Resistance Machines

Equipment: Many different kinds of exercise machines are designed for developing muscle fitness. The machines shown below can be found at many health clubs or purchased from manufacturers.

Technique:

- Proper technique is essential to maximize exercise benefits and prevent injury.

- Movements should be slow and smooth.

- Do not jerk the weights.

- Your goal is to perform 2 sets of 15 repetitions for each exercise.

- A *set* is 15 repetitions completed without pausing. Begin the exercise slowly with very low weights. When you can do 1 set of repetitions without pausing, increase the weight by a small increment (5 lbs) or to a level of resistance where you can do 7 to 8 repetitions without pausing. Work up to 2 sets of 15 repetitions.

- When you have worked up to a weight at which doing 2 complete sets is very difficult, stay at that weight for muscle strength and endurance maintenance.

Exercises for Legs and Hips

This series improves strength, flexibility, and balance. It also assists in walking, climbing, and rising from a sitting position and enhances participation in many recreational activities.

Leg Extensions: Strengthens the front of the thighs (*quadriceps*).

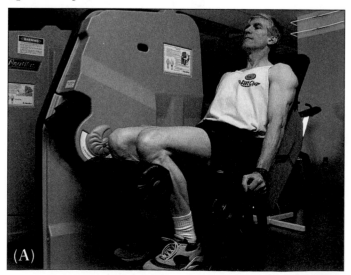

(A)

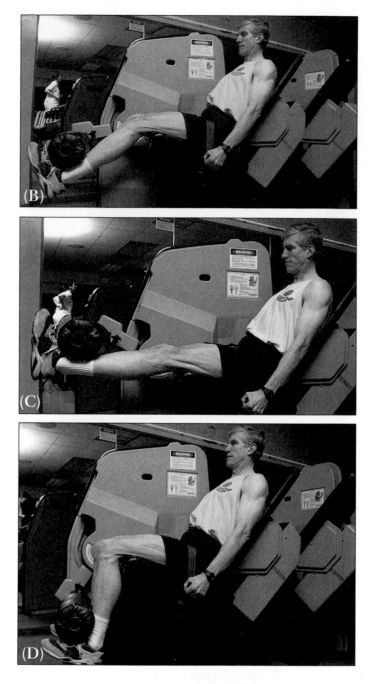

(B)

(C)

(D)

Sit on the seat of the machine with your feet behind the roller pads and your knees just over the front edge of the seat (A). Loosely hold the handles to the sides of the seat. Smoothly push against the roller pads with the front of your ankles until your legs are fully extended (B and C). Slowly lower the weights by lowering the roller pads (D). Be sure your back stays in contact with the seat. Repeat 15 times.

As a variation of leg extensions and leg curls, exercise one leg at a time. Most people favor one side of the body. That side is stronger and tends to carry a larger proportion of the workload during exercise and physical activity. Exercising one leg at a time ensures that you work and strengthen both legs equally. Exercising each leg separately also helps if you have a functional limitation or if you need to build strength in a limb that has atrophied due to bone fracture or some other injury. Use less resistance, reducing the weight to half that you lift with two legs and proceed as shown using only one leg.

Leg Curl: Strengthens the hamstring muscles.

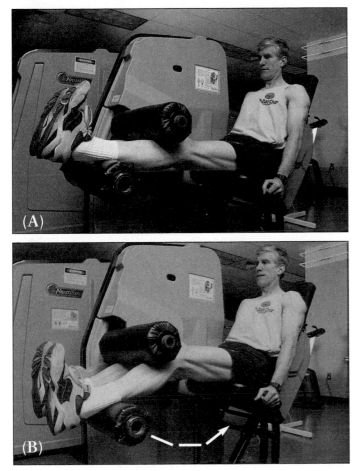

(A)

(B)

Sit on the seat of the machine with your legs extended and your feet between the roller pads. One roller pad should be behind your ankles. The other roller pad should be in front of your shins just below the knees (A). Loosely hold the handles at the sides of the seat. Push in against the roller pads behind your ankles to bring your lower legs up toward your buttocks (B). Slowly return the roller pad to your starting position. Repeat 15 times.

Calf Raises: Strengthens the calf muscles (*gastrocnemius*) and the muscle beneath (*soleus*).

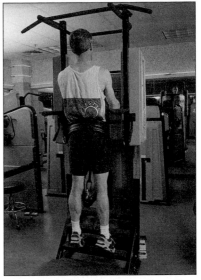

Attach a padded hip belt and adjust it around your hips. Put your toes and the balls of your feet on the front edge of the lowest step. Rise on your toes as high as possible, pause, and lower your heels to your starting position. Repeat 15 times.

Exercises for the Abdomen and Trunk

This series assists with bending, lifting, and carrying. It also helps prevent low back pain.

Abdominal Crunch: Strengthens the abdomen.

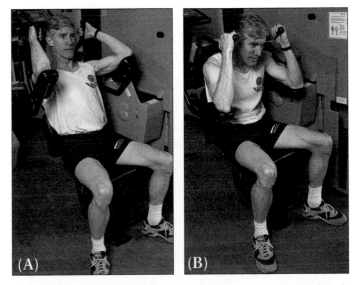

(A)　　(B)

Sit on the seat of the machine with your back straight and your hands gripping the handles above your shoulders. Your palms should be facing in (A). Slowly lean forward using your abdominal muscles to pull your body (B). Return to your starting position. Repeat 15 times.

Caution! Some people have difficulty mastering the technique used in the abdominal crunch. They tend to pull forward with their shoulders instead of their abdominal muscles. This movement stresses the lower back and can cause injury. If you feel a tightness in your lower back when you pull forward, stop and try a lower weight, or ask a fitness instructor about correct technique.

Chest Fly: Strengthens the chest (*pectoralis*).

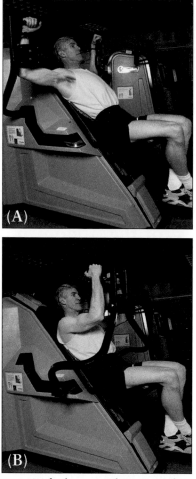

Sit on the seat of the machine with your back straight and your feet crossed at the ankles. Grip the handles above and to the sides of your head and rest your forearms on the weight pads just above your elbows (A). Push your arms together until the weight pads touch (B). Slowly return to your starting position. Repeat 15 times.

Compound Rowing: Strengthens the shoulders (*deltoids*), upper shoulders (*trapezius*), and rib cage muscles (*latissimus dorsi*).

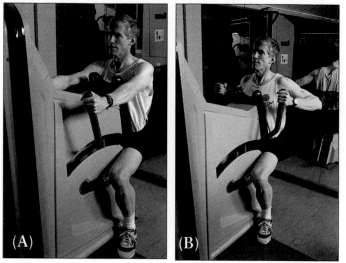

Sit on the seat of the machine with your feet flat on the floor to each side of the machine. Grip the handles so that your arms are parallel or sloping slightly down to the ground (A). Pull the bars back, bending your elbows out from the sides of your body until your hands are at a level with, and close to, your chest (B). Return to your starting position. Repeat 15 times.

Exercises for the Back, Shoulders, and Arms

This series improves strength, flexibility, mobility, and function. It also assists in many daily activities that require lifting objects above your head, carrying, pushing, and supporting yourself as you move or change positions.

Pull-Ups: Strengthens the upper arms (*biceps*) and shoulders (*deltoids*).

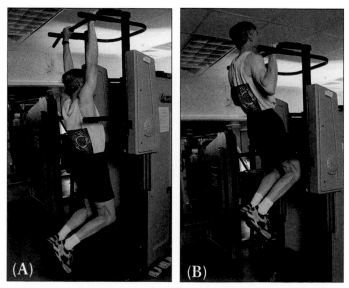

Using the overhand grip, grasp the horizontal bar so that you hang with your arms straight (A). This is your starting position. Pull up until your chin is above the bar (B). Lower yourself slowly back to your starting position. Repeat 15 times.

Overhead Press: Strengthens the shoulders (*deltoids*) and the back of the arms (*triceps*).

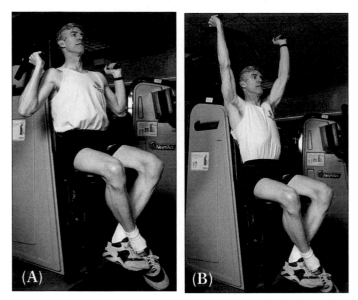

Grip the handles to the sides of your shoulders (A). Push the bar straight up above your head, keeping your elbows wide (B). Do not arch your back, but keep it flat against the seat back. Pause when your arms are fully extended. Slowly return to your starting position. Repeat 15 times.

If you find your back arching as you lift the weights, stop. Either the weight is too heavy or you do not have the flexibility required to lift the bar. Try reducing the weight, and do some stretching exercises *(see Appendix 1 on pp. 289–291)* to strengthen and improve flexibility in the lower back before you return to the exercise.

Arm Curls: Strengthens the upper arms (*biceps*).

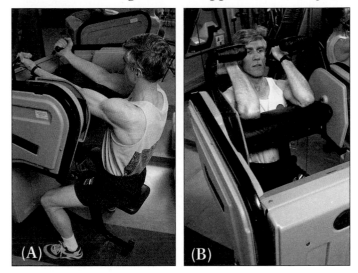

Sit straddling the bench with your feet flat on the floor. Place your elbows on the pad in front of you and grip the handles of the bar so that your upper arms are parallel to the ground (A). Curl both arms to pull the bar toward your chest (B). Slowly lower to the extended position. Repeat 15 times.

Seated Dip: Strengthens the back of the arms (*triceps*).

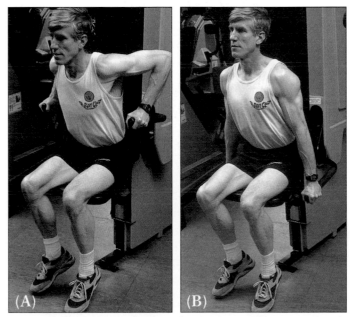

Sit on the seat of the machine with your back straight. Grip the handles of the bar, keeping your elbows bent (A). Push down on the bar until your arms are fully extended (B). Slowly return to your starting position. Repeat 15 times.

INDEX